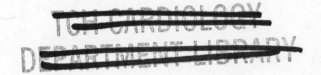

CARDIOVASCULAR FLUID DYNAMICS

VOLUME 1

CARDIOVASCULAR FLUID DYNAMICS

Edited by

D. H. BERGEL

Fellow of St. Catherine's College,
University Laboratory of Physiology, Oxford, England

VOLUME 1

1972

ACADEMIC PRESS

LONDON AND NEW YORK

ACADEMIC PRESS INC. (LONDON) LTD.
24/28 Oval Road,
London NW1

United States Edition published by
ACADEMIC PRESS INC.
111 Fifth Avenue
New York, New York 10003

Library of Congress Catalog Card Number: 79–185200
ISBN: 0–12–089901–9

PRINTED IN GREAT BRITAIN BY
THE WHITEFRIARS PRESS LIMITED
LONDON AND TONBRIDGE

List of Contributors

*B. J. BELLHOUSE, *Magdalen College, Department of Engineering Science, Oxford, England.*

*JAN E. W. BENEKEN, *Research Group on Cardiovascular Physics, Institute of Medical Physics TNO, Da Costakade, Utrecht, The Netherlands.*

*D. H. BERGEL, *St. Catherine's College, University Laboratory of Physiology, Oxford, England.*

*J. R. BLINKS, *Department of Physiology, Mayo Medical School, Rochester, Minnesota, U.S.A.*

STANLEY E. CHARM, *Department of Physiology, Tufts University Medical School, Boston, Massachusetts, U.S.A.*

GARY G. FERGUSON, *Department of Biophysics, Faculty of Medicine, University of Western Ontario, London, Ontario, Canada.*

J. M. FITZ-GERALD, *Department of Mathematics, University of Queensland, St. Lucia, Brisbane, Australia.*

*IVOR T. GABE, *M.R.C. Cardiovascular Unit and Department of Medicine, Hammersmith Hospital, London, England.*

*U. GESSNER, *Department of Biomedical Engineering, Hoffmann-La Roche & Co., A.G., Basel, Switzerland.*

B. S. GOW, *Department of Physiology, University of Sydney, Sydney, Australia.*

*B. R. JEWELL, *Department of Physiology, University College, London, England.*

G. S. KURLAND, *Department of Medicine, Beth Israel Hospital and Harvard Medical School, Boston, Massachusetts, U.S.A.*

C. C. MICHEL, *Queen's College, University Laboratory of Physiology, Oxford, England.*

*CHRISTOPHER J. MILLS, *Cardiovascular Research Unit, Royal Postgraduate Medical School, London, England.*

W. R. MILNOR, *Department of Physiology, Johns Hopkins University School of Medicine, Baltimore, Maryland, U.S.A.*

DALI J. PATEL, *Section on Experimental Atherosclerosis, National Heart and Lung Institute, National Institutes of Health, Bethesda, Maryland, U.S.A.*

MARGOT R. ROACH, *Department of Biophysics, University of Western Ontario, London, Ontario, Canada.*

*K. SAGAWA, *Department of Biomedical Engineering, Johns Hopkins University School of Medicine, Baltimore, Maryland, U.S.A.*

*D. L. SCHULTZ, *St. Catherine's College, Department of Engineering Science, Oxford, England.*

R. SKALAK, *Department of Civil Engineering and Engineering Mechanics, Columbia University, New York, U.S.A.*

RAMESH N. VAISHNAV, *Department of Civil and Mechanical Engineering, The Catholic University of America, Washington, D.C., U.S.A.*

* Contributors to Volume 1.

Preface

The purpose of this book is to make available, in as concise and manageable a form as possible, the results of the intensive study of the fluid dynamics of the mammalian cardiovascular system undertaken in the previous decade. In the ten years that have elapsed since the publication of McDonald's monograph on "Blood Flow in Arteries", so much has been achieved that a new assessment is needed.

I hope that the various chapters will show what is the present situation in this field, and how this point has been reached through experimentation based on a proper understanding of the physical background. The methods and concepts used in this work will be only partly familiar to biologists, physicians and fluid dynamicists. It has been my intention to produce a book which will serve these specialists in introducing them to a very active field of experimental research and will allow them to enter it with a good understanding of the established physical and biological features of the fascinating cardiovascular system.

At this point it is customary for the editor to thank all those who have contributed to the work. I hope it will be clear that my expressions of thanks are a great deal more than conventional. My own contribution here has been quite modest, for although I have myself worked in many of the areas discussed, I have been aware that others are much better qualified now to deal with these subjects. It has been a great privilege to work with so large and varied a team and I can only hope that our friendship will survive the strain. I wish especially to thank all the Oxford authors, and also Dr. Colin Clark, whose continuing criticisms and suggestions have helped me greatly. Finally, the publishers, who have transformed a great heap of paper into what I hope is now a coherent whole; may they never regret the effort.

D. H. BERGEL

Oxford
June, 1972

Acknowledgements

Grateful acknowledgement is made to the following Journals and Publishers, and to the Authors, for permission to use the following figures and tables: Circulation Research and the American Heart Association Inc. for Figs. 21 and 26 in Chapter 5, Fig. 9 in Chapter 7, Figs. 2, 3, 4, 5, 11, 12 and Tables 1, 2, 3, 4 in Chapter 11, and Figs. 11, 13 and 14 in Chapter 12; *Acta Physiologica Scandinavica* for Fig. 7 in Chapter 7; *The American Journal of Physiology* for Figs. 10, 27, 28a and 28b in Chapter 5, Fig. 8 in Chapter 7, Figs. 8 and 9 in Chapter 12; *Pflügers Archiv* for Fig. 31 in Chapter 5; W. B. Saunders Company for Figs. 12, 24 and 25 in Chapter 5, and Figs. 9 and 10 in Chapter 6; Pergamon Press for Fig. 29 in Chapter 5; *The Journal of Applied Physiology* for Fig. 21 in Chapter 6; *Archives Internationales de Physiologie et Biochemie* for Fig. 29 in Chapter 5; The Federation of American Societies for Experimental Biology for Fig. 2 in Chapter 6; *The Journal of Physiology* for Fig. 1, and the Cambridge University Press for Fig. 4 in Chapter 7.

CONTENTS

Chapter 1

Introduction

D. H. BERGEL

Chapter 2

Pressure Measurement in Experimental Physiology

IVOR T. GABE

Chapter 3

Measurement of Pulsatile Flow and Flow Velocity

CHRISTOPHER J. MILLS

Chapter 10
Vascular Input Impedance
U. GESSNER

Glossary

Adventitia	The outermost coat of a blood vessel.
Aneurysm	A localized dilation of an artery.
Angiogram	An X-ray picture in which the contents of the blood vessels have been rendered radio-opaque by the injection of a contrast medium.
Arteriole	The finest subdivision of the arterial tree, typically vessels of 100–200 μm in diameter. The walls are relatively muscular and variations in the activity of this muscle play a major part in the control of the circulation.
Arteries	The vessels carrying the blood from the left or right ventricles to the tissues.
Atherosclerosis, arteriosclerosis	Varieties of degenerative disease of the arteries. Atheroma is a fatty degeneration of the inner layers of an artery; in the early stages intimal plaques of atheromatous material may be visible.
Attenuation	See Decibel, Neper.
Baroreceptors	Areas of the vascular system which function as pressure receptors. Nerve endings in the vessel wall respond to its deformation. The most important systemic arterial baroreceptors are found in the arch of the aorta (near its origin) and near the point at which the carotid artery in the neck divides into two branches, at about the level of the angle of the jaw.
Blood	Blood is a suspension of cells in the fluid plasma. The cells comprise the red cells (erythrocytes), white cells (leucocytes) and the platelets (thrombocytes), the average numbers of each per mm^3 of blood being about 5×10^6, 10^4, and 3×10^5, respectively.
Bode plot	A diagram which presents the frequency response of a system as an amplitude ratio (gain) and the phase shift as functions of frequency, on a logarithmic scale. The unit of gain is the decibel where gain in dB = 20 log (output amplitude/input amplitude).
	For a first-order system (q.v.) the gain is zero up to the corner frequency (q.v.) and falls thereafter with a slope of -20 dB/decade. The phase shift tends towards $-90°$ ($90°$ lag) at high frequencies and has a value of $-45°$ at the corner frequency. For a second-order system the attenuation is -40 dB/decade and the maximal phase shift is $-180°$.
Boundary conditions	Known conditions at one or several of the boundaries of the physical process considered; they are in general required in order to obtain full solutions to the equations governing the process.

Boundary layer (viscous)	Usually a rather thin layer of fluid adjacent to a solid surface in which shear forces due to viscosity predominate and give rise to steep velocity gradients.
Capillary	The finest blood vessels, normally about 5–6 μm in diameter, and about 0·5 mm long in the systemic circulation.
Cavitation	The formation of cavities filled with vapour or gas within a moving liquid due to the local pressure being reduced to below the vapour pressure for the liquid.
Cervical rib	An abnormal small rib in the lower neck.
Coarctation	An isolated narrowing of an artery; generally refers to a congenital defect of the aorta.
Complex number	A complex number is an expression of the form $X = a + ib$, where a and b are real numbers, and i is the imaginary unit $\sqrt{(-1)}$. Such numbers are used to describe time varying quantities which are characterized by an amplitude or modulus ($M = (a^2 + b^2)^{\frac{1}{2}}$), together with a phase relationship with some time reference. They may be visualized as vectors in a Cartesian coordinate system. The projection on one axis has the value a and is termed the real part (Re X), the projection on the other axis is ib, the imaginary part (Im X). A real number, A, can be considered as a vector lying along the real axis, rotation by 90° will result in an imaginary number, iA, with no real part. A further rotation by 90° returns the vector to the real axis but it is reversed, i.e. $-A$. Thus if one rotation is indicated by multiplication by the imaginary operator i, two such rotations are equivalent to multiplying by -1; i can then be seen to be equal to $\sqrt{(-1)}$.
Compliance (distensibility)	A measure of the ability of a hollow structure to change its volume, generally the ratio of volume change to internal pressure change (dV/dP). The inverse of compliance is elastance.
Corner frequency (break frequency)	A frequency analogous to the resonant frequency of a mechanical system. For a first-order system the relation of the corner frequency to the time constant, τ, is $\tau = 1/\omega_0$. where ω_0 is the corner frequency in radians/second. In the electrical analog of a first-order system the product RC has the value $\omega_0/2\pi$.
Decibel (dB)	A logarithmic measure of the ratio between two quantities. The gain of a system may be expressed in dB, where gain = 20 log (output amplitude/input amplitude).
Diastole (atrial or ventricular)	The resting phase of the cardiac cycle.
Drag	A force induced on a solid surface by fluid moving past it, and in the direction of the fluid motion. Drag may be due to viscous shear forces alone, for example, on the

	wall of a pipe, or may also have a component due to relatively low pressures in the wake region behind an immersed body.
Elasticity	A measure of a material's resistance to deformation. See Modulus.
Electrocardiogram (E.C.G.)	A record of the electrical activity of the heart, normally obtained with electrodes on the skin.
Endothelium.	The layer of cells lining the blood vessels.
Energy (ML^2T^{-2})	Unit energy or work is that exchanged when unit force acts through unit displacement in the direction of the force. One joule is the work done when one newton acts through one metre. $(J = 10^7 \text{ ergs.})$
First-order delay (or lag) system	A system whose input-output relationships are those of a parallel resistance-capacitance unit (time constant $= RC$). As such a system is excited with an input of increasing frequency the output becomes reduced and lags progressively with a maximal lag of 90°. The performance of a first-order system depends both on the input function and its first time-differential.
Force (MLT^{-2})	Unit force is that which gives unit acceleration to unit mass. One newton gives an acceleration of 1 m s^{-2} to 1 kg, one dyne gives an acceleration of 1 cm s^{-2} to 1 g. Unit force (gravitational) is the force of gravitation on unit mass in the locality in question and is therefore expressed in mass units. Thus a mass of M grams is attracted to the earth with a force of M grams weight which is equal to Mg dynes, where g is the local acceleration due to gravity in cm s^{-2}. The accepted value for g is $9 \cdot 80665 \text{ m s}^{-2}$.
Haematocrit	The relative volume of the cells in blood, normally about 45 per cent.
Heart	The mammalian heart consists of four chambers, right and left atria, right and left ventricles. The atria are thin walled chambers into which blood flows at low pressure from the veins. Between atria and ventricles are the tricuspid (right) and mitral (left) valves. Blood at high pressure leaves the ventricles by the pulmonary artery (right) and aorta (left); there are valves at the origin of each of these. The blood supply to the heart itself comes from the coronary arteries which spring from the aorta at its origin. Normally both atria beat together a short time before the synchronous beat of the ventricles.
Histology	The microscopic study of tissue structure.
Hookean material	An ideally elastic material for which tensile stress is proportional to strain, i.e. the Young's modulus, E, is constant.
Hypertension, pulmonary or systemic	A condition in which the arterial blood pressure is abnormally high (cf. hypotension, which is low pressure).

Intima	The innermost coat of a blood vessel, comprises the endothelium and a thin connective tissue layer.
Isometric contraction	One in which no change of muscle length is allowed to occur.
Isotonic contraction	One in which the load on the muscle is constant.
Impedance (Z, electrical, acoustic, mechanical, hydraulic)	The resistance to disturbance of a system or material. It is measured as the complex ratio of a force (voltage, pressure, stress) to the resulting change (current, fluid flow, strain) at a specified frequency. An impedance plot shows the impedance as a function of frequency. The hydraulic input impedance is the complex ratio of pressure to flow at the input to a hydraulic system, e.g. the root of the aorta or pulmonary artery, and is both a function of frequency and of position.
Inertia	In fluid flows inertia is represented by the property density and is the force required to accelerate fluid particles, provided by a pressure gradient.
Inlet length (entrance length)	The region of a pipe or channel near the inflow point, in which the thickness of the boundary layer progressively increases. At the end of this region, where the final velocity profile is established, the flow is said to be fully developed.
Karman trail (or vortex steet)	A regular series of fluid vortices in a wake region, in which alternate eddies rotate with opposite sense.
Kinetic energy	The energy associated with the velocity of a material particle or system, and is given by: $\frac{1}{2}$ (speed)^2 per unit mass.
Laminar flow	In laminar pipe flow the fluid velocity remains constant on cylindrical surfaces within the fluid which are concentric with the axis. The flow is well ordered and stable and can be considered as individual cylindrical laminae of fluid sliding over each other.
Laplace transform	The Laplace transform of a function is expressed by an integral formula. This enables the algebraic solution of linear differential equations in terms of initial conditions. For fuller details the reader is referred to the textbooks listed in the references to Chapter 5.
Media	The middle coat of a blood vessel, generally the thickest. It contains the fibrous proteins elastin and collagen, and smooth muscle.
Modulus	The real part of a complex number. Such a number can be visualized as a vector whose length is the modulus and whose angle with the real axis is its phase.
Modulus, of elasticity	A measure of the resistance to deformation of a material, the stress (force/unit area, $ML^{-1}T^{-2}$) required to cause unit strain. The three moduli are the tensile modulus (Young's modulus, E), the shear modulus (G) and the bulk modulus (modulus of compressibility, K).
Murmur (bruit)	An abnormal sound heard over a blood vessel or the heart.

Muscle	Three broad types of muscle are distinguished. Skeletal or striated muscle is normally used for conscious movement and is that commonly referred to as "muscle". Cardiac muscle is the muscle forming the walls of the cardiac chambers. Smooth muscle is a broad term describing the muscle, normally not under voluntary control, which is contained in the walls of the alimentary canal, blood vessels, and other structures. Papillary muscles are strands of cardiac muscle which support the mitral and tricuspid valves and are convenient for studies on the properties of cardiac muscle.
Myocardium	The muscle of the heart.
Neper	A measure of attenuation. If a wave attenuates with distance travelled (L) as $\exp(-\alpha L)$, the attenuation is α nepers/unit length.
Nerva vasorum	The nerves that supply the wall of a blood vessel.
Newtonian fluid	One in which the ratio of shear stress to shear strain is constant.
Nyquist diagram	An alternative to the Bode plot (q.v.) for plotting the frequency response of a system. The transfer function is plotted as a vector with its amplitude representing the gain and the angle with the real axis as the phase shift. The locus of the vector tips at different frequencies is the Nyquist plot. By convention, for a negative feedback system the phase delay at zero frequency is plotted as zero degrees rather than as $-180°$. Thus a delay on this diagram of 180° represents a difference of 360° between input and output. If the plot shows a gain >1 at a phase shift of 180° then the system is likely to be unstable and go into feedback oscillations at the frequency at which the 180° phase shift line is crossed.
Peripheral resistance	The ratio of the mean pressure drop across a circulatory bed to the mean flow through it.
Phonocatheter	A catheter bearing a small microphone for the recording of intravascular sounds.
Plethysmograph	A device for measuring the volume changes of an organ or part of the body.
Polycythaemia	An abnormal increase in the number of red cells in blood.
Potential energy	The energy associated with position in a gravitational field relative to some datum level at which the potential energy may arbitrarily be set equal to zero.
Power ($M L^2 T^{-3}$)	Unit power is that rate of doing work in which unit energy is exchanged in unit time. 1 watt (W) is 1 J s^{-1}.
Power, hydraulic	The energy flux associated with a given flow and having, in general, "pressure", kinetic and potential components.
Pressure ($M L^{-1} T^{-2}$)	A measure of the force per unit area exerted by a fluid. The SI unit of pressure is one newton/sq. metre (N m^{-2}) or one pascal (pa). This is equal to 10 dynes cm^{-2}. The

	conventional millimetre of mercury (mmHg) is equal to $13\cdot5951 \times 980\cdot665 \times 10^{-2}\,\mathrm{N\,m^{-2}}$. One Torr is equal to 1 mmHg to within 2×10^{-7} Torr. One bar is $10^5\,\mathrm{N\,m^{-2}}$.
Pressure gradient	The pressure drop per unit length along a flow channel.
Pressure, static	The pressure measured in still fluid; ideally that also measured in flowing fluid with a device sensitive only to the force perpendicular to the direction of flow. The dynamic pressure is that measured with a device sensitive to force parallel to the direction of flow, and is different from the static pressure by the quantity $\frac{1}{2}\rho V^2$ where ρ is the fluid density and V the local velocity vector.
Pressure, transmural	The difference in pressure between the inside and outside of a hollow structure.
Radian (r or rad)	A measure of angle. An angle of $360°$ is equal to 2π radians, thus $1\,\mathrm{r} = 57\cdot34°$, $1° = 0\cdot017453\,\mathrm{r}$.
Reynolds number (Re)	An important dimensionless group in fluid mechanics defined as the product of a characteristic length and flow speed divided by the kinematic viscosity of the fluid. The magnitude of the number represents the relative importance of inertia forces compared with viscous forces.
Sarcomere	The functional unit of a fibre of striated muscle.
Sarcoplasm	The material in which the contractile apparatus of a muscle cell is embedded.
Second-order system	A system whose transfer function depends on terms up to the second time-differential of the input. Such properties are shown, for example, by a mechanical system containing elements with frictional, elastic and inertial properties.
Stenosis	A narrowing of a blood vesel or of a valve.
Strain	A measure of the deformation of a material relative to some reference dimension. Tensile and volumetric strains are changes in length (along some defined axis) and in volume, respectively. Shear strain refers to a relative displacement of material elements in two parallel planes in a direction within the planes.
Stream function	A measure of the flux of fluid volume; it remains constant along streamlines. Velocity components may be computed as appropriate derivatives of the stream function.
Stress ($M\,L^{-1}\,T^{-2}$)	A measure of the deforming force applied to a material, the units are force/unit area.
Surfactant, pulmonary	A material lining the finest air spaces of the lungs, the alveoli, which is normally present and which lowers the surface tension at the air–fluid interface.
Sympathomimetic drug	A drug whose action is similar to that produced by stimulation of the sympathetic nervous system, this being generally an increase in the rate and force of cardiac contraction and an increase in the peripheral

	vascular resistance. Catecholamines are a chemically defined group of sympathomimetic agents including adrenalin and noradrenalin.
Systemic circulation	The circulation to the body, the term excludes the pulmonary circulation which contains the gas-exchanging pulmonary capillaries.
Systole (atrial or ventricular)	The active part of the cardiac cycle.
Transportation lag (dead time, latency)	If there is a time lag, L, between an input signal change and the alteration in the output the system is said to have a transportation lag. This is often represented in control system engineering by the transfer function $\exp(-sL)$ where s is the Laplace operator.
Transfer function	The transfer function of a control system (or subsystem) is the ratio of the Laplace transforms of its output and input, and so characterizes the response of the system.
Turbulence	Turbulent flows are characterized by random fluctuations of the fluid motions which cannot be predicted in detail. These fluctuations may be superimposed upon a particular average direction of flow as occurs, for example, in pipe flow. This feature is due to the inherent instability of the flow, i.e. induced disturbances will grow with time whereas, in laminar flow, such disturbances would be damped out.
Vasa vasorum	The blood vessels that supply the walls of the larger blood vessels.
Vasomotor control system	A term describing the physiological mechanisms, both nervous and endocrine, which alter the hydraulic resistance of the vascular bed. This is brought about by changes in the activity of the muscle in the vessel walls, thereby altering the size of the vascular lumen.
Veins	The vessels carrying blood from the tissues to the atria of the heart.
Venomotor control system	The physiological control system whereby the compliance of the veins, and hence the volume of contained blood, may be altered by changes in the activity of the muscles in their walls.
Viscoelasticity	A viscoelastic material is one in which both the strain (elastic response) and the rate of strain (viscous response) are functions of the imposed stress.
Viscosity ($M L^{-1}T^{-1}$)	The property of resisting deformation in a fluid, it gives rise to tangential or shear stresses. Kinematic viscosity is the dynamic viscosity divided by density and can be considered as the diffusion coefficient governing the transport of molecular momentum within a fluid. The units of viscosity are the poise (P) and the centipoise (cP), one poise is the viscosity of that material which requires unit shear stress (1 dyne cm^{-2}) to maintain a shear velocity gradient of 1 (cm s^{-1} cm^{-1}) or

	$1\ s^{-1}$. The SI unit of viscosity is the newton second per sq. metre ($N\ s\ m^{-2}$) and is equal to 10 poise. The unit of kinematic viscosity is the Stoke (St). ($1\ St = 10^{-4}\ m^2\ s^{-1}$.)
Windkessel	A term used by Otto Frank in 1899 to describe the elastic reservoir function of the aorta. In the simple windkessel theory the systemic bed was modelled as an elastic reservoir connected to a peripheral hydraulic resistance.
Zero-order system (zero-memory system)	A system in which the output follows the input with no lag. The electrical analogue is an ohmic resistance.

Contents of Volume 2

To Nicolette, Timothy, Stephen, Oliver
and Matthew; with great love

Chapter 1

Introduction

D. H. BERGEL

Fellow of St. Catherine's College, Oxford:
University Laboratory of Physiology, Oxford, England

In the last ten years there have been very rapid advances in our understanding of the physical performance of the mammalian cardiovascular system. Particularly remarkable has been the development of a coherent and useful description of the function of the major arterial system.

The decade may, for convenience, be considered to have begun with the publication in 1960 of McDonald's book "Blood Flow in Arteries". This work introduced to a wide audience a physically reasonable theory of vascular function which avoided various assumptions previously made. While these had undoubtedly led to increased understanding, it seemed then that things were getting to the state where the framework had to be unreasonably distorted to fit the new data. The new wine demanded new bottles.

McDonald's book, despite its title, was written before much was known about actual arterial flow patterns. It appeared just when adequate flowmeters were entering service. Its strength lay in the fact that the theory was available when the data began to accumulate. In the decade that followed it found immediate application and a period of great activity was the result.

While the theoretical basis of the approaches used in the sixties still stands, two things have happened which call now for a reappraisal. The introduction of many new techniques, especially in the measurement of blood flow and velocity, has put much flesh on the theoretical structure put forward earlier. In addition there has been greatly increasing collaboration between engineers and biologists in this area, a collaboration that has led to the establishment of several bio-engineering units and to an enormous increase in the sophistication and depth of analysis. Our understanding of the mechanics of the arterial system has increased enormously. However, in the application of the new tools to other parts of the system where the degree of complexity is very much greater we still have a long way to go. For example, interest is beginning to shift from the major arteries towards investigation of the heart and the smaller vessels. In these parts of the system, active behaviour, as contrasted to the rather passive mechanical reactions of the arteries, complex

1

enough though these are, demands analysis in terms that are still not wholly clear. If progress is to occur this particular ghost must be put back in the machine.

This book is intended to introduce to both biologists and those in the physical sciences some current problems and concepts of mammalian cardiovascular function. The emphasis has been on experimental studies and the first three chapters have been devoted to a review of methods. The mathematical treatment has been kept to the minimum consistent with the aim of clearly demonstrating how particular conclusions have been reached and what simplifying assumptions have been made. Biologists should not fear to be overwhelmed here with mathematics and in all cases the arguments can be followed by those without specialized knowledge; where necessary reference is given to basic textbooks.

The authors have been drawn in equal numbers from biologists and physical scientists. It has always been my experience that engineers respond with enthusiasm to physiological problems and it is my firm belief that progress will only come from the closest collaboration of both groups in the experimental laboratory. It does take time and experience to get the feel of biological materials and acquire the right sense of proportion and biologists need to gain confidence in methods and techniques which, while new to them, have been well tested by the engineers.

Those who have no experience with cardiovascular physiology may find the following brief introduction useful. This will serve to introduce the subject so that one can appreciate the relevance of the problems discussed here.

The general features of the mammalian cardiovascular system have been well known to anatomists for many years. Figure 1 taken from Vesalius (1543) shows the essentials, with one important omission, the capillaries. The heart is composed of four chambers arranged in two pairs. The thin walled atria are each connected through a valved orifice to a thick walled muscular ventricle. Each ventricle connects in its turn to a major distributing artery, the mouths being guarded by a second set of valves. The left ventricle is the thicker and leads to the aorta, in which the average pressure is about 100 mmHg (ca. $1 \cdot 36 \times 10^4$ Nm^{-2}) through which oxygenated "arterial" blood is distributed to the tissues of the body. The aorta has relatively distensible walls and is classed as an elastic artery. With successive subdivisions of the arterial tree the structure of the walls alters, becoming less distensible and more muscular. The muscle concerned is the type known as smooth muscle, its most significant feature is a tendency to sustained and slow contraction, as opposed to "twitch" behaviour; for various reasons it has proved extremely difficult to study. The transition between elastic and muscular arteries is gradual; it is roughly true that the named major branches of the aorta are of intermediate type.

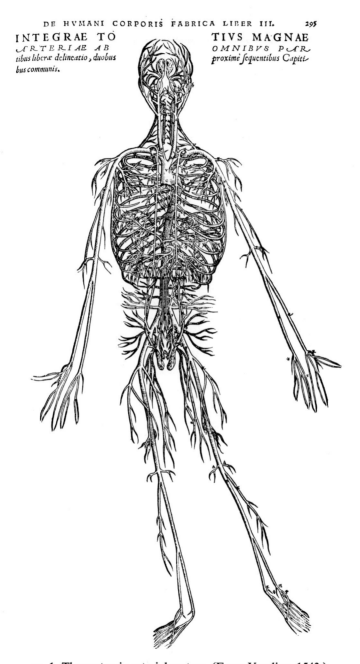

INTEGRAE TO TIVS MAGNAE
ARTERIAE AB *OMNIBVS PAR*
tibus liberæ delineatio, duobus *proximè sequentibus Capiti-*
bus communis.

IG. 1. The systemic arterial system. (From Vesalius, 1543.)

The final subdivisions of the arterial tree may be considered to be the arterioles (see Table 1). These are small (i.d. 30–100 μm) vessels whose wall is almost exclusively composed of circumferentially arranged smooth muscle cells. These vessels give rise to the capillaries, the region in which the exchange

TABLE 1

Some quantities relevant to the circulation

Blood volume	6 litres
Number of red cells	5×10^6 mm^{-3}
Number of white cells	10^4 mm^{-3}
Specific gravity of blood	1·06
Viscosity of blood	Variable. 0·03 poise in large tubes
Cardiac output	6 litres min^{-1}
Heart rate	80 beats min^{-1}
Stroke volume	70 ml
Duration of systole	0·3 s
Duration of diastole	0·5 s

Dimensions of the circulatory bed

Vessels	Pressures (mmHg)	Diameter (cm)	Blood velocity (cm s^{-1})	Contained volume (ml)
Aorta and large arteries	120/80 mean 100	3–1	100/0 mean 25	300
Small arteries	120/70 mean 90	1–0·1	10–1	400
Capillaries	20	0·0008	0·05	300
Small veins	10	0·5	1	2300
Main veins	0–5	4	0/25 mean 10	900
Heart	—	—	—	360 (diastole)
Pulmonary artery	25/10 mean 15	4	50/0 mean 15	130
Pulmonary capillaries	5	0·001	0·02	110
Pulmonary veins	0	1	10	200

The figures are very approximate idealizations for an adult man.

of fluids and metabolites between blood and tissues takes place, and which are discussed fully in Chapter 17.

Blood returns to the heart in the veins. These are generally relatively thin walled vessels of rather greater cross-sectional area than the corresponding division of the arterial bed. Consequently the venous blood, which is at near atmospheric pressure, moves slower than does the arterial blood. Most veins contain valves in their walls.

The two largest veins, the inferior and superior venae cavae, join the right atrium and through them returns all the blood to the heart with the exception of that from the heart itself. This bed, the coronary circulation, largely drains through the separate coronary sinus directly into the right atrium. The venous blood is transferred to the right ventricle and thence to the pulmonary artery, which branches and terminates in the gas exchanging vessels of the pulmonary capillaries. The pulmonary arteries are under less pressure than the systemic arteries, the mean pressure is about 20 mmHg. Their walls are relatively thin and the smooth muscle less prominent at all levels (see Chapter 18). The circle is finally closed by the pulmonary veins which deliver arterial blood to the left atrium.

The heart is a hollow muscular pump. The muscle is a distinct variety known as cardiac muscle with properties in many ways intermediate between those of smooth and skeletal muscle (see Chapter 7). The important features of this muscle is that it beats spontaneously and repetitively of its own accord. The heart is innervated but nervous activity merely modifies the rate and forcefulness of the beat. The contraction of the heart is co-ordinated by an elaborate system of modified muscle cells which ensure that the electrical changes which trigger mechanical contraction are conducted rapidly to the whole ventricular mass. Since these electrical changes involve the co-ordinated change in a large mass of muscle (about 300 g in man) it is possible to detect these changes as electrical potentials on the body surface, the record being the electrocardiogram.

The modern era of cardiovascular physiology may be taken to have begun in 1628 with William Harvey's demonstration of the circulation of the blood. It had been previously held that blood ebbed and flowed in veins and arteries with each heart beat, but Harvey was able, by a combination of experiment and simple arithmetic, to show that it had to circulate or be absorbed and remade at an unbelievable rate. Although the idea that it circulates now seems childishly obvious, a rather similar demonstration concerning the circulation of a type of white blood cell was only achieved, with very fundamental consequences, a few years ago. It is also true that it is often difficult to truly comprehend the consequences of the fact that blood circulates (see Chapter 5).

Harvey was forced to postulate the existence of invisibly fine vascular connections between the arteries and veins; the capillaries were seen by Malpighi in the frog's lung in 1661, following the introduction of the microscope. The new ideas were developed in the century after Harvey's work but undoubtedly the greatest single contribution was made by the vicar of

Teddington, Stephen Hales (1677–1761). As well as being a brilliant experimentalist, albeit that his experiments often appear gruesome to us and to some of his contemporaries,† Hales' work is distinguished by his passionate desire to measure. He measured the arterial blood pressure, estimated cardiac output and came very close to our present concept of the peripheral vascular resistance. (He also made fundamental contributions to the study of sap movements in plants and has a reasonable claim to have been the originator of air conditioning.)

The essential features of cardiovascular function were elaborated in the centuries that followed and incorporated in what may be thought of as the d.c. model of the system. The blood in the arteries is at high pressures and is delivered to the capillaries through the distributing network. The pressure in the major arteries is about 100 mmHg and has fallen to about 30 mmHg at the arterial end of the capillaries and to about 15 mmHg at the other end. Thus the greatest reduction in pressure occurs in the arteriolar section and by analogy with Ohm's law we can say that the hydraulic peripheral resistance is distributed through the tree in direct proportion to the pressure drop over each segment. Thus about 30–40 per cent of the total resistance is placed in the systemic arterioles but by no means all of it. However, this part of the system is very well supplied with smooth muscle and variations in activity (tone) of the muscle in response to local metabolic needs and central nervous commands will significantly vary the distribution of resistance. By these means blood may be preferentially diverted to various organs as required.

The control of peripheral resistance has been extensively studied. The amount of blood to be distributed depends on the heart rate and the forcefulness of each beat. These are also under nervous control but since the output cannot exceed the flow of blood to the heart (the venous return), the characteristics of the venous system become important. The manner in which the interactions of the whole system can be studied, and the results of such studies, are discussed by Sagawa in Chapter 5.

An area of special interest is the so-called microcirculation which includes the smallest arteries and veins and the capillaries. In this region the fact that blood is not a simple liquid becomes of significance. About 45 per cent of blood is made up of gas-transporting red cells which are themselves about the same size as the capillary lumen. Within the capillaries exchange of fluids and solutes occurs across the wall. A balance of forces is established between the hydrostatic and osmotic pressures such that the circulating volume

---

† ... the good Pastor Stephen Hales
  Weighed moisture in a pair of scales,
  To lingering death put Mares and Dogs,
  and stripped the skin from living Frogs.

remains essentially constant and the fluid does not normally leak away in the tissues. This is an extremely difficult region to study and the problems are discussed in Chapters 15, 16 and 17 by Charm and Kurland, Fitz-Gerald, and by Michel.

One idea of great significance advanced by Hales was of the elastic reservoir function of the large arteries. He made an analogy with the air-filled compression chamber used to smooth the flow of water from early fire pumps. This device became the Windkessel in translation and led directly to the first coherent physical interpretation of pulsatile arterial haemodynamics.

This development, which occurred in the last hundred years, was largely the work of the German physiologists. The great improvement in pressure transducers was an essential precursor to this; indeed it is not too fanciful to relate the Windkessel theory to precision manometry and the contemporary developments to the appearance of adequate blood flowmeters. The strengths and shortcomings of the theory have been excellently described in a review by McDonald and Taylor (1959) and more recently by Wetterer and Kenner (1968) and I do not propose to repeat them here, but a brief description is necessary to illustrate the significance of the present concepts.

The original Windkessel theory postulated a short, purely elastic chamber into which blood was abruptly ejected at each heart beat and out of which blood drained, at a rate proportional to the instantaneous pressure, through the peripheral resistance. The pressure waveform would thus show a sharp rising phase in systole and an exponential fall in diastole. It also followed that knowledge of the elasticity of the chamber would allow computation of the volume ejected by the heart, the stroke volume. The advantage to both clinicians and physiologists of the ability to measure the cardiac output on a beat-by-beat basis were, and are, so great that much effort was given to the development of pulse contour methods for the measurement of cardiac output. A recent study of this type, described by Skalak in Chapter 19, shows that fair results can be attained in this way under certain conditions.

Some few years before Frank's first attack on the problem (1899) the relation between elasticity and wave velocity in a fluid-filled tube was established theoretically by Korteweg (1878). In fact the original solution was given by Young (of Young's Modulus fame) in 1888 and had been reached independently by others. Korteweg was able to draw on the experimental work of Moens and it is general to refer to his expression as the Moens–Korteweg equation. The waves described by this are radial expansion waves, often referred to as Young waves to distinguish them from the Lamb waves in which the wall motion is axial.

Thus the wave velocity could be used to estimate aortic elasticity and the number derived used in the original Windkessel expressions which assumed pressure equilibration throughout the whole elastic chamber, i.e. an infinite wave velocity.

The model therefore required modification to allow finite wave speeds and many of the subtleties of the pressure contour were explained as due to interactions with reflected waves arising at the termination of the elastic chamber. Indeed an aortic standing wave was predicted and deduced from experimental records of pressures which were interpreted as showing a node at the level of the diaphragm.

It will be apparent that this analysis is based on the idea of transient excitation of the system with each arterial ejection with subsequent return to quiescent state before the next beat. But the demonstration of reflections led to the suspicion that the disturbances could outlive the pulse interval and that a steady state existed. This idea was vigorously expounded by McDonald and his school. It is best summarized in his book (McDonald, 1960) and has proved very fertile. This is not to say that Windkessel model is wholly false, but the steady state analysis is very much simpler than the transient approach and much more amenable to the incorporation of additional refinements. For example the much debated aortic standing wave would involve the presence of an antinode of flow at the diaphragm. Unpublished studies of my own in conjunction with Dr. Gabe and Mr. Mills have confirmed that there is indeed something of the sort in the dog. However, this can now be interpreted in terms of the properties of the whole arterial tree rather than leading to discussion of the physical limits of the conceptual Windkessel.

McDonald's interest stimulated the work of Womersley and led to the solution (Womersley, 1957) of the linearized Navier Stokes equations for the relation between an oscillatory pressure gradient and the fluid flow. These developments are described in detail by Noordergraaf (1970). The predictions of the oscillatory pressure flow relation in arteries were broadly confirmed by McDonald (1960). Other predictions on the form of the oscillatory flow profile have also been confirmed (see Chapter 9) while Womersley's expressions for wave velocity and damping were extended and tested by Taylor (1959).

Many of the chapters in this book can thus be seen as exploration of the consequences of the steady-state analysis of arterial function. Many problems remain and these are discussed in the chapters that follow. At the risk of being repetitious I intend to emphasize here some that are of personal interest to me.

1 . It is not at all clear to what extent non-linearities in the system have to be taken into account. These aspects are discussed by Skalak and Schultz

in Chapters 9 and 19 where it can be seen that there is a need for detailed comparison of experimental results with non-linear solutions and for a full examination of the combined effects of a number of influences (arterial visco-elasticity, arterial taper, elastic non-linearity, entrance length effects, etc.).

2. Although the Moens–Korteweg equation for wave velocity has been mentioned, substantial modifications are necessary to take account of fluid viscosity, wall viscosity and external tube restraint, and many other factors. Cox (1969) has emphasized the considerable disparities between the many published treatments, and for none of these has truly adequate agreement with experimental results been achieved.

3. A rather similar position exists for the prediction of arterial flow patterns. The most successful measurements of arterial flow from the pressure gradient have been made in the aorta. In this situation inertial forces predominate and blood viscosity may be entirely neglected with little effect on the oscillatory flow pattern. Detailed analysis (Fry et al., 1964) of such flow patterns in the aorta showed discrepancies with the Womersley predictions which have not yet been accounted for. In other regions, say in the femoral artery, no comparison has been made between predicted and observed flow waveforms since those discussed by McDonald in 1960.

4. As far as the heart is concerned ejection is certainly a transient phenomenon, and the aortic valve introduces a discontinuity in the pressure flow relationship. It should now be possible to move towards an understanding of the coupling between heart and aorta. We have rather good data on the input impedance of the aorta and its determinants (see Chapter 10) but almost no idea how to use this information to describe the mechanics of cardiac ejection.

5. The control of the circulation (see Chapter 5) is exercised partly by variations in the activity of the vascular smooth muscle. Although much is known about the passive properties of blood vessels (Chapter 11) we still have a lot to learn about the way in which these may be actively modified, although a start has been made in this direction (see Chapter 12). To make much progress here we will need to know much more of the detailed architecture of blood vessels, the properties of vascular muscle itself and the mechanics of highly deformable anisotropic non-homogeneous visco-elastic structures. Without such advances it will not be possible to reach a full understanding of arterial disease (see Chapters 13 and 14).

Each chapter in these volumes will suggest further problems. That is one function of this work and since many of these questions can now be posed in rather definite terms it would seem that prospects for the future are good.

REFERENCES

Cox, R. H. (1969). Comparison of linearized wave propagation. Models for arterial blood flow analysis. *J. Biomechanics.* **2,** 251–265.

Fry, D. L., Griggs, D. M. Jr. and Greenfield, J. C., Jr. (1964). *In vivo* studies of pulsatile flow: the relationship of the pressure gradient to the blood velocity. *In* "Pulsatile Blood Flow" (E. O. Attinger, ed.), McGraw-Hill, New York.

Hales, S. (1733). Statical essays, containing haemastaticks. Reprinted 1964. Hafner Publishing Co., New York.

Harvey, W. (1628). Exercitatio anatomica de muto cordis et sanguinis in animalibus. Trans. Franklin, K. J., 1957. Blackwells, Oxford.

McDonald, D. A. (1960). "Blood Flow in Arteries", Edward Arnold, London.

McDonald, D. A. and Taylor, M. G. (1959). The haemodynamics of the arterial circulation. *In* "Progress in Biophysics and Biophysical Chemistry" (J. A. V. Butler and B. Katz, eds.), Vol. 9, Pergamon Press, London.

Noordergraaf, A. (1970). Haemodynamcis. *In* "Biological Engineering" (H. P. Schwann, ed.), McGraw-Hill, New York.

Taylor, M. G. (1959). An experimental determination of the propagation of fluid oscillations in a tube with a visco-elastic wall; together with analysis of the characteristics required in an electrical analogue. *Phys. Med. Biol.* **4,** 63–82.

Vesalius, A. (1543). "De Humani Corporis", Basel.

Wetterer, E. and Kenner, TH. (1968). "Grundlagen der Dynamik des Arterienpulses", Springer-Verlag, Berlin.

Womersley, J. R. (1957). An elastic type theory of pulse transmission and oscillatory flow in mammalian arteries. Wright Air Development Center Technical Report WADC-TR-56-614.

Chapter 2

Pressure Measurement in Experimental Physiology

M.R.C. Cardiovascular Unit and Department of Medicine,
Hammersmith Hospital, London, W.12

1. INTRODUCTION

Although the measurement of pressure is now a routine in physiological and cardiac laboratories, there are many practical problems which continue to present difficulties. Obtaining pressure records of the highest quality demands time and care and sufficient time is not usually available in a busy cardiac laboratory investigating several patients each day. There are many outstanding accounts in the literature on physiological pressure measurement, including those of Hansen (1949), Fry (1960), and McDonald (1960). The emphasis here will be on practical problems in manometry but we shall nevertheless discuss theoretical matters in a descriptive way. An investigator will only be able to understand how good his records should be if he understands the underlying nature of the physics involved.

2. THEORETICAL BACKGROUND

The general object of physiological pressure measurement is to record pressure variations faithfully, usually in permanent analogue form. The process will involve a transducer capable of changing pressure signals into a form that is convenient—which normally now means a conversion from mechanical to electrical signals. The transducer will need an amplifier connected to some form of recorder and the whole system is required to behave in such a way that distortion of the pressure information is within acceptable limits. The distortion that can occur may be divided into that related to static or very slowly changing pressures and that connected with dynamic events.

A. STATIC PRESSURE REQUIREMENTS

It is first demanded that proportionality be maintained between steady pressures and the final output over the range of pressure likely to be encountered. Tests for linearity will require some primary means of pressure measurement and this will usually be a water or mercury manometer. Such tests are only possible if the system is sufficiently stable over the period of time taken. Preliminary tests will therefore be needed to show the amount of drift in the output when a steady pressure is applied over a long period. If this is small enough (when expressed in terms of pressure and in relation to final requirements) linearity tests repeated at intervals will show if the system is linear and if the gain is constant. During such tests hysteresis may be observed, i.e. the output levels recorded when steps of increasing pressure are applied are not the same when the pressure steps decrease. Satisfactory transducer systems must clearly show minimal hysteresis—say 1 per cent of full scale deflection or lesss.

A potent cause of baseline drift is change in temperature. With many transducers time must be allowed for thermal equilibrium to be reached after switching on. The warmth of a hand on a transducer may produce significant drift, and the effects of changes in room temperature should be considered.

B. DYNAMIC PRESSURE REQUIREMENTS

If the pressure to be recorded is varying with time the dynamic response of the system will have an important effect on the way in which signals are treated. If the transducer cannot respond quickly to fast changes in pressure than it is clear that there will be distortion. High fidelity requires great care in the choice and use of apparatus. The degree of fidelity needed in any measurement will depend upon the object of the investigation. If only mean blood pressure is of interest it will be pointless to expend great energy on achieving a high frequency response. We need, therefore, to define in a useful way the characteristics of the physiological pressure signal which is to be dealt with.

For the purpose of discussion it will be convenient to have in mind a particular pressure signal. The arterial pressure waveform will serve well for it is widely known and the general principles involved may be readily applied to other waveforms. Let us deal initially with the simplest situation—a regular heart rate and an arterial pressure that repeats exactly with each beat. Fourier theory shows that the waveform can be considered as a mean level together with the sum of a series of sine waves of appropriate amplitude and phase. The lowest frequency sine wave will be that of the heart rate and the other frequencies will be integral multiples of this fundamental frequency. If we are to reproduce this waveform then the apparatus used including the transducer, amplifier and recorder, must be able to deal with the mean level and the harmonic components in such a way that their subsequent summation still yields the original waveform. For perfection, this means that there should be no amplitude or phase distortion. However, there is one condition in which the shape of the original wave will be retained even if the last restriction is not strictly met. If there is no disturbance of the relative amplitudes of the frequency components but their phases are shifted in proportion to frequency, then synthesis from the components will still yield the original waveform although it will be delayed in time by an amount dependent upon the phase shifts.

In practice it is unnecessary to avoid amplitude and phase distortion at all frequencies. The larger harmonics will be at the lowest frequencies and as frequency rises they will decrease in magnitude until they become indistinguishable from the effects of background biological and instrumental noise. Examples of harmonic analyses of pressure waveforms obtained from the heart and great vessels of man may be seen in the study by Patel, Mason, Ross and Braunwald (1965). There is no definite boundary above which biological pressure variations may be ignored, but the effects of omitting harmonics higher than the tenth is, for most purposes, quite small. This means, for example, that if the heart rate is 120 min^{-1} or 2 Hz we need a flat amplitude response to the tenth harmonic or to 20 Hz. At a lower heart rate the frequency range required—or bandwidth—would be less.

There are circumstances in which the demand for fidelity may be greater than this. If the maximum time-derivative of the pressure signal is needed, the problem of the bandwidth required becomes less clear. Differentiation of a signal increases the amplitudes of its frequency components by factors that are proportional to frequency. Thus noise at higher frequencies can become very large on differentiation. The original signal should be as free from noise as possible, i.e. by the use of a low-pass filter set at such a frequency that the derivative of the pressure waveform is not significantly affected. The bandwidth required may be estimated, as before, by Fourier analysis of the time-derivative signal and then making a decision on the number of harmonics which appear to be important. The results of such an approach are given by Gersh, Hahn and Prys-Roberts (1971). It may be useful to consider here a different method that can have general applicability and is simple enough to give immediate estimates of required bandwidth. Figure 1 shows a record

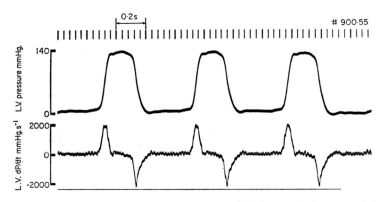

Fig. 1. A record of left ventricular pressure and left ventricular rate of change of pressure in a dog. Left ventricular pressure was measured by an implanted Microsystem 1017 transducer and the first derivative was obtained by an analogue computer.

of the left ventricular pressure and left ventricular rate of change of pressure in a dog. The pressure was measured by an implanted semiconductor device which had been shown to have a flat amplitude response up to 105 Hz, the maximum frequency obtainable from the sinusoidal pressure generator used (Gabe, Guz, Noble and Stubbs, 1970). Let us suppose that our object is to determine values for the maximum rate of change of pressure. We therefore need to reproduce faithfully the heights of the positive peaks in the time-derivative record. The positive wave is preceded by a long quiescent interval and its shape is similar to a cosine-squared pulse.† The relative amplitude spectrum of a cosine-squared pulse may be computed and is shown in Fig. 2. It will be seen that if the base-width of the pulse is T seconds, then the important amplitude components have frequencies less than $2/T$ Hz.

† A cosine-squared pulse consists essentially of a single cosine wave.

This can be shown experimentally by passing a cosine-squared pulse from a signal generator through a variable low-pass filter and displaying the original signal and the filtered waveform on an oscilloscope. The results of such an experiment, for different values of the base-width T, are given in

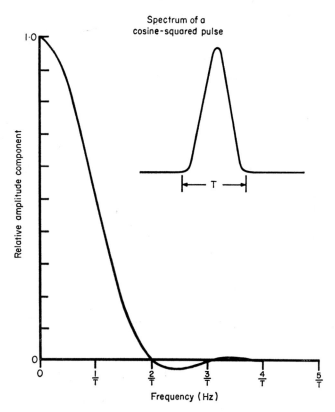

FIG. 2. The spectrum of a cosine-squared pulse of base-width T seconds. The amplitudes have been scaled in relation to the zero frequency term. Note that the significant amplitude components have frequencies of less than $2/T$ Hz. The small portion shown between $2/T$ and $3/T$ is drawn as negative because the phase has changed by 180°.

Fig. 3. The interrupted line shows the bandwidth that was required to include frequencies up to $2/T$ Hz; the error in the level of the peak was difficult to measure but was less than 1 per cent. If an error in the estimation of the peak of 5 per cent is acceptable then the bandwidth required will be less, and is shown by the solid dots and the continuous line in Fig. 3. Thus if the base-width T is 0·08 seconds a bandwidth of 17 Hz will diminish the peak by only 5 per cent while a bandwidth of 25 Hz will bring the error to the 1 per cent level.

The action of a low-pass filter on a signal is such that the frequencies above the nominal cut-off frequency are not attenuated absolutely; the filter used for the experiment shown in Fig. 3 reduced amplitudes by 30 per cent

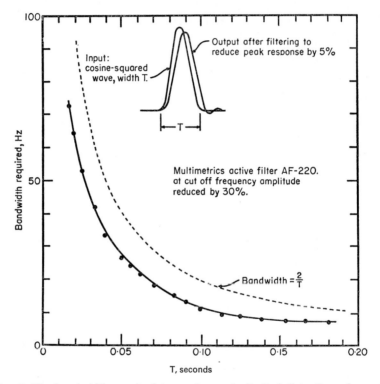

Fig. 3. The bandwidth required to produce only limited distortion of a cosine-squared wave of variable duration (T seconds). A cosine-squared wave from a signal generator was passed through an active low-pass filter, the cut-off frequency of which could be varied. The cut-off frequency needed to reduce the peak response by 5 per cent, at different values of the basewidth T, was determined. The experimental results are shown by the solid dots. The interrupted line shows the predicted bandwidth required to include frequencies up to $2/T$; the error in the peak was then less than 1 per cent.

at the cut-off frequency and thereafter at 24 dB per octave. Another way of visualizing the effect of ignoring frequencies above a given level is by synthesizing the harmonic components of a waveform. The inset of Fig. 4 shows the time-derivative of a left ventricular pressure waveform. Fourier analysis of this yielded the harmonic components. A series of harmonic syntheses including different numbers of harmonics, enabled the error in the estimated peak to be calculated. When eight harmonics were used for the synthesis the height of the peak dP/dt was estimated with an accuracy of 5 per cent. This was achieved using no frequencies above the eighth harmonic at 12·7 Hz.

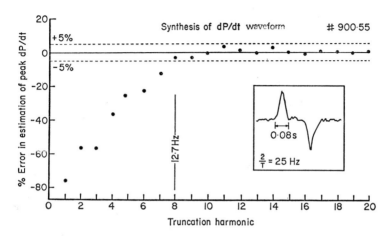

FIG. 4. Synthesis of a $LV\ dP/dt$ waveform (shown inset). The number of harmonics used for the synthesis is plotted against the resultant percentage error in peak dP/dt—in comparison with the original waveform. The estimated basewidth of the positive pulse is 0·08 seconds and this would suggest that it would be reproduced well if frequencies up to 2/0·08 or 25 Hz were included. This criterion is more stringent than it need be for many purposes since the omission of all harmonics above the eighth at 12·7 Hz still results in only a 4 per cent error in the peak produced on re-synthesis.

Since the base-width of the positive wave of left ventricular dP/dt was approximately 0·08 seconds a suggested bandwidth of $2/T$ or 25 Hz is therefore more than generous.

The empirical rule just described enables a working estimate of the bandwidth needed to be arrived at quickly if the object is to record accurately a particular feature of a waveform. If the feature is asymmetric the use of half a cosine-squared pulse is appropriate, as illustrated in Fig. 5. Half a cosine-squared pulse should be fitted to the initial part of the wave; the bandwidth required will then be the reciprocal of the half period. It is implicit that the record used for such an estimate must be made with apparatus capable of dealing with a frequency range larger than that shown finally to be necessary.

It was mentioned above that an initial assumption was that the pressure waveform was exactly periodic. Although this restriction is required if the

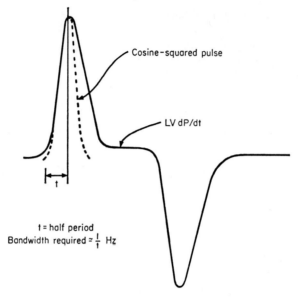

FIG. 5. Estimation of the bandwidth required if the desired pulse is asymmetric. Half a cosine-squared pulse should be fitted to the initial slope. The bandwidth required will then be the reciprocal of the half-period.

results of Fourier analysis are to be interpreted precisely, the basic ideas are not affected by lack of periodicity—although the way in which the spectral content is extracted may have to be modified.

C. THEORETICAL ANALYSIS OF PRESSURE TRANSDUCER SYSTEMS

The essential dynamic properties of a pressure transducer system may be revealed by an analysis of a transducer connected to a rigid needle: this is the analysis of a single degree of freedom system. In many practical situations the results of such a study are of great value—even when a catheter is used instead of a needle. In other situations, when for example the catheter is long, transmission line theory must be invoked to explain the phenomena which are observed. Although the analysis then becomes more complex the basic properties of the system can nevertheless be understood without great difficulty.

(1) *The single degree of freedom system*

This, the simplest system, has been studied by many workers. For those who require the complete analysis, Hansen (1949) and Hansen and Warburg (1950) should be consulted. Since our main concern is with practical problems we shall give only the results. The nomenclature and symbols used by different writers vary considerably; here we shall largely keep to the symbols used by McDonald (1960), whose lucid account of manometer behaviour has helped so many.

Consider a needle of length l and radius r connected to a pressure transducer. Let the pressure–volume relationship of the diaphragm† of the transducer be $E = \Delta P/\Delta V$. We shall suppose that the system is filled with liquid of density ρ and viscosity μ. The mass of fluid within the needle is thus coupled to the elastic diaphragm and the phenomena of resonance will therefore arise. It can be shown that the natural frequency, f_0, of the system is given by

$$f_0 = \frac{1}{2\pi} \sqrt{\frac{\pi r^2 E}{\rho l}} \qquad (2.1)$$

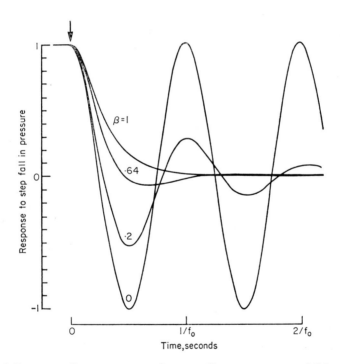

FIG. 6. Response of a pressure transducer-needle system to a step fall in pressure. Results are shown for four values of the damping factor, β: 0, 0·2, 0·64 and 1·0. The time scale is in terms of the reciprocal of the undamped natural frequency, f_0.

† Only displacement of the diaphragm will be useful for the measurement of pressure, but liquid over the diaphragm is compressible and the performance will depend on the total compliance.

The natural frequency is the frequency at which the system would resonate in the absence of any viscous losses or damping. The amount of damping, termed here the damping factor, β, may be calculated from

$$\beta = \frac{4\mu}{r^3} \sqrt{\frac{l}{\pi E}} \qquad (2.2)$$

When the pressure applied to the needle is suddenly changed from one level to another the system will resonate at the damped resonant frequency

Statham P23 Gb transducer. Needle I.D. 0·495mm, length 31 cm

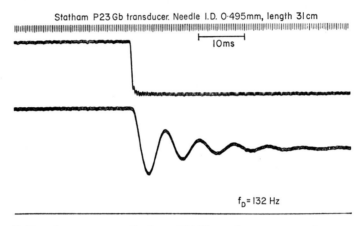

10ms

$f_D = 132$ Hz

FIG. 7. Transient test on a Statham P23Gb strain-gauge transducer connected through two stopcocks to a needle, i.d. 0·495 mm, 31 cm long. The damped resonant frequency, f_D, was 132 Hz. As in Figs. 10 and 12, the upper trace is the pressure at the input recorded directly by a second P23Gb transducer, while the lower trace is the transient response of the system. Records were made initially on a Precision Instruments tape recorder at 37·5 in s^{-1}; the tape was played back at 0·375 in s^{-1} on to a Cambridge Instrument Company photographic recorder. By this means a relatively slow recorder (100 Hz oil damped galvanometers) could be used to reproduce events faithfully up to the kHz range.

—a frequency less than the undamped resonant frequency. The characteristics of such a response are illustrated in Fig. 6. When the value of the damping factor is zero (a physically unrealizable state) the diaphragm will vibrate sinusoidally and the oscillations will continue indefinitely. When the damping factor is unity the diaphragm will return exponentially to its equilibrium position as quickly as it can without overshooting; the amount of damping is then said to be "critical". If the damping factor is less than unity there will be some overshoot and the oscillations that occur take the form of a damped sinusoid. An example of a transient test on a Statham P23Gb strain-gauge transducer connected to a needle, 31 cm long and i.d.

0·495 mm, is shown in Fig. 7. The damped resonant frequency is 132 Hz. Using (2.1) the predicted undamped resonant frequency is 145 Hz.

The way the system behaves to a transient change in pressure is of great value in testing the performance of a transducer. Practical problems in transient testing will be dealt with later. Equally important is the response to sinusoidal oscillations. If a sinusoidal pressure is applied to the needle we would like the displacement of the diaphragm to be of constant amplitude

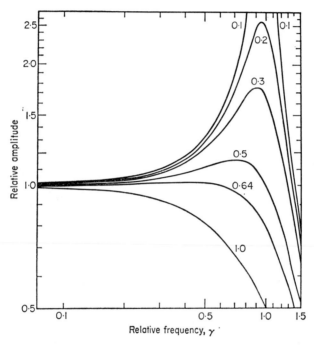

FIG. 8. The amplitude response of a pressure transducer to a sinusoidal pressure signal of unit amplitude. Relative frequency (logarithmic scale) is the ratio of the forcing frequency to the undamped natural frequency of the system. Response curves are shown for systems with a damping factor, β, of 0·1, 0·2, 0·3, 0·5, 0·64 and 1·0.

at any frequency; ideally, too, there should be no phase difference between the two oscillations. However, a single degree of freedom system cannot behave in this manner. The way in which the amplitude of the diaphragm oscillations vary with frequency and damping factor is shown in Fig. 8. In this diagram relative frequency, γ, is the ratio of the forcing frequency to the undamped natural frequency. It will be seen that for low values of the damping factor the amplitude rises to a peak with an increase of frequency, before then decreasing again. At critical damping, when $\gamma = 1\cdot0$, the relative amplitude falls continuously as frequency rises. Figure 9 shows the phase-lag of the diaphragm behind the forcing oscillation.

Figures 8 and 9 enable some estimates to be made of the frequency range over which a pressure transducer system can be held to be accurate. If we have a system in which the damping factor is 0·2 then we can say that the relative amplitude will be correct to within 5 per cent up to a relative frequency of 0·2. Also, the phase-lag is very nearly linear with frequency over

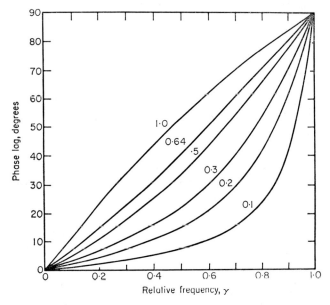

Fig. 9. The phase-lag of a pressure transducer behind a sinusoidal pressure signal for different values of the damping factor, β. Relative frequency is the ratio of the forcing frequency to the undamped natural frequency of the system.

this range. Hence signals which contain frequencies of significant amplitude in this range only will be little distorted, although they will be delayed by a time interval dependent on the phase shift. The useful frequency range can be extended by raising the amount of damping—but the phase-lag will then be increased. For many purposes a damping factor of 0·64 is desirable; the error in the amplitude is then less than 2 per cent up to 67 per cent of the natural frequency and the phase-lag is tolerably linear over this range. When β is 0·64 the amount of overshoot in the transient test is 7 per cent, as shown in Fig. 6. If more exact estimates are required than are shown in Figs. 8 and 9, the Tables in Hansen (1949) should be consulted.

The simple analysis of the transducer-needle system as one with a single degree of freedom rests on a series of assumptions, the most significant of which concerns the fluid flow in the needle. If viscosity is ignored it can be assumed that the fluid in the needle moves as a single solid mass, with a flat velocity profile. Damping is introduced by assuming that viscous losses in the needle are those that would be expected if the flow were steady and the velocity profile was parabolic, as predicted in the Poiseuille–Hagenbach equation. In fact, flow is not steady but oscillatory, and from this two effects follow. First, the effective mass of fluid in the needle—the fluid inertance—is higher than would be expected, but falls asymptotically as frequency rises. Secondly, the viscous losses are also higher, but rise with increase in frequency. More exact analysis is necessarily more complex and was first carried out by Lambossy (1952). The improvement in prediction produced thereby is, however, marginal. The matter is discussed in McDonald (1960).

Another assumption in the simple theory is that the liquid in the needle is incompressible and that pressure changes at one end of the needle will be transmitted instantaneously to the other end. In fact, the transmission of pressure along the needle will occur very nearly at the velocity of sound in water (about 1400 m s^{-1}) and the time taken for pressure waves to travel down needles less than 1 m long is small in relation to the period of the resonant frequency. If a long catheter is used this may no longer be so and the analysis becomes more difficult.

(2) *Transmission line theory*

That the analysis of a transducer–catheter system as a single degree of freedom system is not always justified is indicated by the result of transient test shown in Fig. 10. The catheter was a No. 7 cardiac catheter, i.d. 0·117 cm, 125 cm long, and the transducer was a Statham P23Gb strain-gauge. Great care was taken to eliminate air-bubbles from the system. The resonant frequency was 83 Hz but the form of the oscillation was not that of a damped sinusoid—although if it had been recorded with a slower time scale the departure from a damped sinusoid might have been ignored. The time taken for the fall in pressure to travel from the end of the catheter to the transducer was approximately 2·1 ms and the velocity of propagation along the 125 cm length was therefore 595 m s^{-1}. The phenomena that are here observed can be interpreted in terms of transmission line theory. This was done by Hansen (1949), by Fry (1960) and more recently by Latimer (1968) and Latimer and Latimer (1969). Detailed analysis requires a mathematical account which, for many, may obscure rather than illuminate. Here we shall try to present the essential ideas with the important results that follow. It will simplify matters if, provisionally, we ignore the viscous losses along the catheter.

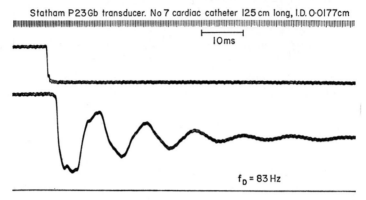

Statham P23Gb transducer. No 7 cardiac catheter 125 cm long, I.D. 0·0177cm

10ms

$f_D = 83\,Hz$

FIG. 10. Transient test on a No. 7 cardiac catheter (U.S.C.I.) i.d. 1·17 cm, 125 cm long, connected to a Statham P23Gb strain-gauge transducer. Note that the oscillations, occurring at 83 Hz, do not now take the form of a damped sinusoid and that therefore it cannot be maintained that the transducer and catheter form a simple single degree of freedom system.

We now represent the catheter as an elastic tube of radius r and length l, containing a liquid of density ρ. The compliance, C, per unit length of catheter is $\Delta V/\Delta P$, where ΔV is increment of internal volume of catheter and ΔP is increment of pressure. The inertial effects of the fluid in the catheter may most usefully be quantitated by the fluid inertance, L, per unit length, $\rho/\pi r^2$. (We ignore, for simplicity, the fact that the velocity profiles are not flat: this follows from the assumption that viscous effects may be neglected.) The essential quantities to be considered when a catheter is treated as a transmission line are the compliance and the fluid inertance per unit length. Both these are distributed evenly along the catheter.

Suppose now that the catheter is infinitely long. If the pressure at one end is suddenly raised there will be a certain flow of fluid into the lumen. Thus the catheter will appear to have a certain resistance, R_0, and its magnitude is given by

$$R_0 = \sqrt{(L/C)} \qquad (2.3)$$

R_0 is known as the characteristic resistance of the catheter. (If viscous effects are taken into account there will be, in general, phase differences between pressure and flow and characteristic impedance is the term then used instead of characteristic resistance.) The catheter behaves as a fixed resistance, R_0, no matter how long it is. At each point the travelling wave of pressure sees ahead of it, as it were, more catheter of characteristic resistance R_0. If at some point the catheter were cut and attached to a pure fluid resistance of value R_0 the wave would dissipate itself in the viscous resistance. However, if the resistance inserted were not equal to R_0, complete dissipation would not be possible and at least part of the wave would then be reflected back to the origin.

The velocity, c, with which a wave is propagated along the catheter is given by

$$c \simeq \frac{1}{\sqrt{LC}} \tag{2.4}$$

From this an estimate of the compliance per unit length may be derived:

$$C = \frac{1}{c^2 L} \tag{2.5}$$

It will be helpful to translate these expressions into numerical terms in a special case—that shown in Fig. 10. For a No. 7 cardiac catheter of internal radius 0·0585 cm, the fluid inertance per cm is $1/(0·0585^2 \times \pi) = 93·0$ dyn s^2 cm^{-6}. From Fig. 10 the velocity of propagation is 595 m s^{-1} and therefore the compliance per cm is $1/(59\,500^2 \times 93) = 3·04 \times 10^{-12}$ dyn^{-1} cm^4. We now calculate the characteristic resistance of the catheter:

$$R_0 = \sqrt{(L/C)} = 5·53 \times 10^6 \text{ dyn s cm}^{-5}.$$

The catheter used for Fig. 10 was 125 cm long and was terminated in a strain-gauge transducer, the dominant element of which is a compliant diaphragm. This cannot dissipate energy and hence must reflect waves back along the catheter. The reactance, X_t, of the diaphragm at the resonant frequency of the system is

$$X_t = \frac{1}{2\pi f C} \tag{2.6}$$

which gives $X_t = 6·31 \times 10^8$ dyn s cm^{-5}. Thus the reactance of the diaphragm is larger than the characteristic resistance of the catheter by two orders of magnitude and the catheter is, in effect, terminated by an absolute obstruction.

We may now picture, in a qualitative way, what happens when a transient pressure change passes down a catheter connected to a stiff diaphragm. The events are illustrated in Fig. 11. As the pressure falls at the open end of the catheter a forward-going pressure wave, F_1, starts to travel to the closed end. It arrives after a delay t_d but no flow can occur at the point of obstruction and a backward-going pressure wave, B_1, is produced of the same magnitude and sign as F_1: the sum of F_1 and B_1 is a pressure fall of twice the size of either. B_1 arrives at the open end after a further delay t_d, or $2t_d$ after the initial transient. At the open end no pressure changes can occur and a second forward-going pressure wave F_2 is generated of equal magnitude but opposite sign to B_1, so that the sum of the two is zero. F_2 will arrive at the closed end after another delay t_d and will there generate yet another backward-going wave B_2. It will be seen from Fig. 11 that the

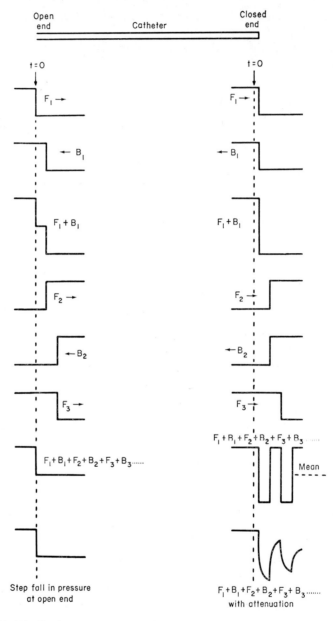

FIG. 11. Idealized representation of the transmission of a step fall in pressure from the open end of a catheter to the other end, closed here by a very stiff membrane. The initial fall in pressure at the open end results in a forward pressure wave, F_1, travelling to the closed end. There it will be reflected as an identical

process will repeat itself indefinitely. At the open end the sum of all the waves will be such that a single step fall in pressure is produced; at the closed end there will be a series of square wave oscillations. It can be shown that the frequency of the oscillations will be at $c/4l$ Hz. The effects of viscosity in the fluid and in the elastic wall have been neglected and the oscillations will not continue for ever in reality. They will tend to take the form shown in the lower right-hand diagram in Fig. 11; their resemblance to Fig. 10 is clear. Thus oscillations are possible in a system in which the compliance of the diaphragm is entirely ignored. Even with a needle similar phenomena must occur. The elasticity per unit length of needle will derive largely from the compressibility of water. The velocity of propagation will be approximately that of sound in water. The natural resonant frequency of a closed-end needle, 30 cm long, will be approximately $140\,000/(4 \times 30)$ or $1\cdot2$ kHz. In this case the diaphragm will not be stiff in relation to the needle and the system becomes simplified into a single lumped inertance in the needle and a single compliance at the diaphragm—that is to say, into a single degree of freedom system.

Shortening a catheter will diminish the delay due to wave travel and may make the system approximate to one with a single degree of freedom. Figure 12(a) shows the transient response of a Statham P23Gb transducer connected to 125 cm of PTFE tubing, i.d. 0·89 mm. The measured wave velocity was 460 m s^{-1}. Considered as a lossless transmission line with a closed end the resonant frequency expected is $46\,000/(4 \times 120) = 96$ Hz. The actual resonant frequency was 87 Hz and the transient response was not that of a pure damped sinusoid. When the catheter was shortened to 30 cm, Fig. 12(b) was recorded. Some sharp vibrations may be seen early in the transient; their frequency is approximately 1·6 kHz and their origin is not clear. They are possibly the result of longitudinal wave transmission in the catheter wall. When the same record was filtered at 1 kHz and these fast vibrations removed, Fig. 12(c) resulted. The resemblance of the oscillation to a damped sinusoid is clear. The resonant frequency was 208 Hz; the frequency to be expected from a corresponding closed end transmission line is 383 Hz, considerably more.

---

backward-going wave, B_1. The sum of F_1 and B_1 at the closed end will result in the pressure drop doubling in magnitude. The backward-going wave B_1, will reach the open end after some delay and its reflection will this time produce a forward-going wave F_2 of opposite sign. The generation of successive forward- and backward-going waves will result in the single step fall in pressure at the open end and a series of pressure oscillations at the closed end. In a real system there will be attenuation of the waves as they travel along the catheter and the final pressure changes at the closed end will tend to have the appearance shown in the lower right-hand curve (cf. Fig. 10). Note that such oscillations will occur even if the diaphragm closing the end of the catheter is infinitely stiff.

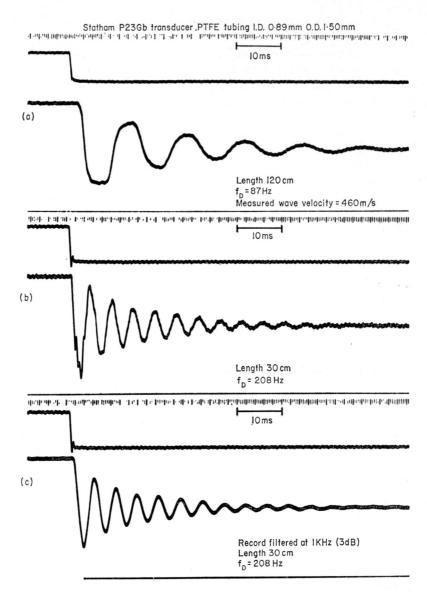

Statham P23Gb transducer .PTFE tubing I.D. 0·89mm O.D. 1·50mm

10ms

(a)

Length 120 cm
$f_D = 87$ Hz
Measured wave velocity = 460 m/s

10ms

(b)

Length 30 cm
$f_D = 208$ Hz

10ms

(c)

Record filtered at 1KHz (3dB)
Length 30 cm
$f_D = 208$ Hz

Fig. 12. Transient response of a P23Gb strain-gauge transducer connected to PTFE tubing, i.d. 0·89 mm, o.d. 1·50 mm. In Fig. 12(a) the length of catheter was 120 cm and the measured wave velocity was 460 m s^{-1}. The resonant frequency was 87 Hz. When the catheter was shortened to 30 cm the record shown in Fig. 12(b) was made. The dominant oscillation was at 208 Hz but sharp vibrations at approximately 1·6 kHz can be seen early in the record. When the record was filtered electrically at 1 kHz (effectively; because of the tape speed changes the actual filtering frequency was at 10 Hz) the trace shown in Fig. 13(c) was produced. The resemblance to a damped sinusoid is now strong.

The actual departure of transducer–catheter systems used in cardio-vascular investigation from those with a single degree of freedom may be quite small even when the catheter is relatively long. The reason for this is that the frequency range required for pressure records extends only to about 20 Hz. At that frequency the catheter is likely to be much shorter than the wavelength. The wavelength is the ratio of wave velocity to frequency, for a wave velocity of 500 m s^{-1} the wavelength at 20 Hz will be 25 m; at lower frequencies it will be even longer.

The extension of the frequency range by transmission line matching technique has been suggested by Ranke (1952), van der Tweel (1957), Latimer (1968) and others and will be discussed later in the section on damping.

3. Types of Transducers

Few will now have need to make their own pressure transducers and we shall here describe only briefly the principles underlying the main types of transducer used. Nearly all contain a diaphragm of some sort, the displace-ment of which is arranged to be proportional to the steady pressure applied. If the transducer is external to the vascular system it is desirable for the diaphragm to be stiff in order to achieve an adequate frequency response. By far the greatest need is for single-sided pressure transducers, where the pressure recorded is compared with constant atmospheric pressure. If the difference between two varying pressures is demanded, either a differential manometer will be required or the electrical difference between two single manometers must be taken.

A. STRAIN-GAUGE MANOMETERS

At the present time the manometers most widely used in cardiovascular laboratories are of the strain-gauge type. They depend upon the fact that a change in the length of a wire produces a change in its resistance (see Chapter 4). The principle can be applied to measure the displacement of a diaphragm. The diaphragm is coupled to wire elements which themselves form the arms of a Wheatstone bridge. Strain-gauge manometers are stable and rugged and their volume displacements can be as small as those available in other types of external transducers. The strain-gauge manometer with the smallest compliance in general use now is the Statham P23Gb, which has a volume displacement of 0·01 mm^3 per 100 mmHg (or $E = 1·33 \times 10^{10}$ dyne cm^{-5})—a figure worth remembering so that the specifications of other gauges can be immediately compared. There is little justification for using, in cardiovascular work, a gauge with a volume displacement of greater than 0·04 mm^3 per 100 mmHg.

The wire strain-gauge transducer normally occupies sufficient space to make it necessary that it be connected to the vascular system by a needle or catheter. However, in the Statham SF–1 transducer the strain-gauge is mounted at the end of a cardiac catheter and the resonant frequency in fluid is at least 1 kHz. Unfortunately, the life expectancy of an SF–1 is very much less than that of an external transducer and few laboratories can afford to use them regularly.

High precision differential manometry with strain-gauges has most commonly been achieved by differencing electrically two single-sided, balanced strain-gauges (Greenfield and Fry, 1962); similar precision was obtained by the strain-gauge differential manometer described by Porjé and Rudewald (1961). Commercially available differential pressure transducers are apt to be disappointing in their dynamic and even sometimes in their static performances.

The development of semiconductor techniques has resulted in a new set of devices, still using the resistive effects of strain. Silicon has a gauge factor (defined as the ratio of the proportional change in resistance to the proportional change in length) about 50–60 times as large as that of the metals usually used in strain-gauges. This means that the resistance change for a given deformation of the diaphragm can be much greater when silicon is used, with a corresponding decrease in the requirements of the amplifier.

The devices can be miniaturized and mounted on the end of needles or catheters; some are designed to be implanted in blood vessels and ventricles (the left ventricular pressure record shown in Fig. 1 was made with such a transducer). The frequency response is then far greater than that required for biological purposes.

B. CAPACITANCE MANOMETERS

The property of capacitance can be used to determine the displacement of a diaphragm. A plate is held a short distance from the diaphragm and the combination constitutes a capacitor. The dielectric used may be air or oil. Variations in the spacing between diaphragm and fixed plate can be recorded by measuring the electrical impedance of the device. By using high frequencies very small changes in capacitance, and therefore in displacement, can be detected. The capacitance manometer made by Lilly (1942) had a volume displacement of only 0·001 mm^3 per 100 mmHg. The construction and properties of a capacitance manometer are described in detail by Hansen (1949).

In spite of the sensitivity of the capacitance manometer the method is not much used at the present time. Unless particular care is taken in the design of the manometers and the electronic apparatus they can be unstable.

C. INDUCTANCE MANOMETERS

Variations in the inductance of a coil, or in the inductive coupling between two coils, can form the basis for the detection of the motion of a diaphragm. Such transducers are commercially available but the volume displacements of the external gauges are larger than those which can be obtained by other methods, although there is no necessary reason why this should be so. The principle is compatible with miniaturization and a catheter-tip inductance manometer was devised first by Wetterer (1943). Gauer and Gienapp (1950) improved on Wetterer's design and the instrument, subsequently developed by the Telco Company, France, can be obtained commercially. The frequency response extends well into the sonic range so that intracardiac sounds and murmurs can be recorded.

D. OPTICAL MANOMETERS

The use of a light beam to detect diaphragm displacement has a long history in physiology, but it is seldom employed now. Frank described his optical manometer in 1924 (although it was used for many years before that) and similar but improved devices were produced by Wiggers (1914) and Hamilton, Brewer and Brotman (1934). In these and other instruments a light beam was reflected from a mirror mounted on a diaphragm and then passed over a distance of several metres to a moving photographic film. The long optical lever removed the need for electronics, but necessarily made the apparatus bulky and sensitive to vibrations. The use of a photocell (Müller and Shillingford, 1954) can reduce the size of the apparatus but its stability is still less than that that can be obtained by other techniques.

Recently catheter-tip transducers employing an optical method have been described (Ramirez, Hood, Polanyi, Wagner, Yankopoulos and Abelmann, 1969; Lindström, 1970). A light guide of glass fibres inside a catheter conducts light from an external source to the catheter-tip. At the tip a diaphragm reflects a variable amount of light into a second light guide leading to an external photodetector. The performance was excellent, both in stability and in frequency response.

E. SERVO-MANOMETER

The measurement of pressure in the microcirculation poses considerable technical problems. The microinjection pressure measuring technique, described by Landis (1926, 1966) gives information intermittently on slowly changing pressures. The microcannulae which are necessary severely limit the frequency response attainable with most pressure transducers. Bloch (1966) has given an account of modifications to a Lilly capacitance transducer which enable it to be used satisfactorily with cannulae of 35 μm bore;

improvements to a Statham P23Gb strain-gauge for a similar purpose are
described by Levasseur, Funk and Patterson (1969b). The system introduced
by Wiederhielm (1966) differs from others in principle and can be used
with micropipets of only 0·5 μm–5 μm diameter. A micropipet is filled with
2 M solution of sodium chloride, the conductance of which is greater than
that of body fluids. It is arranged that the micropipet forms one arm of a
Wheatstone bridge. If the pressure in the blood vessel is higher than that in
the micropipet, fluid enters the tip and the bridge becomes unbalanced,
producing an error signal. This is amplified and used to drive a bellows which
increases the pressure in the system and returns the micropipet to its original
state. The pressure in the hydraulic system should therefore follow the
pressure in the medium surrounding the tip and can be recorded with a
gauge of relatively large volume displacement. The effective volume displacement of the system is very low and the usable frequency range extends to
about 20 Hz.

4. PRACTICAL PROBLEMS IN MANOMETRY

Even with the best equipment the making of good pressure records with
external transducers requires more care than can often be given. The use of
catheter-tip transducers would avoid most of the difficulties—but for econo-
mic reasons their day has not yet come and most investigators will continue
to use external gauges for the bulk of work. This is a matter for regret, since
the problems of using external transducers to the limit of their capacity
continue to be large. In principle high quality records can be made; in
practice a busy cardiac laboratory investigating three or four patients daily
will not be able to attain even half the frequency range possible. The usual
resonant frequency of the systems in such laboratories is about 10–14 Hz. It
can be argued that for most purposes the limitation of frequency range
does not matter; and that may well be so. But the contrast between technical
possibility and everyday practical achievement is almost absurdly great.
With enough care and time this gap can be closed.

A. SELECTION OF PRESSURE TRANSDUCER AND ASSOCIATED APPARATUS

In general the choice of apparatus will not be free but will be determined
by what is available in the laboratory. Every effort should be made to see
the specifications of the apparatus but it would be wise to test for oneself
what one can and to assume the minimum. I have personal knowledge of
three transducers introduced by different manufacturers which dynamic
testing showed to have volume displacements 2–4 times larger than was
claimed. None of the makers had tested the gauges adequately. One had
correctly estimated the volume displacement of the diaphragm but had

forgotten that this was effectively doubled because of the compression of water in the rather large dome.

The main features of any transducer which will have to be tested are sensitivity, linearity, hysteresis, stability and volume displacement. The sensitivity obtainable must be considered in relation to the object of the investigation, e.g. whether venous or arterial pressures are to be measured and how much noise will be acceptable. Linearity tests will require the application of known pressures from a water or mercury manometer or from the kind of apparatus shown in Fig. 13; the measurements should be made on the recorder which will be used. It may seem unlikely that transducers now sold will exhibit significant hysteresis, but large hysteresis was in fact found recently on testing a new miniature transducer. Tests on hysteresis and stability require the system to be run with the recorder going at a slow speed and with a series of constant pressures applied to the transducer. Changes in ambient temperature may be important in long-term stability. The volume displacement can most easily be measured by the dynamic tests described below.

At the end of such tests the adequacy of the manometer system for the purpose in mind should be clear. It is important to be conscious of the frequency range required for the investigation. Whether the transducer will be adequate will often depend on the catheter or needle which can be used and a preliminary calculation of the natural frequency of the system, using (2.1), and making the assumption of a single degree of freedom system will give an immediate rough idea of what can be obtained. Increasing the diameter of the catheter will, initially, at least, increase the frequency response, but the size must be a matter for compromise. The shorter the catheter the better. The common practice in cardiac laboratories of using a second catheter to connect the first to the transducer should be avoided whenever possible.

Any transducer will require stopcocks so that the catheter or needle can be flushed easily and calibrating pressures applied to the diaphragm. Transducers are expensive devices and the tendency to employ cheap stopcocks is a natural one. The use of such stopcocks is the source of much trouble and is indeed a false economy. Plastic taps are extremely variable in their performance and should not be used. The best stopcocks manufactured are, in my opinion, those made by Elema-Schonander† and Ole Dich‡.

B. PREPARATION OF THE APPARATUS

When the transducer and the associated apparatus have been chosen, preparation should begin by cleaning and re-greasing the stopcocks indivi-

† Elema-Schonander, Stockholm, Sweden.
‡ Ole Dich, 18 Avedoereholmen, 2650 Hvidovre, Denmark.

dually. Pipe cleaners are indispensable for cleaning the passages in the stop-cocks: it is particularly important that excess grease is not left to block the free flow of liquid. If a tap leaks there may be two main effects. First, the damping in the system will increase, perhaps significantly. Secondly, blood may pass up the catheter towards the leak and clotting may then occur. The presence of leaks may be quickly established after the stopcocks have been assembled on the transducer by pressurizing the gauge, recording the output and turning all the stopcocks so that the transducer is isolated from outside pressure. In principle the pressure within the transducer should then be maintained. In practice the pressure will probably fall slowly unless the stopcocks are well made and properly greased. If the gauge has a small volume displacement only a small volume will have to leak away before the diaphragm is displaced.

The actual arrangement of stopcocks on a transducer will depend to some extent on the object of the investigation. The arrangement in our laboratory, which works well, consists of two three-way stopcocks attached to the central Luer connector of the dome of a Statham P23Gb strain-gauge transducer. One stopcock is connected to the catheter and is used also for flushing saline through the catheter. The second stopcock is used for applying calibration pressures to the transducer. A two-way stopcock is attached to the side Luer on the dome and is semi-permanently connected to a plastic tube leading from an aspirator bottle which holds water for flushing the system.

The most difficult part of the preparation for manometry is filling the transducer with water so that it is free from bubbles. Modern transducers have small volume displacements and even fine bubbles in the system increase the total compliance considerably and decrease the resonant frequency. If the dome of the transducer is transparent bubbles may be actually seen, but often they lie in the catheter and in the metal connectors (Luer connectors are frequently traps for bubbles and the elimination of some of these connectors in the Elema-Schonander and Ole Dich stopcocks is of great value). Many cardiac catheters, while having the advantage of being very stiff, are made with a weave next to the lumen and this has a natural attraction for bubbles. Removal of bubbles from such catheters is particularly difficult.

Since air bubbles may not be visible it is important to have some means for testing the dynamic performance of the system after filling. An essential and very simple piece of apparatus is a needle of which the internal radius and length have been measured with care. This can be connected to the transducer so that the natural frequency of the system can be determined and compared with theoretical expectation. The needle must be sufficiently long and narrow to place the natural frequency (calculated from (2.1)) within the working frequency range of the recorder and amplifier. If the comparison is good it may be assumed that bubbles are absent from the transducer and the stopcocks. It may be necessary to obtain a long length of narrow, stainless steel, hypodermic tubing and solder it to a suitable end connector. Trouble should be taken to clean the bore of the needle with a strong agent such as acid dichromate.

The methods used to fill a transducer with water vary greatly. In our laboratory, after trying many techniques, our practice is to pass boiled distilled water slowly through the transducer until the transient performance with a needle of known dimensions gives the expected resonant frequency. The distilled water, with a small quantity of a surface active agent such as Detergicide† added, is boiled in a 2-litre flask and transferred to an aspirator bottle. The arrangement is a permanent one, so that a supply of air-free water is available with little trouble. The initial filling of the transducer with water is carried out under only a few cm head of water by connecting it to the aspirator bottle with a plastic tube and holding it just below the surface of the water in the bottle. Any attempt to fill an instrument quickly will lead to the entrapment of bubbles; similar entrapment is liable to occur if a syringe is used for filling. The transducer itself should be clean inside and preliminary wetting with Detergicide may be helpful if it has not been used for some time. Even after filling in this way it is uncommon for the expected resonant frequency to be achieved immediately. If the system is being filled for use the next day it is then flushed very slowly with the air-free water until required; the flow rate through the system will only be about one drop every 3 or 4 sec. Often, flushing in this manner for 2 to 3 h will eliminate the bubbles; it is unusual for flushing to be required for more than 24 h. The transient responses shown in Figs. 7, 10 and 12 were made by flushing the transducer and catheters for 24 h and establishing that no further improvement occurred after subsequent flushing. The mechanism by which the bubbles are removed is presumably solution in the flowing air-free water. The efficacy of the technique is surprising. Leaving the system with no flow is highly ineffective.

Once the transducer, with its stopcocks, has been shown to be free from bubbles our practice is to leave it filled until the stopcocks need re-greasing. We use plastic catheters and, with a suitable choice of connector, bubbles can usually be flushed out of these tubes without difficulty. Each time the transducer is used again a needle of known dimensions is attached first and the absence of bubbles demonstrated by a transient test.

It is clear enough that the method just described will not be practical for everyone. In a cardiac laboratory there are problems of sterility to consider

---

† United States Catheter and Instrument Corporation, Glen Falls, New York, U.S.A.

which will require the technique to be modified. There may not be time to flush a system slowly. It is probably true that there is no certain way of eliminating bubbles from a system quickly. One may be lucky; more often one is unlucky and time has to be spent. One is more apt to be satisfied if no dynamic tests are carried out.

Some transducers can be sterilized by boiling and this is an excellent and certain way of removing bubbles. All the stopcocks should be left in the open position. An alternative method is to fill the system with carbon dioxide and then to replace this with freshly boiled distilled water or with sodium citrate solution. Bubbles of carbon dioxide which are left are absorbed more quickly than those of air.

C. STATIC CALIBRATION

If tests show that the output of the transducer–amplifier–recorder system is linear with change in steady pressure, static calibration may be carried out with sufficient accuracy by applying two known pressures. The calibrating pressures must be measured in relation to the reference level chosen for the investigation. Commonly, the reference level selected in supine patients is 5 cm below the costochondral junction. It is simplest if one of the calibrating pressures is taken from a fluid-filled bottle adjusted to this level. The other can be applied by turning a stopcock to another column of known height above the reference level, or to a water or mercury manometer system. The apparatus used in our laboratory employs a precision dial manometer (at the suggestion of Dr. D. L. Schultz). The model used is the FA 145, manufactured by Wallace and Tiernan Limited.† The dial is $8\frac{1}{2}$ inches in diameter but the pointer covers full scale in two revolutions so that the total scale length is as long as 45 inches. The accuracy is 0·1 per cent of full scale and in our model this is equivalent to 0·2 mmHg. Such accuracy would be difficult to achieve with an ordinary water or mercury manometer and indeed is rather better than we are likely to require. Figure 13 shows the apparatus used. The system is pressurized by the sphygmomanometer bulb; fine changes in pressure are made by adjusting the metal bellows. The apparatus is secured to a wall and the air pressure line is led to a bottle containing water which is connected to one or more transducers. The water level is held at the reference level so that only one stopcock need be used for calibration. If it is desired to suppress zero pressure two higher calibrating pressures can very easily be generated with accuracy.

The calibration of catheter-tip transducers requires the use of an external gauge connected to the catheter lumen provided. The sensitivity of the external and internal gauges are made equivalent by testing before the catheter is

† Wallace and Tiernan Limited, Priory Works, Tonbridge, Kent, England.

introduced; if the external gauge is properly filled the waveforms obtained by both instruments should be similar. If possible the catheter should be advanced to the ventricles where the pressure excursions are maximal. The internal gauge may be subject to drift and its calibration can be checked in this way.

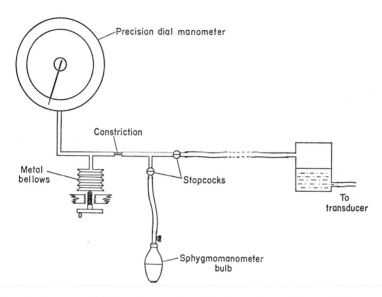

FIG. 13. An assembly for the static calibration of transducers. The pressure is read from a precision dial manometer. Pressure is raised to any desired level by the sphygmomanometer bulb; final adjustment of pressure can be made by fine compression of the metal bellows. The constriction protects the dial manometer against sudden accidental decompression.

The static testing and calibration of differential manometers requires thought and care. An account of some of the problems is given by Greenfield and Fry (1962). Fundamental is the requirement of a small static imbalance. A perfect differential manometer should give no output if the same static pressure is applied to both sides of the system. In fact there will be some change in the output. Let us suppose that the instrument will be used over a range of 200 mmHg. The recorder deflection, d mm, produced when 200 mmHg is applied steadily to both sides should be measured. The pressure on both sides is returned to zero and a small pressure, p mmHg, is applied to one side—giving, say, a recorder deflection of D mm. The deflection d mm will therefore be equivalent to $p.d/D$ mmHg and the static imbalance will be $(p.d/200D) \times 100$ per cent. The requirement for static imbalance when the pressure gradient technique is used to measure the blood velocity is of the order ± 0.1 per cent, a figure not achieved by many commercial differential transducers.

D. DYNAMIC TESTING OF TRANSDUCER SYSTEMS

If the frequency response of a transducer system is of importance at all in an investigation the importance of dynamic testing will be clear. Two

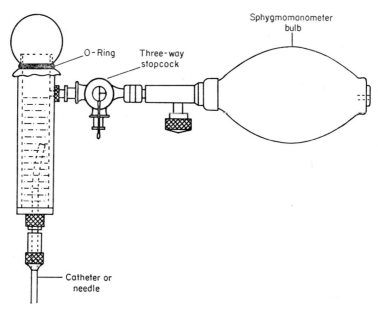

FIG. 14. Simple arrangement for transient testing of pressure transducer systems. The open end of the catheter or needle is sealed in a methacrylate tube by means of an adaptor which compresses a rubber washer. Excess flushing fluid is discharged through the stopcock. After sealing the top of the tube with a rubber membrane and an O-ring, the chamber is pressurized with the sphygmomanometer bulb.

methods are available, the transient and the sinusoidal, and since the transient technique requires least in terms of apparatus, it is this that could most widely be used. Unfortunately, there are too many laboratories in which the "pop" of a transient test is never heard.

(1) *Transient testing*

The object of this method is to apply a sudden change in pressure to the transducer system. A simple apparatus for doing this is shown in Fig. 14. The catheter or needle is sealed in a methacrylate tube by means of a screw adaptor. The system is flushed and excess fluid passes out through the stop-cock. When the test is to be performed a rubber membrane (a surgical glove is excellent) is drawn taughtly over the upper end of the tube and held in position with an O-ring. The pressure within the system is raised by means of the sphygmomanometer bulb and, with the recorder going at an adequate speed, the balloon is punctured with a burning match or a hot soldering iron. An example of a transient test is shown in Fig. 7. The damped resonant frequency is then calculated and compared with what should be attained theoretically. If the frequency observed is low then the almost invariable cause is the presence of bubbles in the system.

The damping factor can be calculated from data measured as shown in Fig. 15. In Fig. 15(i) the equilibrium line is drawn and the distances $d_1, d_2, d_3 \ldots$ are measured. These are plotted on semilogarithmic paper and a line of best fit drawn in by eye. From this the best estimate of d_1/d_3 is made and the logarithmic decrement, Λ, is then calculated as

$$\Lambda = \ln (d_1/d_3) \tag{4.1}$$

If T_D is the period of one complete oscillation the damping factor, β, is given by

$$\beta = \frac{\Lambda}{\sqrt{4\pi^2 + \Lambda^2}} \tag{4.2}$$

and the undamped natural frequency, f_0, may be derived from

$$f_0 = \frac{\sqrt{4\pi^2 + \Lambda^2}}{2\pi T_D} \tag{4.3}$$

A slightly simpler method of measurement is shown in Fig. 15(ii). This does not require measurements from the equilibrium line—only the measurements $D_1, D_2, D_3 \ldots$ from successive peaks. Again, semilogarithmic plotting of $D_1, D_2, D_3 \ldots$ will allow the best estimate of the ratio D_2/D_1 or D_{n+1}/D_n to be made (although for rough estimates plotting will probably not be necessary). The damping factor, β, may then be derived directly from Table 1 and a slightly awkward calculation avoided. The undamped resonant frequency, f_0, may be calculated from the observed damped resonant frequency, f_D, by multiplying f_D by the ratio f_0/f_D found against the appropriate value for D_{n+1}/D_n in Table 2. Finding the undamped resonant frequency is necessary when Figs. 8 and 9 are used, especially when the damping is not low.

If the system has a damping factor greater than unity there will be no free vibrations on transient testing and the methods just described for the calculation of β will not be applicable. If it is desired to calculate the damping factor in such a system the technique given by Warburg (1949) may be used.

It requires the measurement of the times taken to reach 0·4 and 0·9 of full deflection after the start of the transient. The value of β can be read from a table after calculating the ratio of these two times. The recording paper

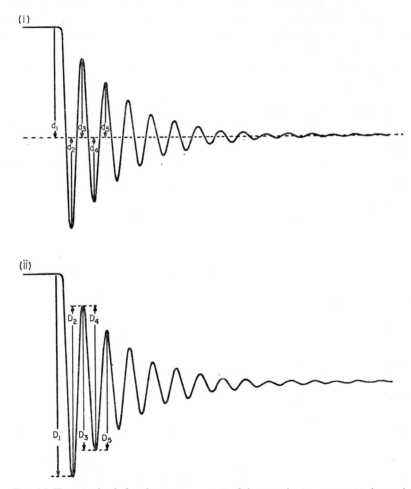

FIG. 15. Two methods for the measurement of the transient response to determine the amount of damping. In (i) the distances of successive peaks from the final equilibrium position are measured, i.e. $d_1, d_2, d_3 \ldots$ In (ii) it is not necessary to draw in the equilibrium level as the distances $D_1, D_2, D_3 \ldots$, between successive peaks are measured.

must be run fast enough to allow accurate timing. It is unlikely that there will be many occasions when the exact damping of such systems will be needed.

TABLE 1
Determination of the damping factor, β, from the transient response of
a single degree of freedom system

D_{n+1}/D_n	β	D_{n+1}/D_n	β	D_{n+1}/D_n	β	D_{n+1}/D_n	β
0·000	1·000	0·250	0·404	0·500	0·215	0·750	0·091
0·005	0·860	0·255	0·399	0·505	0·213	0·755	0·089
0·010	0·826	0·260	0·394	0·510	0·210	0·760	0·087
0·015	0·801	0·265	0·389	0·515	0·207	0·765	0·085
0·020	0·780	0·270	0·385	0·520	0·204	0·770	0·083
0·025	0·761	0·275	0·380	0·525	0·201	0·775	0·081
0·030	0·745	0·280	0·376	0·530	0·198	0·780	0·079
0·035	0·730	0·285	0·371	0·535	0·195	0·785	0·077
0·040	0·716	0·290	0·367	0·540	0·192	0·790	0·075
0·045	0·703	0·295	0·362	0·545	0·190	0·795	0·073
0·050	0·690	0·300	0·358	0·550	0·187	0·800	0·071
0·055	0·678	0·305	0·354	0·555	0·184	0·805	0·069
0·060	0·667	0·310	0·349	0·560	0·181	0·810	0·067
0·065	0·656	0·315	0·345	0·565	0·179	0·815	0·065
0·070	0·646	0·320	0·341	0·570	0·176	0·820	0·063
0·075	0·636	0·325	0·337	0·575	0·173	0·825	0·061
0·080	0·627	0·330	0·333	0·580	0·171	0·830	0·059
0·085	0·617	0·335	0·329	0·585	0·168	0·835	0·057
0·090	0·608	0·340	0·325	0·590	0·166	0·840	0·055
0·095	0·600	0·345	0·321	0·595	0·163	0·845	0·054
0·100	0·591	0·350	0·317	0·600	0·160	0·850	0·052
0·105	0·583	0·355	0·313	0·605	0·158	0·855	0·050
0·110	0·575	0·360	0·309	0·610	0·155	0·860	0·048
0·115	0·567	0·365	0·305	0·615	0·153	0·865	0·046
0·120	0·559	0·370	0·302	0·620	0·150	0·870	0·044
0·125	0·552	0·375	0·298	0·625	0·148	0·875	0·042
0·130	0·545	0·380	0·294	0·630	0·146	0·880	0·041
0·135	0·538	0·385	0·291	0·635	0·143	0·885	0·039
0·140	0·531	0·390	0·287	0·640	0·141	0·890	0·037
0·145	0·524	0·395	0·284	0·645	0·138	0·895	0·035
0·150	0·517	0·400	0·280	0·650	0·136	0·900	0·034
0·155	0·510	0·405	0·276	0·655	0·133	0·905	0·032
0·160	0·504	0·410	0·273	0·660	0·131	0·910	0·030
0·165	0·498	0·415	0·270	0·665	0·129	0·915	0·028
0·170	0·491	0·420	0·266	0·670	0·126	0·920	0·027
0·175	0·485	0·425	0·263	0·675	0·124	0·925	0·025
0·180	0·479	0·430	0·259	0·680	0·122	0·930	0·023
0·185	0·473	0·435	0·256	0·685	0·120	0·935	0·021
0·190	0·467	0·440	0·253	0·690	0·117	0·940	0·020
0·195	0·462	0·445	0·250	0·695	0·115	0·945	0·018
0·200	0·456	0·450	0·246	0·700	0·113	0·950	0·016
0·205	0·450	0·455	0·243	0·705	0·111	0·955	0·015
0·210	0·445	0·460	0·240	0·710	0·108	0·960	0·013
0·215	0·439	0·465	0·237	0·715	0·106	0·965	0·011
0·220	0·434	0·470	0·234	0·720	0·104	0·970	0·010
0·225	0·429	0·475	0·231	0·725	0·102	0·975	0·008
0·230	0·424	0·480	0·228	0·730	0·100	0·980	0·006
0·235	0·419	0·485	0·224	0·735	0·098	0·985	0·005
0·240	0·414	0·490	0·221	0·740	0·095	0·990	0·003
0·245	0·409	0·495	0·218	0·745	0·093	0·995	0·002

TABLE 2
Determination of f_0/f_D from the transient response of a single
degree of freedom system

D_{n+1}/D_n	f_0/f_D	D_{n+1}/D_n	f_0/f_D	D_{n+1}/D_n	f_0/f_D	D_{n+1}/D_n	f_0/f_D
0·000	∞	0·250	1·093	0·500	1·024	0·750	1·004
0·005	1·961	0·255	1·091	0·505	1·023	0·755	1·004
0·010	1·774	0·260	1·088	0·510	1·023	0·760	1·004
0·015	1·669	0·265	1·086	0·515	1·022	0·765	1·004
0·020	1·597	0·270	1·083	0·520	1·021	0·770	1·003
0·025	1·542	0·275	1·081	0·525	1·021	0·775	1·003
0·030	1·499	0·280	1·079	0·530	1·020	0·780	1·003
0·035	1·462	0·285	1·077	0·535	1·020	0·785	1·003
0·040	1·432	0·290	1·075	0·540	1·019	0·790	1·003
0·045	1·405	0·295	1·073	0·545	1·018	0·795	1·003
0·050	1·382	0·300	1·071	0·550	1·018	0·800	1·003
0·055	1·361	0·305	1·069	0·555	1·017	0·805	1·002
0·060	1·342	0·310	1·067	0·560	1·017	0·810	1·002
0·065	1·326	0·315	1·065	0·565	1·016	0·815	1·002
0·070	1·310	0·320	1·064	0·570	1·016	0·820	1·002
0·075	1·296	0·325	1·062	0·575	1·015	0·825	1·002
0·080	1·283	0·330	1·060	0·580	1·015	0·830	1·002
0·085	1·271	0·335	1·059	0·585	1·014	0·835	1·002
0·090	1·260	0·340	1·057	0·590	1·014	0·840	1·002
0·095	1·250	0·345	1·056	0·595	1·014	0·845	1·001
0·100	1·240	0·350	1·054	0·600	1·013	0·850	1·001
0·105	1·231	0·355	1·053	0·605	1·013	0·855	1·001
0·110	1·222	0·360	1·052	0·610	1·012	0·860	1·001
0·115	1·214	0·365	1·050	0·615	1·012	0·865	1·001
0·120	1·206	0·370	1·049	0·620	1·012	0·870	1·001
0·125	1·199	0·375	1·048	0·625	1·011	0·875	1·001
0·130	1·192	0·380	1·046	0·630	1·011	0·880	1·001
0·135	1·186	0·385	1·045	0·635	1·010	0·885	1·001
0·140	1·180	0·390	1·044	0·640	1·010	0·890	1·001
0·145	1·174	0·395	1·043	0·645	1·010	0·895	1·001
0·150	1·168	0·400	1·042	0·650	1·009	0·900	1·001
0·155	1·163	0·405	1·041	0·655	1·009	0·905	1·001
0·160	1·158	0·410	1·039	0·660	1·009	0·910	1·000
0·165	1·153	0·415	1·038	0·665	1·008	0·915	1·000
0·170	1·148	0·420	1·037	0·670	1·008	0·920	1·000
0·175	1·144	0·425	1·036	0·675	1·008	0·925	1·000
0·180	1·139	0·430	1·035	0·680	1·008	0·930	1·000
0·185	1·135	0·435	1·035	0·685	1·007	0·935	1·000
0·190	1·131	0·440	1·034	0·690	1·007	0·940	1·000
0·195	1·127	0·445	1·033	0·695	1·007	0·945	1·000
0·200	1·124	0·450	1·032	0·700	1·006	0·950	1·000
0·205	1·120	0·455	1·031	0·705	1·006	0·955	1·000
0·210	1·117	0·460	1·030	0·710	1·006	0·960	1·000
0·215	1·113	0·465	1·029	0·715	1·006	0·965	1·000
0·220	1·110	0·470	1·028	0·720	1·005	0·970	1·000
0·225	1·107	0·475	1·028	0·725	1·005	0·975	1·000
0·230	1·104	0·480	1·027	0·730	1·005	0·980	1·000
0·235	1·101	0·485	1·026	0·735	1·005	0·985	1·000
0·240	1·098	0·490	1·025	0·740	1·005	0·990	1·000
0·245	1·096	0·495	1·025	0·745	1·004	0·995	1·000

The estimation of the damping factor by the transient technique assumes that the system may be regarded as one with a single degree of freedom. However, even where this is probably not a good approximation, a high resonant frequency in relation to the highest frequency considered to be important is evidence that the distortion over the range of interest will be small. Thus the transient response shown in Fig. 10 (from a Statham P23Gb transducer and a No. 7 cardiac catheter) is not that seen in a single degree of freedom system. But the resonant frequency of 83 Hz is a factor of 5 greater than 15 Hz, which may reasonably be regarded as above the highest pressure frequency of significance in man. Hence the distortion should be small—with one proviso. Disturbance of the catheter within the vascular system can produce artefacts, usually at around resonant frequency. The phenomenon is often termed catheter "whip". It may be produced by the tapping of a heart valve on the catheter or by actual acceleration of the catheter. If the catheter is moved back and forth longitudinally with each beat there will be no change in the mean pressure if there is no net change in the position of the catheter but the accelerations will produce transient effects. If the catheter is moved from side to side through an arc there will also be an effect on the mean pressure, although probably only a small one.

The transient test described here is easy to perform and should be carried out at the beginning and end of every investigation where the dynamic performance is believed to be of importance. Doing it once or occasionally is not satisfactory quality control since a transducer system cannot be assumed to be bubble-free every time it is used. The test apparatus should be readily available at the end of the procedures. Simple modification of the system shown in Fig. 14 will enable more than one transducer to be tested simultaneously. Some care should be exercised in the practice of transient testing by connecting the catheter to a syringe and rapidly withdrawing the piston. The negative pressure so produced can be large and at least one diaphragm has been torn from its seating by this method. A pressure generator for making repetitive squarewaves has been described by Levasseur, Funk and Patterson (1969a) and this could be of particular value when damping adjustments are being made.

It may sometimes be necessary to correct recorded waveforms of pressure for the distortion produced by the transducer system. If it can be shown that amplitude changes are small over the working frequency range and that the phase-lag is linear with frequency, then the original waveform will only be delayed. If the undamped resonant frequency and the damping ratio are calculated from the transient test then the range over which the phase-lag is linear can be estimated from Fig. 9. Within this range it will be seen that at, say, f Hz the phase-lag is ϕ degrees. The time delay for a waveform containing significant information within this frequency range will be $\phi/360.f$

seconds. Hence, correction will consist in advancing the waveform in time by this amount.

If constancy of amplitude and linearity of phase-lag with frequency cannot be assumed, then correction can be carried out on the harmonics of the waveform, derived by Fourier analysis; if necessary, synthesis of the corrected harmonics will then yield the original undistorted waveform. If a harmonic term consists of $A \cos 2\pi ft + B \sin 2\pi ft$, where A and B are the cosine and sine coefficients at the frequency, f, then the corrected coefficients A' and B' will be

$$A' = (1 - \gamma^2)A + 2\beta\gamma B$$
$$B' = (1 - \gamma^2)B - 2\beta\gamma A$$

$$(4.4)$$

where $\gamma = f/f_0$, the ratio of the frequency considered to the undamped natural frequency and β = the damping factor.

The need for Fourier analysis is clearly inhibiting for many applications. Given that a better transducer system cannot be obtained, corrections to the waveform may be carried out by analogue means. This is discussed by Fry (1960). Devices which can produce corrections have been described by Liu and Berwin (1958) and Noble and Barnett (1963).

(2) *Sinusoidal method*

The apparatus needed to generate sinusoidal pressure waveforms is necessarily more complex than that for the creation of transients. Ideally, the pump should produce sinusoidal pressure waveforms which do not vary in amplitude with frequency or with changes in fluid flow out of the pump. The magnetic pump described by Hansen (1949) was elaborate and few would now wish to use the same principle. Simpler electromagnetic devices have been described by Noble (1959), Vierhout and Vendrik (1961), Stegall (1967) and Shelton and Watson (1968). Linden (1959) used the piezo-electric effect to generate pressure waveforms, employing a barium titanate strain-gauge. A purely mechanical pump is described in detail by Yanof, Rosen, McDonald and McDonald (1963). That used by Ball and Gabe (1963) compresses an air chamber sinusoidally by means of a bellows. Most of the pumps described are used with a monitor pressure transducer because the pressure waveforms are not exactly constant in amplitude with change of frequency. This is usually because of the physical characteristics of the pump itself but it may also result if the mechanical source impedance of the pump is too high in relation to the input impedance of the catheter–transducer system. This means that it tends to be a constant flow generator rather than a constant pressure generator. For example, if the pump consists of a small fluid-filled chamber compressed sinusoidally and the amount of fluid which enters the catheter varies with frequency then the pressure amplitudes generated will not be constant. The effect is discussed by Vierhout and Vendrik (1965). Provided a monitor transducer is used, however, and the system is linear, useful measurements can still be made with such pumps.

Some practical details on the use of pressure pumps are worth noting. If a catheter is inserted into a pump and the pump chamber opened to air near the point of insertion then in principle no pressure change should be recorded by the transducer at any frequency. In practice pressure waves will usually be seen at least over some range of frequencies. These result from vibration of the mechanical structure of the pump itself, causing accelerations of the catheter. The effect should be looked for and if present to a significant degree it may be diminished by changing the mounting of the generator. Vibrations of the catheter itself may be reduced by suspending from it some wet swabs. Care should be taken to reduce direct transmission of vibrations along the bench from the pump to the transducer, e.g. by positioning them on benches which are isolated from one another.

One advantage of testing transducer systems with a sinusoidal generator is that precise corrections can be determined for amplitude and phase distortion over the range of frequencies of interest without invoking, for example, the assumption of a single degree of freedom system. The corrections are tedious to carry out by hand, but a digital computer makes this relatively easy.

Most commonly, a sinusoidal pressure generator will only be used to detect the major resonance of the system; if this is high enough then the system will be considered satisfactory. With catheter systems more than one resonance may be seen; a good example is shown in Fry et al. (1957). Such a finding indicates that the system has more than one degree of freedom and that transmission line phenomena are present.

E. ADJUSTMENT OF DAMPING

The amount of damping in a transducer system can profoundly affect the shape of a recorded waveform and there are attractive arguments in favour of adjusting the damping to increase the range of useful frequency response. Thus, with a single degree of freedom a damping factor of 0·64 will mean that there will be less than 2 per cent error in amplitude up to 67 per cent of the natural frequency, with a nearly linear phase-lag (see Figs. 8, 9). Unfortunately, there are considerable problems in achieving and maintaining precise amounts of damping.

The way in which hydraulic damping is usually applied in a single degree of freedom system is by creating a constriction between the catheter and the transducer; the damping is then in series with the inertial element in the needle and the compliance in the transducer. The constriction must be great to produce an adequate viscous effect. Although in principle the necessary constriction for 0·64 damping is calculable for a given system it will only apply if the system does not change. Using the same constriction on each occasion will require that all air bubbles be removed every time. More frequently, the damping resistance may be varied with a needle valve. The amount of damping is then adjusted until satisfactory square wave performance is achieved before the catheter is inserted. Alternatively, the constriction is altered until the pressure waveform from the vascular tree looks "right", a subjective judgment which may be difficult to justify formally. The amount of constriction which is needed may mean that only very slow flushing of the catheter is possible unless a special arrangement of stopcocks is employed. It is most important to remember the consequences of a leaking stopcock on the transducer side of the damping resistance. Because the resistance is high even a slow flow of fluid through it will produce a pressure drop and the mean pressure sensed by the transducer will be less than the mean pressure at the open end of the catheter.

Placing the damping resistance at the open end of the catheter has been advocated for many years and Latimer (1968) has justified it in terms of transmission line theory. If the value of the terminal hydraulic resistance is made equal to the characteristic resistance of the catheter then desirable effects should follow. For example, suppose there is a step fall in pressure at the open end of the resistance. Pressure will fall by 50 per cent across the resistance and this reduced pressure step will travel along the catheter towards the transducer. There it will be reflected as a backward-going wave with consequent doubling of the amplitude. Thus the pressure sensed at the transducer will be that at the open end of the resistance. The backward-going wave will return to the damping resistance and will be completely adsorbed by it so that there will be no further reflection. Again, however, there seem to be formidable practical problems. Maintaining a stable matched resistance at the end of a catheter is far from easy, although on the laboratory bench it may be possible. We may roughly estimate the size of constriction needed in a specific system by calculating the Poiseuille resistance required to match a No. 7 cardiac catheter with a characteristic resistance of 93 dyn cm^{-6}: a tube 2·2 cm long with internal diameter 0·2 mm would be suitable. Through such a resistance the flushing with saline, essential to prevent clotting of blood in the lumen, would be difficult.

A more promising solution is "parallel" damping, described by van der Tweel (1957). A needle valve is placed in parallel with the transducer and adjusted so that it approximates to the characteristic resistance of the catheter. Waves travelling from the open end than meet not the high reactance of the transducer but the matching parallel resistance termination and are not reflected. The frequency range is correspondingly increased. Instead of a constriction, Ranke (1952) suggested the use of a very long catheter as a terminating resistance. Once more, with parallel damping, the problem of flow along the resistance presents difficulties. The open side of the resistance must be pressurized to prevent retrograde flow of blood—but too great a forward flow of saline may disturb the mean pressure sensed by the transducer as there will be a pressure drop along the catheter itself.

The substitution of electrical damping for hydraulic damping is often practiced. If the damped resonant frequency is high then a low pass filter will markedly diminish resonant effects in the records without much distortion, although there will be an additional time delay. If the resonant frequency is only, say, 10 Hz, electrical damping will produce effects which should be measured in the individual case with a sinusoidal pump if fidelity is important.

The solution of adding no damping to the system has much to be said for it. The attainment of a high resonant frequency is important; it should be five times or more the highest frequency considered to be important in the original waveform. If the damping factor is low the phase-lag over the low frequency range is small and linear (Fig. 8) and the amplitude error will also be small (Fig. 7).

F. SUGGESTED PROCEDURE FOR BEGINNERS

It may help to state briefly the action which should be taken by someone starting to make high quality pressure recordings for the first time. One has in mind a postgraduate student not easily daunted and not given to compromise without good reason. What is suggested may not always be necessary; the investigator must be the judge of that. The procedures mentioned are described in greater detail in previous sections.

(1) *Apparatus required*

(a) A pressure transducer, amplifier and recorder.

(b) High quality stopcocks. These should contain a minimum of Luer connectors. Each stopcock should be dismantled in turn for cleaning and greasing. Excess grease should be removed from the bore with a pipe cleaner.

(c) A supply of boiled distilled water. It is worth making a system which will produce several litres without too much trouble.

(d) A needle of known bore and length. Calculation from (2.1) will give the dimensions of the needle necessary to produce, with the transducer, a resonant frequency sufficiently low for the amplifier and recorder used. A special needle may have to be made.

(e) A system for producing transient changes in pressure, as shown in Fig. 14. If more than one transducer at a time is to be tested it will be worth making it larger and fitting additional catheter adapters.

(2) *Initial tests and procedures*

(a) The stopcocks should be attached to the transducer, which should then be filled with boiled distilled water as described previously. The efficiency of the stopcocks should be tested by pressurizing the system and closing the stopcocks while the output is recorded. If the pressure falls within a few seconds then there is a significant leak. The stopcocks may need lapping. Static tests do not require that air bubbles be removed from the system and so time need not be spent on this at first.

(b) The transducer, amplifier and recorder should be tested for noise, linearity, stability (including temperature stability) and hysteresis. The results of these tests should be expressed in terms of input pressure and decisions made on the adequacy of the apparatus for the study in mind.

(c) Dynamic testing should now be carried out. An essential preliminary is the calculation, from (2.1), of the resonant frequency to be expected with the testing needle and the transducer. If it is not known what should be obtained with the system it will be impossible to assess what is achieved. The needle should be attached to the transducer stopcock, flushed, and the transient response recorded. If the resonant frequency is not within 10 per cent of that predicted then continued slow flushing of the system should be undertaken until the performance is adequate. It may be necessary for the slow flushing to continue for 24 h or more.

(d) The needle may now be removed from the system and replaced by the catheter which it is proposed to use in the investigation. If this is a cardiac catheter with an inner weave it is likely that prolonged flushing will again be necessary before the best frequency response is obtained. Knowing the length and bore of the catheter, it is worth calculating the resonant frequency that would be expected if the system had only one degree of freedom. This will be a useful guide.

(e) The transient test should regularly be carried out at the end of the procedure.

5. CONCLUSION

In spite of significant technical advances, it is difficult not to have some misgivings over the state of manometry in physiology and cardiology. Great hope has arisen over the development of intravascular transducers and, given proper care, they are indeed capable of producing high fidelity records with comparative ease. But their lives are not long in relation to their cost and it is probable that external transducers and catheters will be used for many years yet. What has been suggested about the management of external manometers is practicable in the physiology laboratory but in the setting of a cardiac laboratory the problems of high fidelity remain large. I do not know how three or four external transducers can be filled each day by personnel who are not personally committed to getting the best out of each instrument. There is still an excess of art in electro-manometry; the challenge is to remove from the measurement of pressure the need for both thought and skill.

REFERENCES

Ball, G. and Gabe, I. T. (1963). Sinusoidal pressure generator for testing differential manometers. *Med. Electron. Biol. Eng.* **1**, 237–241.

Bloch, E. H. (1966). Low compliance pressure gauge. *In* "Methods in Medical Research" (R. F. Rushmer, ed.), Vol. 11, Year Book Medical Publishers, Inc., Chicago.

Fry, D. L. (1960). Physiologic recording by modern instruments with particular reference to pressure recording. *Physiol. Rev.* **40**, 755–788.

Fry, D. L., Noble, F. W. and Mallos, A. J. (1957). An evaluation of modern pressure recording systems. *Circ. Res.* **5**, 40–46.

Gabe, I. T., Guz, A., Noble, M. I. M. and Stubbs, J. (1970). Measurement of left ventricular pressure and its first time derivative. *J. Physiol.* **208**, 48–50.

Gauer, O. H. and Gienapp, E. (1950). Miniature pressure-recording device. *Science, N.Y.* **112**, 404–405.

Gersh, B. J., Hahn, C. E. W. and Prys-Roberts, C. (1971). Physical criteria for measurement of left ventricular pressure and its first derivative. *Cardiovasc. Res.* **5**, 32–40.

Greenfield, J. C., Jr. and Fry, D. L. (1962). Measurement errors in estimating aortic blood velocity by pressure gradient. *J. Appl. Physiol.* **17**, 1013–1019.

Hamilton, W. F., Brewer, G. and Brotman, I. (1934). Pulse contours in the intact animal. *Amer. J. Physiol.* **107**, 427–435.

Hansen, A. T. (1949). Pressure measurement in the human organism. *Acta Physiol. Scand.* **19**, Suppl. 68, 1–227.

Hansen, A. T. and Warburg, E. (1950). A theory for elastic liquid-containing membrane manometers. General part. *Acta Physiol. Scand.* **19**, 306–332.

Lambossy, P. (1952). Manomètres à l'observation des variations de la pression sanguine. *Helv. Physiol. Acta* **10**, 138–160.

Landis, E. M. (1926). The capillary pressure in frog mesentery as determined by microinjection methods. *Amer. J. Physiol.* **75**, 548–570.

Landis, E. M. (1966). Microinjection pressure measuring technic. *In* "Methods in Medical Research" (R. F. Rushmer, ed.), Vol. 11, Year Book Medical Publishers, Inc., Chicago.

Latimer, K. E. (1968). The transmission of sound waves in liquid-filled catheter tubes used for intravascular blood pressure recording. *Med. Biol. Eng.* **6**, 29–42.

Latimer, K. E. and Latimer, R. D. (1969). Measurements of pressure-wave transmission in liquid-filled tubes used for intravascular blood pressure recording. *Med. Biol. Eng.* **7**, 143–168.

Levasseur, J. E., Funk, F. C. and Patterson, J. L., Jr. (1969a). Square wave liquid pressure generator for testing blood pressure transducers. *J. Appl. Physiol.* **27**, 426–430.

Levasseur, J. E., Funk, F. C. and Patterson, J. L., Jr. (1969b). Physiological pressure transducer for microhaemocirculatory studies. *J. Appl. Physiol.* **27**, 422–425.

Lilly, J. C. (1942). The electrical capacitance diaphragm membrane manometer. *Rev. Sci. Instr.* **13**, 34–39.

Linden, R. J. (1959). Method of determining the dynamic constants of liquid-containing membrane manometer systems. *J. Sci. Instr.* **36**, 137–140.

Lindström, L. H. (1970). Miniaturized pressure transducer intended for intravascular use. *IEEE Trans. Bio. Med. Eng.* **BME17**, 207–219.

Liu, F. F. and Berwin, T. W. (1958). Extending transducer transient response by electronic compensation for high-speed physical measurements. *Rev. Sci. Instr.* **29**, 14–20.

McDonald, D. A. (1960). "Blood Flow in Arteries", Edward Arnold, London.

Noble, F. W. (1959). A hydraulic pressure generator for testing the dynamic characteristics of blood pressure manometers. *J. Lab. Clin. Med.* **54**, 897–902.

Noble, F. W. and Barnett, G. O. (1963). An electric circuit for improving the dynamic response of the conventional cardiac catheter system. *Med. Electron. Biol. Eng.* **1**, 537–545.

Patel, D. J., Mason, D. T., Ross, J., Jr. and Braunwald, E. (1965). Harmonic analysis of pressure pulses obtained from the heart and great vessels of man. *Amer. Heart J.* **69**, 785–794.

Porjé, I. G. and Rudewald, B. (1961). Haemodynamic studies with differential pressure technique. *Acta Physiol. Scand.* **51**, 116–135.

Ramirez, A., Hood, W. B., Jr., Polanyi, M., Wagner, R., Yankopoulos, N. A. and Abelmann, W. H. (1969). Registration of intravascular pressure and sound by a fibreoptic catheter. *J. Appl. Physiol.* **26**, 679–693.

Ranke, O. F. (1952). Registrierung laufender Wellen als Registrierprinzip. *Arch. Kreislaufforsch.* **18**, 99–107.

Shelton, C. D. and Watson, B. W. (1968). A pressure generator for testing the frequency response of catheter/transducer systems used for physiological pressure measurement. *Phys. Med. Biol.* **13**, 523–528.

Stegall, H. F. (1967). A simple inexpensive sinusoidal pressure generator. *J. Appl. Physiol.* **22**, 591–592.

van der Tweel, L. H. (1957). Some physical aspects of blood pressure, pulse wave, and blood pressure measurements. *Amer. Heart J.* **53**, 4–17.

Vierhout, R. R. and Vendrik, A. J. H. (1961). Hydraulic pressure generator for testing the dynamic characteristics of catheters and manometers. *J. Lab. Clin. Med.* **58**, 330–333.

Vierhout, R. R. and Vendrik, A. J. H. (1965). On pressure generators for testing catheter manometer systems. *Phys. Med. Biol.* **10**, 403–406.

Warburg, E. (1949). A method of determining the undamped natural frequency and the damping in overdamped and slightly underdamped systems of one degree of freedom by means of a square wave impact. *Acta Physiol. Scand.* **19**, 344–349.

Wetterer, E. (1943). Eine neue manometrische sonde mit elektrischer transmission, *Z. Biol.* **101**, 332–350.

Wiggers, C. J. (1914). Some factors controlling the shape of the pressure curve in the right ventricle. *Am. J. Physiol.* **33**, 382–396.

Wiederhielm, C. A. (1966). Servo micropipet pressure recording technic. *In* "Methods in Medical Research" (R. F. Rushmer, ed.), Vol. 11, Year Book Medical Publishers, Inc., Chicago.

Yanof, H. M., Rosen, A. L., McDonald, N. M. and McDonald, D. A. (1963). A critical study of the response of manometers to forced oscillations. *Phys. Med. Biol.* **8**, 407–422.

Chapter 3

Measurement of Pulsatile Flow and Flow Velocity

CHRISTOPHER J. MILLS

*Cardiovascular Research Unit, Royal Postgraduate Medical School,
Ducane Road, London, W.12*

1. INTRODUCTION

Pulsatile flow measurement presents several challenges. The three idealized blood flow waveforms from the aorta in Fig. 1 show many different features apart from the mean flow changes. Firstly, flow is not unidirectional even with normal heart valves, thus a directionally sensitive instrument is required as the degree of reverse flow can be used to quantitate the insufficiency of a leaking heart valve (Fig. 1b). Peak flow rate and acceleration of the blood can be used to access the contraction of the heart. Figure 1c shows the decreased peak flow and acceleration in a patient with a myocardial infarction. The need to measure acceleration requires a wide frequency range. Pulsatile pressure and flow recorded simultaneously have led to a much clearer picture of the vascular system (O'Rourke, 1967; Mills *et al.*, 1970; see also Chapter 10). Blood flow waveforms have also been of great

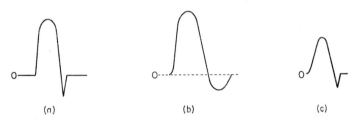

(a)   (b)   (c)

FIG. 1. An idealized set of blood flow waveforms from the ascending aorta, to illustrate the requirements in a measuring device. (a) Normal pattern, a quick upstroke (high acceleration) and a brief but sharp flow reversal. (b) An incompetant valve produces a high peak flow rate and a pronounced period of flow reversal. (c) A depressed heart; low acceleration and low peak velocity.

help in assessing vascular disease (Cappelen and Hall, 1967). Blood flow measurements have been fraught with many practical difficulties which have often vitiated the rigorous theoretical design of many pieces of apparatus. It is the purpose of this chapter to discuss three methods in detail; Electromagnetic, Ultrasonic and Thermal. These seem likely to dominate for some time at least and I shall point out sources of error and how to overcome some of them. Before the methods are discussed the difference between a flowmeter and velocity probe or velometer must be made clear.

A true flowmeter is one whose output is proportional to the total volume which flows through the vessel in a given time, irrespective of the velocity profile. An ideal flowmeter has to possess many other virtues, e.g. to be non-invasive, have a high frequency response and directional sensitivity unaffected by haemotocrit and vessel wall properties. Unfortunately, at the present time there is no such instrument available or this chapter would be unnecessary. However, accurate results can be achieved if the instrument and the principles of its use are not abused. In velocity probes or velometers the output is proportional to the velocity of blood passing the probe and no account is taken of vessel size. Ideally, the velocity should be measured at a point with no disturbance to the flow. This involves the use of extremely small devices or, ideally, of non-invasive techniques. The application of these devices is in the study of velocity profiles and instantaneous velocities in jets and at junctions. Another application is as a substitute for a flowmeter, here the velocity profile is assumed to be flat and that any reading in the cross section will be proportional to the flow rate, only the vessel size being needed to convert velocity to flow.

2. THE ELECTROMAGNETIC FLOWMETER

A. PRINCIPLE OF OPERATION

An historical account of the development will not be given here as many reviews have appeared which deal with this since Kolin (1936) and Wetterer (1937) demonstrated it as a method for measuring flow in blood vessels. Those interested in the history can obtain much information on the electromagnetic technique from the reviews by Wetterer (1963), Wyatt (1968b) and Jochim (1962) and on the basic theory from Shercliff (1962).

Cannula   Perivascular   Intravascular
                                            catheter tip

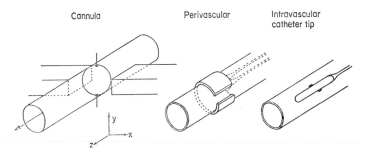

FIG. 2. The three types of electromagnetic transducers. (a) The cannula instrument. Blood flows through an insulated pipe in a magnetic field. A signal proportional to the flow rate is detected by two electrodes, orthogonal to both the magnetic and flow axis, and inserted through the wall to make contact with the fluid. (b) A perivascular transducer. The blood vessel is placed within a "cuff". The cuff contains windings to produce a magnetic field across the vessel. Electrical contact between the electrodes and the blood is through the conducting vessel wall. (c) An intravascular catheter probe. The magnetic field and electrodes are within the vessel.

The electromagnetic flowmeter is the most widely used instrument for pulsatile flow measurement. There are basically three types of electromagnetic flow transducer: (1) "Cannula" instruments which are inserted between the cut ends of a blood vessel or used extracorporeally; (2) perivascular, usually as a "cuff" which slips around an intact vessel, the electrodes being in contact with the vessel wall and not directly with the blood; and (3) intravascular or catheter probes which are inserted into a blood vessel and moved to the site where the measurement is to take place. Figure 2 shows each type schematically. The principle behind the electromagnetic flowmeter dates back to Faraday, and utilizes his laws of electromagnetic induction. Until recently it was only by very careful application (and devotion) that the true potential of the instrument could be reached. Meticulous care in setting up the flowmeter and in positioning the flow probe was required, and base-line stability was often poor. Considerable work on causes of these errors has come from Kolin (1941b, 1960), Wyatt (1961b, 1966a, b, 1968a), Gessner (1961), Hill (1960) and Spencer and Denison (1959) and the effects of changing various parameters have been described.

The electromagnetic flowmeter depends upon measuring the potential difference generated across the flow channel when a conducting fluid passes through a magnetic field. The output V from a cylindrical flowmeter with a uniform magnetic field and uniform velocity across the cross section is given by

$$V = B\bar{u}d \quad \text{(volts)}, \tag{2.1}$$

where d is the tube diameter (m), $\bar{u}$ is the average axial velocity (m s^{-1}) and

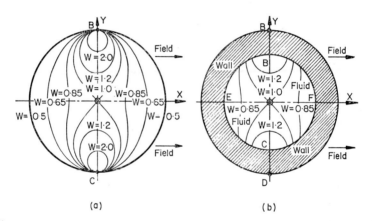

(a)   (b)

FIG. 3. The relative contribution of flow at different locations within a flow head to the output can be represented by the relative value of weight functions (w). (a) For an insulated pipe, electrodes in contact with the fluid. (b) The reduced effect produced by a conducting lining of the same conductivity as the fluid; a similar effect would be produced by a blood vessel wall. (Figure reproduced from Shercliff, 1962.)

B is the magnetic field (Wb m^{-2}). Normally fluid moves faster on the axis than peripherally, as in laminar flow, and higher voltages will be generated here, with current flow between the high and low potentials. It is then very fortunate that for *axially symmetric velocity profiles* the output voltage from a cylindrical flowmeter is proportional to the average velocity over the cross section and is thus proportional to the flow through the pipe.

The cylindrical flowmeter equation can thus be written.

$$V = \frac{4BQ}{\pi d} \quad \text{(volts)}, \qquad (2.2)$$

where Q = flow rate ($m^3 s^{-1}$).

To calculate the effects of non-symmetrical flow, Shercliff (1962) introduced weight functions to determine the contribution of flow at any point to the output. It can be seen from this (Fig. 3a) that the output is twice as sensitive to velocities near the electrodes than at the centre. A low-volume-flow high-velocity jet near one electrode could thus mask the effect of the major flow, even producing negative outputs in the presence of a positive true flow rate. At the sides, away from the electrodes, the sensitivity is one half the central value. These results have been experimentally confirmed by Goldman et al. (1963). The presence of a stationary conducting layer such as a vessel wall between the moving fluid and the electrodes considerably reduces these effects (Fig. 3b). However, if jets are suspected where flow is to be measured, it is well worth while to rotate the probe around the circumference of the vessel and note any change in the flowmeter output. If no change occurs then either there is no jet or the effect is negligible and flow measurements can be made. As a general rule it is advisable to try and measure flow as far away as possible from branches so that the profile is either flat or axis-symmetric.

B. VESSEL WALL AND HAEMATOCRIT EFFECTS

The effect of the vessel wall upon the flowmeter output can be evaluated with axially symmetric flows. This is of great importance as most manufacturers calibrate their flow heads in cannula form. Hill (1960), Gessner (1961), Shercliff (1962), Ferguson and Landahl (1966) and Wyatt (1968a) have all dealt with this theoretically; Gessner and Wyatt also took into account the presence of a conducting layer of fluid surrounding the vessel. Their results seem to predict opposite effects. This is because Gessner takes a flowmeter and increases its size to accommodate the vessel and fluid layer, whereas Wyatt inserts the blood vessel and fluid layer, within the flow head. Assuming the wall thickness is 10 per cent of the diameter, and the conductivity ratio of blood to vessel wall is between 5 and 1, the maximum error is 12 per cent, with a 20 per cent wall thickness it is less than 20 per cent. This is an *increase* in sensitivity; the resistance of the wall is greater than the resistance of of the blood so that the circulating currents and voltage loss will be less than if the area were occupied by stationary blood. The effect of fluid between the outside of the vessel wall and the flow head will be to lower the sensitivity, for this fluid is normally saline and less resistive than blood. This can in fact cancel the effect of the vessel wall which may well explain why Beck *et al.* (1965) found no change in sensitivity when a vessel wall was introduced. It might be thought then that a calibration error of less than 10 per cent might be difficult to achieve, however if a 10 per cent wall thickness is taken into account when calibrating a flow head the error can be reduced to about ± 5 per cent, assuming a value for the blood to wall conductivity ratio of ca. 2 : 1. This will hold if all factors remain constant, but vessel wall thickness or conductivity may change during the period of measurement, especially if the probes are chronically implanted. On the other hand, the conductivity of blood may change, for example if the haematocrit changes. During the course of an experiment it would be most unusual for the haematocrit to change by more than a factor of ± 50 per cent and for the conductivity to alter by a similar factor. Thus the ratio of conductivities might change by ± 50 per cent, in our example above the limits would now be 10–0·5, and the sensitivity changes would be <15 per cent. Again, this can be considerably reduced if the effect of a 10 per cent wall thickness and a conductivity ratio of 2 is taken into account in the initial calibration. Haematocrit changes also influence the non-uniform conductivity of flowing blood, due either to redistribution of red cells across the vessel cross section at different flow rates, or to the changes in the orientation of the red cells. Dennis and Wyatt (1969) found changes of less than -5 per cent for haematocrits between 0 and 66·5 per cent and flows from 0 to 2000 ml/min, including both laminar and turbulent flows. These results were obtained in a uniform magnetic field, a greater effect can be expected in a non-uniform field.

Changes in conductivity alone have been investigated, but the large changes in sensitivity reported with cannulating flow heads are confusing (Spencer and Denison, 1959; Case *et al.*, 1966; Dedichen and Schenk, 1968; Brunsting and Ten Hoor, 1968). The effects of cell distribution and magnetic field inhomogeneity cannot be distinguished as the same probes were not used as cuffs and cannulae. Therefore the effect of changing the conductivity ratio of blood and vessel wall is not clear. The study by Case *et al.* (1966), who used dialysis tubing and sections of aorta and vena cava showed little effect on sensitivity.

Brunsting and Ten Hoor (1968) found changes in sensitivity of up to 15 per cent when changing the haematocrit from 0 to 20 per cent with a cannulating probe and of up to 50 per cent when using a non-cannulating probe. Both these results are beyond the range expected from conductivity changes alone, and the explanation could lie in the actual flow heads and electronic apparatus used. Clearly the experimental results could have been influenced by spatial conductivity changes within the fluid due to red cell distribution, a non-uniform magnetic field, the input impedance of the flow-meter, and the state of the electrodes.

C. SPATIAL VARIATIONS IN MAGNETIC FIELD

The basic equation (2.1) requires a uniform magnetic field, but the use of Helmholtz coils to produce this (Yanof et al., 1963) results in a large inefficient design, not suitable for clinical or physiological use. Practical designs have a far from uniform magnetic field and the effects of this have been studied (Wyatt, 1961b; Kolin and Wisshaupt, 1963; Kolin and Vanyo, 1967; Kanai, 1969; Shercliff, 1968; Clark and Wyatt, 1968). Clark and Wyatt (1968) were able to show, using a large range of non-uniform magnetic fields with axi-symmetric flow, that the change in sensitivity as flow changed from laminar to turbulent was between $-3\cdot5$ and $+5\cdot5$ per cent. This explains why Kolin and Wisshaupt (1963) and O'Rourke (1965), with less sophisticated apparatus, could find no changes. Rummel and Ketelsen (1966), Shercliff (1968) and Bevir (1969) have shown that by tailoring the magnetic field in the region of the electrodes one can make the flowmeter less sensitive to changes in flow profile even if asymmetry exists. The ideal solution of complete independence does not, however, seem possible. Magnetic field variations along the flow axis (Wyatt, 1961b; Shercliff, 1962; Ferguson and Landahl, 1966) also reduce the signal from the flow head by allowing longitudinal circulating currents to flow within and outside the flow head. The transducer must be long enough to avoid this, or the effect taken into account in calibration.

D. TIME VARIATIONS OF THE MAGNETIC FIELD AND ZERO STABILITY

Equation (2.1) only holds for a steady magnetic field, for example from a permanent magnet. However, polarization effects and amplification of small d.c. voltages introduce many problems and for reasons of stability and convenience alternating magnetic fields are used. These introduce other problems associated with the rate of change of the magnetic field, mainly the "transformer effect"; this is a signal at the electrodes induced in the conductive loop containing the wiring and the fluid both inside and outside the flow head. These can be eliminated to a large extent by careful design of the flow head but not entirely as changes in the circulating currents around the probe will alter its magnitude. Various methods have been tried to reduce transformer effects, most involve different waveforms for the magnet current such as square, triangular or trapezoidal waves and pulsed fields. None of these eliminate the transformer action but they change its waveform relative to the flow signal so that the latter can be extracted simply (see Section 2, I), but only in the ideal case.

Unfortunately there are numerous ways in which this unwanted signal can be converted into one indistinguishable from the flow signal to produce baseline error or zero offset. Zero offset is the difference between the output from the flowmeter when the magnet is not energized and that when the magnet is energized but the flow through the probe is zero. Wyatt (1966a) has discussed the cause of and solution to many baseline troubles in sine wave instruments in considerable detail. The most serious problems arise when earth electrodes are used; elimination of earth points on the flow head will considerably reduce errors, quite apart from the resulting increase in safety. Suitably platinized cavity electrodes reduce electrode effects considerably and provided the electronic apparatus is suitably stable baseline errors of less than 2 per cent of full scale (10 μV) can be achieved (Wyatt, 1966b).

With square wave energization the problem is different, yet several common features arise. There should be no transformer effect during the sampling period (see Fig. 7) however, polarization of the electrodes by the circulating currents causes the prolongation of interference into the sampling interval, with resulting zero offset. Hognestad (1966) was able to reduce this considerably by using high resistance electrodes and a very high input impedance amplifier with high common-mode rejection. Cavity electrodes would have produced the same result without the disadvantage of higher noise levels, but Hognestat believed this impracticable. Various balancing arrangements have been used (Kolin, 1941a, 1952; Olmsted, 1959; Folts, 1970) to achieve better zero stability but are of limited use as the interfering voltages will be variable and long-term stability poor. The best cure is minimization by probe design and construction with further reduction in the electronic apparatus.

Current leakage from the magnet windings to the electrodes can obviously cause a false signal. The input impedance of an electromagnetic flowmeter should be of the order of 10^6 Ω at least to avoid errors should the source resistance change. The signal applied to the magnet windings is some 10^6 times higher than the flow-induced signal, thus the resistance between coil and electrodes should be 10^{12} Ω to avoid a leakage signal of the same order as the flow signal. If the leak is symmetrical to each electrode this can be eliminated by the common mode rejection of the pre-amplifier; since it may be asymmetrical the resistance between coil and electrode should be increased, this is extremely difficult even with modern materials, and the use of a screen between coil and electrodes is recommended (Kolin, 1960; Spencer and Barefoot, 1968; Wyatt, 1961b, 1966a) so that any leakage does not pass to the electrodes.

E. CALIBRATION

It is possible to design a cannulating flow head to produce a flow signal within 1 per cent of the theoretically predicted output if all the above sources of error are taken into account. However, commercially available heads have in the past been found to be very much more loosely calibrated, and a need for accurate calibration remains.

A cannulating probe can be relatively easily calibrated if an accurately known flow rate can be generated, but this is not often the case. With a steady flow the bucket and stopwatch method can be used, but due to errors in collection and timing, errors <5 per cent are rarely achieved. A more accurate method is to withdraw or pass a known volume of blood through the flow head, recording the output with accurate timing. The output signal can then be integrated and equated to the volume passed. The time taken can be obtained from the record and the mean signal equivalent to the mean flow can be found. Care must be taken to ensure adequate withdrawal rates and a sufficiently large signal for accurate area determination. The provision of a calibration signal on the flowmeter greatly facilitates subsequent use of the transducers. The calibration signal should be independent of the gain setting so that all is required in calibration is to switch to "calibrate", record a steady output, and multiply the gain setting by the probe calibration factor to obtain the calibration in ml s^{-1} represented by the output. To use a constant signal applied to the input is not as accurate for it will have to be small enough to allow the highest gain setting and will be too small on lower gain ranges. However, if a calibration facility is not available on the flowmeter in use, then a constant input device is easy to build (Bergel and Makin, 1968). With this the process of calibration can be further simplified. The calibrating signal is fed from the output of the flowmeter to an integrator in parallel with the recorder. The integrator output will rise, after a known time (T), to V (volts). This is converted to V s^{-1} by dividing by the time, $(C = V/T)$. A known quantity of blood A (ml) is now passed through the transducer and the integral B (volts) recorded and equated to the quantity of blood passed, i.e. $A/B = K$ ml/volt. Thus the flow rate equivalent to the calibration signal can be obtained:

$$\text{Calibration signal} = \frac{AV}{BT} = KC \quad (\text{ml s}^{-1}). \qquad (2.3)$$

This is easier than using a constant pressure head to achieve a constant flow (e.g. Bond, 1967), and can be applied for *in vivo* calibration of cuff transducers (Cappelen and Hall, 1967). For this the cuff is left on the vessel which is occluded distally, preferably at a point 2–5 diameters downstream, making sure there are no branches between the transducer and occlusion site. A known volume of blood is drawn through the probe with a needle and syringe, or a known volume collected by bleeding the vessel through the probe into a graduated container. The output from the flowmeter is integrated during this time, and related to the calibrating signal.

When working with larger probes on the aorta and pulmonary artery this is a much more difficult procedure and calibration against indicator dilution curves measurements of cardiac output is probably preferable, but the accuracy now depends upon the accuracy of the indicator method. Weber *et al.* (1968) have described their experience with this method and have found that it is accurate for the pulmonary artery, as did Lauridsen *et al.* (1968), for the aorta there was an error of 10 per cent when zero was taken as the average level during diastole. This is not explained by coronary flow for the error would be in the other direction. This rather unexpected result was not found by Guz (1968a), who reported no significant difference in calibration against dye dilution between the pulmonary artery and the aorta. Bond (1967) suggested calibration against a previously calibrated extracorporeal flowmeter so that the effects of changes in haematocrit could be studied. He also suggested that, since only mean flows were required, constriction of up to 50 per cent to produce a good fit of the transducer on the vessel could be tolerated. This constriction would undoubtedly thicken the vessel wall, thus the transducer would have a different sensitivity than when used on a vessel with less constriction. Bergel and Gessner (1966) suggest *in vivo* calibration against dye dilution curves for the larger trans-ducers and *in vitro* calibration for the small ones. Their *in vitro* preparation, like that of many others, consisted of an excised vessel with the transducer around it, all being immersed in a bath of saline. The vessel is stretched to its normal length and distended to normal pressure, a steady flow estab-lished and the mean output from the flowmeter compared to the mean flow determined by collecting the volume over an accurately known period of time. This method has its drawbacks in that the vessel rapidly takes up saline from the surrounding fluid, resulting in conductivity changes (Ferguson and Landahl, 1966), and the large bath around the probe does not simulate the fluid around a flow probe in normal use today (though it may well have done so for earlier instruments which dissipated so much heat it was neces-sary to cool them!). A modern flow transducer should not dissipate more than 0·5 W and this method should not therefore be necessary. Bergel and Makin (1968) described a method which overcomes the problems related above by pumping the vessel with known flows *in situ*. The advantage of this method is that if the descending aorta is exposed over a long section and all branches tied, a whole range of probes can be calibrated at one session.

F. INTRALUMINAL DEVICES

There are basically two types of intraluminal probe: those which measure true flow and those which are velocity sensitive devices. A flowmeter must compensate for the effects of the velocity profile, and the criteria are as for the external flowmeter. The velocity probe detects flow close to its surface and is little affected by changes further away. The principle of the latter type was described by Kolin in 1944 and used by Mills (1966), Mills and Shillingford (1967) and Bond and Barefoot (1967). The orientation of magnetic field and electrodes is different in each case.

Mills used a coil wound along the long axis of the catheter so that its magnetic field was as shown in Fig. 4a, b. Flow passing over the probe surface cuts the maximum concentration of field lines at right angles. The electrodes are placed at right angles to both field and flow axes, where the

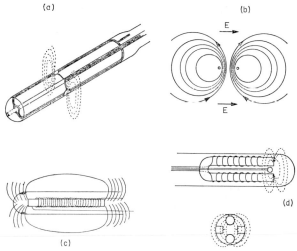

FIG. 4. Schematic diagrams of catheter tip velocity probes. (a) The Mills and Shillingford (1967) design. The magnetic field generated by the parallel wires is shown dotted. Blood flows outside the probe parallel to its long axis. The voltage detected between the two electrodes is proportional to the blood velocity. The probe is long compared to its width to avoid end shorting. (b) The magnetic field in a section through the electrodes, showing a similar voltage generated above and below the probe. As these voltages are in parallel, elimination of one by the probe lying along a non-conducting wall would not influence the output. In practice a blood vessel wall reduces the signal by 5 per cent. (c) The design of Barefoot (1970) shows the field emanating as from a solenoid. Maximum signal will only result from flow past the tip at right angles to the probe and to the plane of the paper. (d) The later design (in fact published earlier) of Spencer and Barefoot (1968) showing a similar field pattern to (a). Most of the magnetic field passes between the poles of the magnet and not through the blood. The signal depends therefore on the fringing of the magnetic field and the design is inefficient.

radial component of the magnetic field is zero. As the voltage induced is in the same direction above and below the probe (Fig. 4b), it is not necessary for the probe to lie against a vessel wall. If this does occur it only affects the signal (provided the velocity profile is reasonably flat) if an electrode actually touches the wall. Thus maximum signal is obtained with this design. In the Barefoot (1970) design the coil is wound around the long axis (Fig. 4c) as a solenoid. The electrodes are placed near the leading end, thus to sense any voltage proportional to velocity it is necessary that the probe lies against the vessel wall to prevent the signal shorting itself out. It is not clear whether the patented design was ever successful, as the construction used by Warbasse et al. (1969) and Spencer and Barefoot (1968) is different (Fig. 4d). Here a horseshoe magnet is used at the catheter tip and the signal is sensed by electrodes situated midway between the poles. The main magnetic field will pass between the poles where there is no blood flow. Its operation depends on the fringing of the magnetic field at the tip, most of the field being wasted. This probe need not lie against the vessel wall. The electrodes are close to the tip of the probe in a region where the velocity profile is disturbed.

The sensitivity to velocity falls rapidly with distance away from a catheter probe. Bevir (1971), in an analysis of the Mills probe, showed the sensitivity to fall off as r^{-4}, so that it is affected only by blood moving close to its surface. Flow can be calculated if the cross sectional area is known and if the velocity profile is flat.

A variation on the velometer which can measure flow in some vessels has been described by Stein and Schuette (1969). This has a guide tube which directs a sample of blood over the face of the probe, producing a signal proportional to the flow through the tube. If the tube completely seals the vessel in which it is placed it will measure the true flow in that vessel. If the sealing is not absolute, then the flow recorded will be a fraction of the total flow. Total flow might be calculated from the relative cross sectional areas of vessel and guide tube, assuming a flat velocity profile.

The first of a series of intraluminal devices described by Kolin (1967) and Kolin et al. (1967) were true flowmeters for the whole flow to a branch was collected by sealing the lumen of a catheter-mounted flowmeter around the opening of the branch, using a spring arrangement in the parent vessel. Flow had then to pass from the parent vessel through the flowmeter lumen to reach the side branch. Calibration could be performed as for an extra-vascular flowmeter, and zero stability checked by positioning the flowmeter away from a branch so that no flow passed through it. This device has to be at least as big as the vessel in which flow is to be measured, thus size becomes the dominant factor, greatly affecting the ease of insertion.

A proportional flowmeter (Kolin et al., 1968) using the same principle was described for use in a main vessel. The catheter was bent by means of a wire to lie across the flow, thus a portion of the total flow would pass through the lumen. The size and the need for a wire to bend the tip limit its use to animals. Kolin (1969) designed a flexible catheter probe with a longitudinal coil as in the Mills design but it could be expanded within the vessel to touch both walls. The magnetic field, although non-uniform, spanned the cross section of the vessel and a flowmeter with sensitivity varying predictably with vessel size was produced. Flexible wires carrying the relatively large magnetic current are not, however, to be encouraged for use in man; this led to an external magnetic field being used with a similar electrode design (Kolin, 1970a).

Extreme reduction in size now seems possible with the use of an external magnetic field. Kolin (1970b) has used a simple bent tube; the two electrodes in contact with the internal vessel wall are not on the same cross-section, but as the magnetic field is uniform over more than the length of the sensor, it should be capable of measuring total blood flow, provided the magnetic field is known at the point and that no motion of the catheter relative to the magnetic field takes place. This is the smallest flowmeter designed to date, being only 0·5 mm in diameter, and is easily inserted through a hypodermic needle.

G. CALIBRATION OF VELOCITY PROBES

The easiest way to calibrate a velocity device is to move it in a bath of fluid and record the output. The diameter of the bath should be at least thirty times the diameter of the probe. This can be done either by towing the sensor through a bath at a constant known rate, or by oscillating it

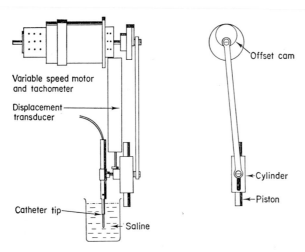

FIG. 5. Calibration rig for catheter probes. The variable speed motor drives the catheter up and down sinusoidally in a bath of saline. The motion is monitored by a displacement transducer. The peak to peak velocity is given by $2\pi fd$, where f is the frequency of oscillation and d is the total displacement of the catheter.

up-and-down sinusoidally. If the displacement (d) and frequency (f) are known it is a simple matter to calculate the peak-to-peak velocity from $V = 2\pi fd$. The signal obtained can be compared with an electrical signal applied at the input amplifier in place of the flow signal. This signal can then be equated to a velocity and used for subsequent calibrations. Mills and Shillingford (1967) have shown that *in vitro* calibrations with saline can be used *in vivo* with little change; the output not being greatly affected by conductivity changes in the fluid or the presence of a conducting wall. Kolin (1969) has also found with the expandable probe that the effect of the vessel is negligible. This method is simpler than placing a probe in a tube and passing fluid past it, as fluid velocities and probe angulation must be accurately measured. Figure 5 shows the calibration apparatus used.

H. MEASURING APPARATUS

The apparatus to measure the small voltages from the electrodes and provide the magnet drive is often called the flowmeter but this term should be reserved for the whole system, transducer and electronic apparatus. The various systems used have received much more attention in the quest for zero stability than have the transducers whereas in fact the major problems lie in the transducers themselves. However, to achieve the best results from the very small signal generated a great deal of thought must still be given to the electronic system.

Many systems have been described since the original permanent magnet arrangements. These were fraught with difficulties, even with non-polarizable electrodes. The introduction of an alternating sine wave current technique (Kolin, 1938) solved some problems yet introduced many more which are only just being understood and dealt with. The use of an alternating current resulted in two signals being detected at the electrodes. One, proportional to fluid flow rate and magnetic field strength, is in phase with the magnet current: the other is ideally in phase-quadrature (90° out of phase) to the current, and proportional to the rate of change of the magnetic field. The quadrature signal is generated by transformer action between the magnet current loop and the electrode loop, i.e. the path between the electrodes through the fluid and the electrode leads themself. This has led to the effect being described in the literature as the quadrature or transformer effect. It is the flow proportional signal that is required and a great deal of effort has been put into the elimination of the transformer signal. This has led to the use of complex magnet current waveforms which have been used to describe flowmeter "types" such as square wave, triangular wave, trapezoidal wave and pulsed systems.

In the sine wave instrument the quadrature component is present throughout the cycle (Fig. 6) and, provided the factors mentioned earlier under zero stability have been taken into account, the transformer effect will indeed be 90° out of phase with the flow signal and small; it will, however, vary in magnitude. It is for this reason that elimination (Kolin, 1938) cannot be relied upon and a gating procedure must be employed. Kolin (1941b)

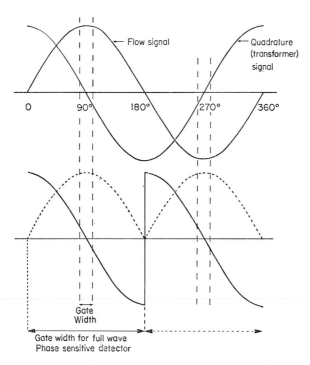

FIG. 6. Sine wave excitation. The relationship between the flow signal and quadrature (transformer) signal. The gate can sample at a time when the flow signal is maximum and the quadrature signal passes through zero, so that the average over the gated period is only flow dependent. Sampling can occur either once or twice per cycle if the algebraic sign is taken into account. When the gate spans the whole cycle with appropriate sign changes every half cycle then full wave phase sensitive detection results.

used a photographic technique to register the flow signal only when the quadrature signal passed through zero. Various electronic methods to do the same have since been reported. The square wave instrument, which required less accuracy in positioning the gate then came to the fore (Denison *et al.*, 1955). It was thought that all unwanted signals related to transformer action would be over before sampling took place (Fig. 7). This has, however, not been entirely successful and with improved phase stability and automatic quadrature rejection the sine wave instrument has re-emerged (Wyatt, 1964).

The gated sine wave phase sensitive detector can either gate once or twice per cycle. A half-wave or full-wave detector can either hold the signal until the next sample (peak detection), or average over the cycle (mean

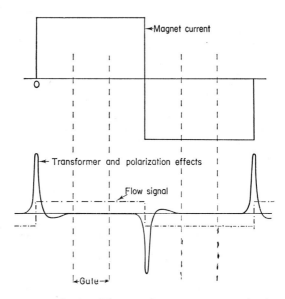

FIG. 7. Square wave excitation. The use of square wave energization only partially removes unwanted signals. The transformer signal should appear as high narrow spikes, but due to eddy currents and polarization they are prolonged, and the sampling period has to be reduced.

detection). Wyatt (1966b) has discussed the relative merits of these, concluding that full wave detection sampling for the entire half period is superior in all aspects apart for a.c.–d.c. conversion efficiency. To sample over the full period (Fig. 6) the signal is inverted for the second half-cycle and the mean over the entire cycle reduces the transformer signal to zero.

I. AUTOMATIC QUADRATURE REJECTION

Automatic quadrature rejection has been used on industrial flowmeters for some years (Hutcheon and Harrison, 1960). Wyatt (1964) has used it in blood flow measurement to lessen the need for phase stability in amplifier and detector. Basically, another detector is used, phased so as to detect the quadrature and reject the flow signal. The output is smoothed and the d.c. level used to modulate an internally generated signal which is fed back into the input in such a way as to reduce the incoming quadrature signal, using a null-detection feedback loop. The flow detector now has little quadrature signal to reject and very high quadrature rejection is achieved. This system gives the best signal-to-noise ratio and stability to date.

J. SQUARE WAVE FLOWMETER

Denison et al. (1955) realized that one way to eliminate quadrature effects was to use square wave energization of the magnet so that all quadrature effects would be over before sampling occurred (Fig. 7). Both half-wave and full-wave versions have been used. Unfortunately the sampling period cannot be as long as was first anticipated, due to the rise time of the current waveform and the delayed decay of the quadrature spike due to polarization effects at the electrodes. The spikes will also charge any coupling capacity used in the input stage, which will further increase the duration of the transformer spike. This can be overcome by using high differential-input impedance (Goodman, 1969), or a d.c. amplifier, but care must be taken that residual electrothermal effects from the electrodes do not overload the amplifier. Another method employs a d.c. amplifier with switched gain. Gain is low during the period when transformer spikes are present and high for the rest of the cycle (Hognestad, 1966). Hognestad also describes in great detail the cause and reduction of eddy current polarization of electrodes in square wave electromagnetic flowmeters; he concludes that a high input impedance (100 MΩ) and the use of high resistance electrodes can substantially reduce the influence of the transformer effect.

Goodman (1969) has designed a square wave unit which gates out the transformer induced signals after wide band amplification. He then converts the resulting wave to a near sine wave by passing it through a bandpass filter, and then employs full-wave phase sensitive mean detection thus achieving quadrature rejection and mean detection without the phase stability required of a sine wave unit. This results in a good square wave instrument, but signal-to-noise ratio and signal-to-input power ratio cannot be as good as in the sine wave designs. The trapezoid wave flowmeter (Yanof, 1961) seems to offer little but a reduction in power for a given sensitivity compared to the square wave instrument; the signal-to-noise ratio cannot be as high as for a sine wave system with the same power dissipation. The same is also true for square wave instruments.

K. PULSED SYSTEMS

Pulsed systems offer the advantage that the current to the magnet windings is only applied for a small fraction of the cycle, thus a large current pulse can be applied to give a high magnetic field and a large flow signal. The average power is thus kept low and the efficiency is high, especially if peak detection is used. Another advantage is that multiple systems can be used at the same basic magnet frequency. Each probe is energized at different times in the cycle, and one probe will not be affected by the magnetic field from a close neighbour. The need to sample the input wave during the short period of the magnet current pulse to avoid transformer and polarization effects, further reduces the period per cycle during which the flow signal is sampled. Thus the signal-to-noise ratio is reduced, offsetting the high signal-to-power ratio previously achieved.

The choice is difficult therefore between systems with different energization waveforms. For low power and high signal-to-noise ratio the modern sine wave instrument is difficult to beat, now that automatic quadrature rejection and elimination of manual gate setting has been achieved. Zero stability now depends upon the probes used and not on adjustment of the electronics, thus the advantages the square wave device once enjoyed have been eliminated and its efficiency in converting magnet drive into a flow proportional signal makes the sine wave device the best one.

The pulsed system only appears to have advantages when close proximity of transducers is required, especially if air cored probes are to be used, as the magnetic field is not contained within the probe. Using the flow heads of Clark and Wyatt (1969) or of Kolin and Vanyo (1967), with a sine wave instrument, the effect of proximity should be small as the magnetic field is essentially contained within the transducer.

L. FREQUENCY RESPONSE

This subject has been much discussed. Ferguson and Wells (1959a) suggested that 8 harmonics were necessary to represent flows in the femoral artery. For the aorta (1959b) they found 21 harmonics were required. Guz (1968b) showed that 12 harmonics were insufficient to record accurately the flow reversal in the aorta of a dog. It would seem that a frequency response to at least 100 Hz would be desirable. The response of many commercial flowmeters often falls short of this and all too often the need for a linear phase response is overlooked. This is essential if an undistorted waveform is required. Frequently the response of a flowmeter is stated as d.c.–X Hz, with no mention of the attenuation of the signals at X Hz and within the range. The practice in electrical engineering is to state the -3 dB frequency which means virtually nothing to most in the medical field. This means that if, for example, the output at f_1 Hz (a very low frequency) is taken as 100 per cent and if the frequency is increased until the output is 70·7 per cent at f_2 Hz, then f_2 is the -3 dB frequency (calculated from dB $= -20 \log V_1/V_2$, where V_2 is the output at f_2 and V_1 the output at f_1. A much clearer picture is given if the response is stated as being flat within y per cent from d.c.–X Hz, and the phase shift is stated to be linear with frequency. A suitable range of filter positions for blood flow measurement is 10, 20, 40, 80 and 120 Hz, responses being flat within ± 5 per cent to these frequencies and with phase shift linearly related to frequency. A separate output giving the mean signal is also desirable. The fall off, the way the signal attenuates at frequencies above the nominated frequency, should be sharp; response should fall to one-tenth amplitude at three times the nominated frequency. The amount of phase shift is not so important, provided it is linear it is very easy to correct as it amounts to a simple time delay.

Filters suitable for use with electromagnetic flowmeters have been described by Wyatt (1960, 1961a) and Goodman (1968). The response of many commercial flowmeters has been given by Bergel and Gessner (1964), O'Rourke (1965), Philips and Davila (1965) and Hainsworth et al. (1968). These data are often omitted from the manufacturer's handbook. It is necessary to test the whole flowmeter rather than just the output filter as interstage filters may have been used. To produce a suitable input a modulation technique must therefore be used. An analogue multiplier is recommended since

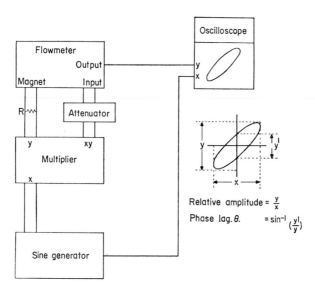

FIG. 8. Frequency response measurement. This uses a multiplier fed by a signal in phase with the magnet current (resistor R is similar in value to the magnet coils of the flow transducer). The modulation signal is fed to the multiplier from a signal generator. The multiplier output is suitably attenuated to provide a signal to the flowmeter input. The flowmeter output is fed to the Y input of an oscilloscope and the X input is connected to the signal generator to obtain a Lissajous presentation (not available on all oscilloscopes). The amplitude and phase response can then be obtained by simple measurements at appropriate frequencies.

solid state multipliers are relatively cheap. The block diagram in Fig. 8 shows a typical arrangement for measuring frequency response. The multiplier can either be of the semiconductor four quadrant variety or a Hall multiplier. An oscilloscope capable of Lissajous reproduction is used, the output from the flowmeter being displayed against the input, from which amplitude and phase errors can be measured.

M. SAFETY

The increasing use of flowmeters in clinical studies had led to more stringent demands for safety in these instruments. In the magnet drive there is a potentially very dangerous supply of electrical energy which must be taken into account in cuff, and especially in catheter designs. The magnet coils should be screened not only for zero stability but so that any leakage from the coil will go to the flowmeter ground. The flowmeter should be isolated so that leakage to any other apparatus can be avoided. The leakage from electrodes should also be reduced, either by using an isolation transformer (Wyatt, 1965) as in sine wave instruments or double capacitors in square wave units. Where the screens on the electrode leads are driven the driving potential should be protected so that, if a screen touches an electrode

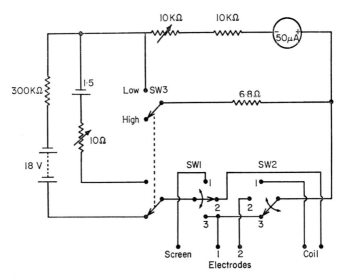

Fig. 9. Circuit diagram of the meter to test the insulation of transducers before use. With SW3 set on "high", the insulation between screen, electrodes and coil can be checked by rotating SW1 and SW2. With SW3 set on "low", the resistance of the coil can be checked. With SW1 and SW2 both set to 3, the meter is zeroed with the variable resistors.

wire, lethal currents (which can be less than 10 μA) will not flow through the patient. Earth electrodes on flow heads should be avoided and the use of multiple earths prevented.

A simple device to which a flow transducer can be connected (Fig. 9) has been in use in this laboratory for several years. It tests the insulation between electrodes and screen, coil and screen, coil and electrodes, and electrode and electrode. Eighteen volts are applied in the test, with a 50 μA meter calibrated to 100 divisions, a reading of 1 division represents 36 MΩ. Resolution to 0·2 of a division is simple; thus a leakage of 0·1 μA can be readily detected, representing a resistance of $1·8 \times 10^8$ Ω. If even a current as small as this is seen, the probe is not used. The device also enables the coil resistance to be measured (switched to low and coil–coil) which ensures that the probe is fully operational before use. It is also of great help in checking flow transducers during chronic implantation, when small current leaks can cause serious offsets and noise.

3. ULTRASONIC FLOWMETERS

Ultrasonic flowmeters, like the electromagnetic devices, are available in cuff, cannula and catheter tip varieties. An ultrasonic beam is passed through the vessel and information on the velocity of blood within the vessel is detected from the difference in time taken for the ultrasound to pass in one direction as opposed to the other (transit time technique), or from the frequency of the sound scattered from the moving red cells (Doppler principle). The Doppler instrument can also be used transcutaneously on vessels close to the surface and on certain deeper sites. Catheter probes using both methods have been developed for use in deeper vessels.

A. TRANSIT TIME TECHNIQUE

Transit time ultrasonic flowmeters, first described by Franklin *et al.* (1962), have been overshadowed in recent years by the Doppler shift instrument which initially appeared the simpler and could give qualitative results transcutaneously for vessels close to the surface. The transit time instrument has been very well described by Baker (1966) and was evaluated by Gessner (1969) for complex velocity profiles. Only a brief description will be given here. A pulse of ultrasound is emitted simultaneously from two crystals on either side of a vessel (see Fig. 10a). If the pulse is short compared with the transit time of sound across the vessel each transmitter can also act as a receiver for the pulse from the opposite side. The difference in transit time is given by:

$$\Delta t = \int_0^l \left(\frac{1}{C + U(x)\cos\theta} - \frac{1}{C - U(x)\cos\theta} \right) dx \qquad (3.1)$$

where l = distance between the crystals, $U(x)$ = blood velocity as a function of x, C = velocity of sound in blood, and θ is the angle between the flow axis and the line joining the crystals.

If $U(x) \ll C$, then

$$\Delta t = \frac{2 \cos \theta}{C^2} \int_0^l U(x)\, dx \qquad (3.2)$$

where

$$\int_0^l U(x)\, dx$$

is the integral of blood velocities through which the beam passes. For wide crystals covering the whole width of the vessel this would closely represent the true average velocity, $\bar{u}$ but for narrow crystals it approaches the average across a diameter, which is not the same as $\bar{u}$.

One may measure either the time difference or the phase difference $\Delta\phi$ between the two received signals if they were originally emitted in phase, since $\Delta t = \Delta\phi/2\pi f$. Thus for $U = 1 \text{ m s}^{-1}$, $\theta = 45°$; $C = 1\cdot5 \text{ km s}^{-2}$ and $l = 3$ cm we have $\Delta t = 30$ ns. If $f = 10$ MHz then $\Delta\phi = 40°$. For a resolution of 1 cm s^{-1} a difference of $0\cdot4°$ must be detected and accurate matching of crystals and stability of the measuring apparatus are required. Both Baker and Gessner show that with a parabolic velocity profile and a narrow beam of ultrasound an overestimate of velocity of 33 per cent is made, for the instrument takes the average velocity across a diameter, rather than across the whole volume of blood contained in the vessel. Baker pointed out that with wider crystals this error could be reduced considerably. Gessner (1969) and Kivilis and Reshetnikov (1965) also showed that even with the blunted velocity profile encountered in turbulent flow (McDonald, 1960) the error would amount to an overestimate of 5–8 per cent.

Gessner extended this study to oscillating flow and showed that for α† greater than 10, the error in amplitude was less than 10 per cent and in phase less than 5°. For $\alpha = 5$ the errors are 20 per cent and 7·5°. Thus on small vessels where α is low the errors are appreciable and corrections should be made.

A catheter tip device using the transit time method (Scheu et al., 1965) was placed in the ascending aorta of a dog, where α is high, and compared with an external electromagnet probe with satisfactory results. Further evaluation (Fricke et al., 1970), and a description of the apparatus and in vitro performance (Studer et al., 1970) have showed that this instrument is one capable of accurate measurement. It is small (2·3 mm diameter), has a linear output between -40 cm s^{-1} and $+180 \text{ cm s}^{-1}$ and has an adequate

---

† α (see McDonald, 1960) is a dimensionless number which characterizes the nature of oscillatory fluid flow. It is discussed further in Chapter 19, Section 4.

frequency response. The determination of flow zero is uncertain with this device and it has been used only where it is known that flow is zero for part of the cycle.

B. DOPPLER METHOD

The reason for the great interest shown in the Doppler technique since its first introduction by Franklin *et al.* (1961), is that it can record signals transcutaneously (Baker *et al.*, 1964; Stegall *et al.*, 1966).

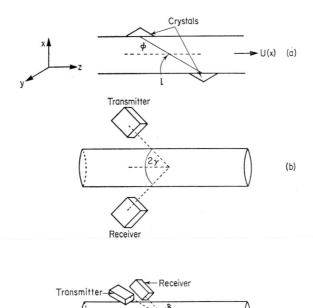

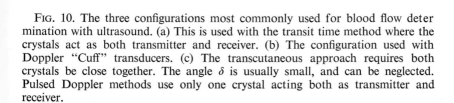

FIG. 10. The three configurations most commonly used for blood flow deter mination with ultrasound. (a) This is used with the transit time method where the crystals act as both transmitter and receiver. (b) The configuration used with Doppler "Cuff" transducers. (c) The transcutaneous approach requires both crystals be close together. The angle δ is usually small, and can be neglected. Pulsed Doppler methods use only one crystal acting both as transmitter and receiver.

The Doppler principle states that if there is relative motion between a transmitter and receiver there will be a change in the frequency of a wave detected by the receiver. If the wave is reflected from the receiver back to the transmitter, or to another receiver stationary with respect to the trans-

mitter, there will be a further shift in frequency. Consider the arrangement
in Fig. 10b; then

$$f' = f[(C - U \cos \gamma)/C] \qquad (3.3)$$

where f' is the frequency seen by the reflector (red cell) moving at velocity U,
f is the emitted frequency, C the velocity of sound in the medium, and γ
is the angle between the emitted sonic beam and the flow axis. Furthermore

$$f'' = f' \left[\frac{C - U \cos \gamma}{C} \right] \qquad (3.4)$$

and

$$f'' = f \left[\frac{C - U \cos \gamma}{C} \right]^2 \qquad (3.5)$$

where f'' is the frequency seen by the receiver. Therefore

$$\Delta F = f - f'' = \frac{2fU \cos \gamma}{C} - \frac{U^2 f \cos^2 \gamma}{C^2} \qquad (3.6)$$

In general $(U \cos \gamma/C)^2 \ll 1$ and we may write

$$\Delta F = \frac{2fU \cos \gamma}{C}. \qquad (3.7)$$

Thus for $\gamma = 45°$, $C = 1.4$ km s^{-1}, $f = 10$ MHz and U varying between
0 and 2 m s^{-1}, we find $\Delta F = 0$–20 kHz.

In a transcutaneous instrument the crystals are usually arranged as shown
in Fig. 10c; the angle δ is very small and can be neglected, but γ can
approach $0°$ (Light, 1969) and the range of ΔF now extends to $\simeq 30$ kHz.
These figures serve as a guide to the expected Doppler shift. As the attenuation of an ultrasonic beam is greater at higher frequencies (Wells, 1969)
a 2 MHz beam is often used for longer distances. The Doppler band is now
reduced to 6 kHz, but the reduced resolution does not seem to be critical.

It must be stressed that (3.7) only applies if all reflectors within the beam
are *moving at the same velocity:* in practice a spectrum will be received.
Flax *et al.* (1970) predict the spectrum (Fig. 11) produced by two types of
velocity profile and with the ultrasonic beam either wider or narrower
than the vessel. Their predictions were confirmed experimentally. As the
spectrum changes both with velocity profile and the width of the ultrasonic
beam, the question arises as to what is actually being measured by a Doppler
flowmeter. The usual technique is to feed the signal into a zero crossing
detector after previous high pass filtering (at 100 Hz) to remove low frequency
signals, which could be caused by vessel wall movement, and the large
non-Doppler shifted coupling frequency which could overload the detector.
Low pass filtering ($\simeq 15$ kHz) is used to remove high frequencies which

could increase the noise level. The effect of the low pass filter is to limit the highest velocity that can be recorded. In most commercial instruments this has been set to about 100 cm s^{-1} which may well be too low for many systemic arteries, especially in cases of valvular disease.

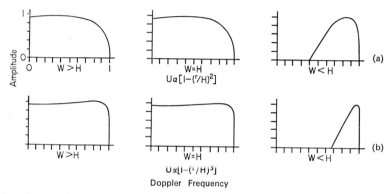

Fig. 11. Predicted spectra for two different velocity profiles and different widths of the ultrasonic beam relative to the radius of the flow tube. W is the width of the ultrasonic beam and H the radius of the pipe. (a) For a parabolic velocity profile. (b) For plug flow. Redrawn from Flax et al. (1970).

The effect of the high pass filter is to set a threshold below which the velocity is assumed zero. At first sight this may seem a trivial restriction, for it is usually around 2 cm s^{-1}, but it also introduces a marked non-linearity around zero and a zero offset which will be in opposite directions for forward and backward flow. This offset amounts to about 1 cm s^{-1} (Fig. 12).

This is not troublesome in most applications of transcutaneous Doppler instruments where many other errors can arise. It should, however, be borne in mind when extravascular cuff probes and catheter tip devices are used and compared with other methods of flow detection. The problem manifests itself in directional devices where the "S" shaped sensitivity curve effectively compresses the low velocities, making calibration difficult.

The zero crossing detector converts the frequency information to an analogue voltage output. This is done by producing a narrow pulse every time the input signal crosses through zero in either a positive or negative going direction or in both. The resulting series of pulses is low-pass filtered to produce the desired analogue voltage. This is very simple to visualize for pure tones but for random frequencies things are much more complex. Rice (1944, 1945) predicted the number of zero crossings from the spectral content of the signal. Flax et al. (1970) used this to determine the output expected from their predicted spectra. They concluded that the output would be proportional to the maximum frequency, i.e. maximum velocity, present in the spectrum. In practice the spectrum received is not well defined due to noise. This extends the range beyond the predicted maximum frequency so that a high signal-to-noise ratio is required for accuracy. The highest velocity seen will depend upon the velocity profile and the Doppler device tends to be a maximum velocity sensor. Thus calibration in terms of flow will require knowledge of the profile, and in the circulation different

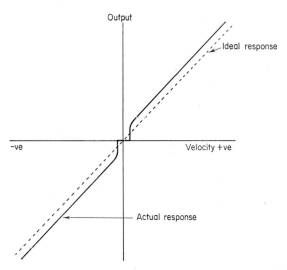

FIG. 12. The deviation from linearity produced by inserting a high pass filter to remove low velocity wall motion artefacts and the large non-Doppler shifted energization signal.

calibrations will apply for different vessels. In addition the spectrum will change if the vessel is larger or smaller than the beam width. Disturbed flow, around an atheromatous plaque, for example, could create severe problems. As the signal received by the transducer may well be 10^5 times lower than that emitted, great care must be taken in amplification to reduce background noise, and efficient transducers used. Since attenuation of an ultrasonic wave is proportional to frequency and distance, lower frequencies are required for deep vessels if accuracy is to be maintained.

Flax et al. (1970) extended their analysis into the accuracy of measurement when the variance of zero crossing intervals was taken into account. They showed that to reduce the variance considerably low pass filtering after detection was required. This rendered the system accurate for mean flows, but unable to follow pulsatile waveforms. They suggested improvements to overcome this either by probe design so that the axial velocities are in the ultrasound beam or "with a dynamic band pass filter to track the Doppler signal". Other workers have been unhappy with the zero crossing detector (Light, 1969; Gosling, 1970) and have concentrated on observing the frequency spectrum itself.

One of the early criticisms of the Doppler flowmeter, its inability to detect flow direction, was overcome by McLeod (1967) An instrument employing his technique was used by Chiche *et al.* (1968) on veins and peripheral arteries. It produced waveforms very similar to those seen with electro-magnetic flowmeters but no quantitative tests have been described and personal experience with a similar device has shown it to lack in frequency response and linearity in the range of interest. A question arising with directional Doppler instruments is; what do positive and negative outputs represent? In pulsatile flow the inner and outer fluid shells may be going in different directions (McDonald, 1960; and see Chapter 9) at the same time. The volume in the shells will be different yet equal weight will be given to both so that equal velocities will result in a false zero output. As this situation is likely to occur around zero flow both amplitude and phase distortion will occur around this level.

This unprecise measurement of volume and the effects of the profile on flow measurements has led to the more complex pulsed ultrasonic flowmeter (Peronneau *et al.*, 1969). This uses one crystal instead of the usual two, and emits 8 MHz ultrasound at repetitive frequencies of 20–33 kHz in pulses of 0·3–3 μs duration. For the remainder of the cycle, the transducer acts as a receiver. The received signal is sampled only when a narrow "gate" is opened after a predetermined delay from emission. Since the sound wave will have had time to go and return a known distance before the gate is opened, the distance to the reflecting point can be found. Resolution on this is stated to be 0·5 mm.

The signal coming through the gate has been frequency shifted by the Doppler effect. As it returned from a small volume of blood moving at approximately uniform velocity, the simple Doppler equation (3.7) is approximately valid. The signal received $(f+f'')$ is fed to a beat detector and mixed with a signal F_0 $(=f+f_r)$ to give an output f_r-f'' which is fed to a frequency meter. If the beam strikes a stationary object, i.e. vessel wall, then $f'' = 0$ and the output proportional to f_r is the reference zero. This method can be further improved (Peronneau *et al.*, 1969) by locking f with the Doppler shift f'', thereby increasing accuracy at low velocities, but the leakage of the emission frequency or direct reflection from stationary objects with no Doppler shift must be kept very small. Another method of extracting the velocity signal (Peronneau *et al.*, 1969) is similar to that used by McLeod (1967). Two separate detecting systems are used in which the Doppler shifted signal is mixed with signals at the transmitted frequency which are

90° out of phase with each other. Comparison of the resulting signals indicates whether the Doppler shift, and hence the direction of flow, was positive or negative.

The great advantage of the gating method is that it should be possible to measure velocity profiles without any intrusion into the vessel and zero can easily be obtained electronically. The vessel diameter can also be found by moving the timing of the gate to receive the signal from each wall and translating this time shift to distance. At the present time the method is complex but development over the next few years may result in gated ultrasonic devices replacing continuous emission instruments.

Considerable use has been made of the ultrasonic method in the study of vascular disease. Interesting and useful information can be obtained, but so far no quantification is possible and serious errors can be made if the area of the vessel is not known. For example, suppose that an atheromatous plaque is to be removed. Velocity measurements before removal may show higher values than after surgery for the luminal area will be increased. The total flow must rise considerably to compensate for this and this increase will depend upon the ratio of the resistance of the plaque to the resistance peripheral to its site. Thus great care must be taken in interpreting such results.

Catheter tip ultrasonic Doppler probes have been used to study the circulation in places not accessible transcutaneously (Stone *et al.*, 1967; Kalmanson *et al.*, 1969; Benchimol *et al.*, 1969). These devices will prove extremely valuable when the problems of detection and response have been overcome.

4. THERMAL DEVICES

A. PRINCIPLE OF OPERATION

As this chapter is concerned with pulsatile flow measurement reference will only be made to thermal devices which have a sufficiently good frequency response. Thermal devices used in this application depend upon the heat loss from a heated element being related to the velocity of blood flowing past it. The heated element can be fed from a constant current source; as the temperature changes due to heat lost to the moving fluid the resistance of the element will change, and the voltage change across it can be measured. The element is usually mounted in a balanced bridge formation, changes in temperature caused by flow will change its resistance, offsetting the bridge and giving an output related to flow velocity. Since the temperature must first change the response is limited by the thermal time constant of the element and the substrate on which it is mounted. It has proved impossible to reduce this sufficiently, consequently this technique does not have an adequate frequency response for pulsatile blood flow determination.

A modified technique maintains the heated element at a constant temperature by use of a positive feedback bridge (Fig. 13) and measures the power to keep it constant. This reduces the thermal time constant greatly. This is the constant temperature or constant resistance technique. Adjustment of the variable resistor allows the temperature of the thermistor (or thin film, see later) to be set above the temperature of the fluid. Heat loss to the fluid cools the thermistor, increases its resistance and unbalances the bridge.

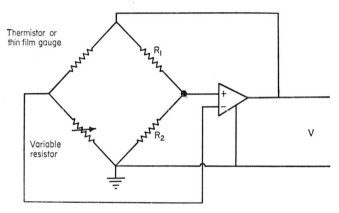

Fig. 13. Schematic diagram of a constant temperature (or resistance) feedback bridge.

Bridge and amplifier are arranged in such a way that the output of the amplifier is increased and more current flows through the thermistor, heating it and restoring both temperature and bridge balance. If the gain of the amplifier is high then the thermistor remains virtually at constant temperature. The device now has a high frequency response dependent upon the gain-bandwidth product of the amplifier.

Thermistors were used as the heating or sensing element in the feedback bridge arrangement of Katsura et al. (1959). They were unable to obtain sufficiently high frequency response for arterial flow measurement, and the device was not directionally sensitive. Grahn et al. (1968) increased the response to over 150 Hz, and by using three thermistors were able to obtain a stable, directionally sensitive device. They found that the power required to maintain constant temperature varied linearly with the logarithm of the fluid velocity, i.e. $\propto V^x$; thus by taking the anti-logarithm of a signal proportional to power a linear relationship to velocity was achieved. The mounting of the thermistors in this design resulted in unequal sensitivities to forward and backward flows and corrections had to be applied. The device exhibited high frequency response but was affected by its position in the vessel. Due to the distorted response to low velocities there were uncertainties at around zero level.

Grahn *et al.* (1969) changed their 1968 design to overcome the problems encountered in direction sensing and position sensitivity. Three thermistors were used, two sensing velocity (R_{F1} and R_{F2}) and one (R_{T1}) for temperature compensation (Fig. 14). The velocity sensing thermistors were mounted

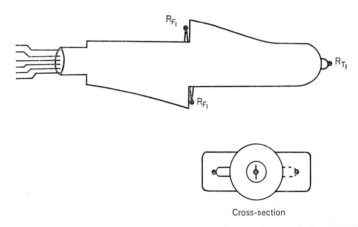

Cross-section

Fig. 14. A directionally sensitive thermal probe can be made by shielding the thermistors so that one is influenced only by forward flow and the other only by reverse flow. Redrawn from Grahn *et al.* (1969).

on a former in such a way that one was sensitive to forward and the other to reverse velocities. These were connected to separate constant temperature bridges, independently compensated for blood temperature by the third thermistor and an ingenious seven thermistor complex mounted in the instrument. The power to each bridge was measured and compared to a reference level; the anti-log of the difference was taken to get signals proportional to the forward and backward velocities. Finally, the difference between these signals was taken to obtain a directionally sensitive output. Comparisons with electromagnetic flow measurements were very good, showing no discontinuity at flow reversals. Comparison in the ascending aorta showed nothing to suggest the device was very sensitive to movement. The size of the catheter is that of a No. 6F cardiac catheter (2·3 mm o.d.), and the former was shaped so that its largest diameter was the same as the diameter of the catheter.

Measurements with constant temperature anemometry of blood velocity were developed from aeronautical measurements with hot wire gauges. The wire has been replaced by a thin heated film of platinum or gold, evaporated or vacuum sputtered on to a dielectric substrate, or a platinum-silver suspension painted on to a suitable surface. Devices incorporating these techniques have been reported by Ling and Atabek (1966), Bellhouse et al. (1967), Ling et al. (1968), Bellhouse and Bellhouse (1968) and Seed and Wood (1970). The difference between thin metal and thermistors is that thermistors usually have a negative temperature coefficient, that is, resistance falls as temperature rises while metals have positive temperature coefficients and resistance rises with temperature. This presents no problem: the bridge circuit is connected differently. For thin film anemometers, as the film begins to cool, the resistance *drops* and the output must rise to reheat the film. Thus for thin film gauges the connections to the amplifier in Fig. 13 must be reversed.

The relationship between the output voltage, V, and the velocity U is

$$\frac{V^2}{\Delta T} = A + BU^{\frac{1}{2}} \qquad (4.1)$$

where A and B are constants depending upon the initial conditions and ΔT is the overheat of the film above blood temperature. This awkward relationship is inconvenient for practical applications and the voltage signal is passed through an electronic linearizing circuit to produce a signal directly proportional to velocity. The equation shows that sensitivity is a function of the overheat. A figure of 5 °C overheat seems to have been accepted by workers in this field both for thermistors and thin films since it provides adequate sensitivity and frequency response, and the temperature is not high enough to cause fibrin deposition or red cell damage (the same criteria limit the power dissipation in electromagnetic probes). As sensitivity is proportional to overheat, stability of temperature is essential. With thin film sensors operating initially at 5 °C overheat, a 1 °C change in ambient temperature can produce a change in sensitivity of 13 per cent (Ling et al., 1968). Automatic temperature compensation has not been used with thin films as it has in the thermistor designs of Grahn et al. (1968), and frequent checking of the temperature and re-adjustment of the overheat, if necessary, are required. Calibrations in steady flow have shown dependence (Seed and Wood, 1970) upon the position of the film relative to the tip. Ling et al. (1968) placed the film at 90° to the flow axis either on the apex of a cone at the end of a needle or 20° back from the apex when an insertion angle of 70° was used to reduce flow disturbances due to the shaft of the needle. Thus the sensitivity altered with the direction of flow. Another problem with this type of probe was found by Seed and Wood (1970). The separation point of the fluid on the probe is dependent on the velocity; on a cone or sphere it moves forward towards the leading edge as velocity increases. Separation should not reach the films but this does cause reduced sensitivity at a velocity which depends on the size of the probe. Seed and Wood (1970) found with a design similar to that of Ling *et al.* (1968) that this velocity was about 25 cm s^{-1}. Mounting the film ahead of the apex or angulating the probe would help, but only for flow in one direction. Bellhouse *et al.* (1969) used a straight probe but mounted the film on its side back from the tip of the needle. The needle could be rotated so that forward and backward velocities could be resolved.

Bellhouse and Bellhouse (1968) used an L-shaped probe (Fig. 15). This avoids the separation problem and, depending on how close to the leading

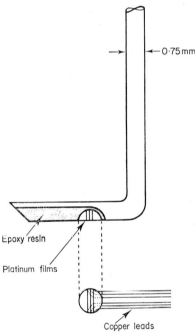

FIG. 15. A thin film needle velocity sensor showing the position of the three films for sensing velocity and flow direction. From Bellhouse and Bellhouse (1968).

edge the film is, a nearly equal response in both directions is achieved. This shape was used by Schultz *et al.* (1969) and in most of the studies by Seed and Wood (1970).

B. PERFORMANCE IN OSCILLATORY FLOW

Apart from fluid dynamic effects there seems to be an instrumental effect in some apparatus. Seed and Wood (1970) found that the response to small oscillations of the probe was dependent upon the degree of overheat and apparatus used. When this effect was eliminated by working at a 5 per cent (i.e. 5 per cent absolute temperature) overheat rather than at 1 per cent, the steady and oscillatory calibrations were the same, provided there was no backflow.

As with all thermal devices thin films are not directionally sensitive. Auxiliary films must be added as direction sensors, these merely serve to show the direction in which heat is transmitted from the heated film. One such film would be enough, but in the presence of turbulent flow two sensors on either side of the hot film were found to be more satisfactory (Schultz et al., 1969). They can be used to indicate flow direction (Bellhouse et al., 1967) or to switch and invert the signal automatically as with the thermistor devices, but due to the response at low velocities this operation is doubtful. The frequency response of a hot film is satisfactory so long as the quantity $fx/U \ll 1$ (Schultz et al., 1969), where f is the frequency, x the distance of the film from the leading edge and U the velocity. Thus at low velocities the response is degraded. This explains why on many records taken with non-directional devices the signal does not return to zero before rising again when flow reversal occurs. Automatic phase switching will cause errors as too high a forward velocity will be transposed to too high a reverse velocity (Fig. 16). The dynamic response would depend on whether or not a steady flow was present. Bellhouse and Bellhouse (1968) showed no difference between static calibration and that obtained by shaking the probe in a static bath. However, Seed and Wood (1970) found errors independent of frequency but dependent upon the amplitude of oscillation if the probe was oscillated in still fluid. This could amount to as much as a difference of 20 per cent from the steady calibration. This seems likely to stem from the position of the heated element relative to the leading edge of the probe, for Seed and Wood (1970) found they could reduce the error by moving the film nearer the tip. Whether this affects the sensitivity to different flow directions is not, however, discussed.

There is also some difference of opinion in the literature as to whether there is a difference between calibration in water and blood. Ling et al. (1968) used whole blood with an oscillating flow and found changes in sensitivity with haematocrit changes suggesting there would be a difference between water and blood calibrations. Seed and Wood, in preliminary tests, found variations between blood and water calibrations, whereas Bellhouse and Bellhouse (1968) and Schultz et al. (1969) did not.

The ideal instrument to measure either pulsatile blood flow or blood velocity does not exist. The electromagnetic perivascular transducer seems to offer the best solution if blood flow is to be measured accurately and exposure of the vessel is acceptable. Ultrasound does not seem to offer any advantage over the modern electromagnetic device in this requirement, unless telemetry from free ranging animals is contemplated; but in fact the total power required for a modern electromagnetic system can be less than 1 W, and the improved accuracy offsets the little extra power required. Ultrasound comes into its own when non-invasive techniques are required: it is the only method. Considerable interest and continued improvement is to be expected which will increase the accuracy and frequency response. The next few years may well see greater advances in this method than any other.

In the accurate measurement of velocity profiles, pulsed ultrasound, used non-invasively, seems very attractive, and as this technique is only in its

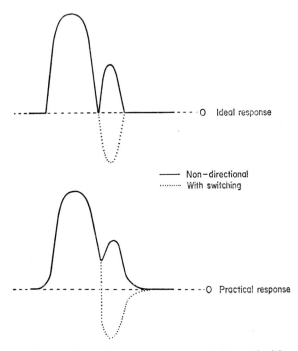

FIG. 16. The effect of low frequency response at low velocities on thin film devices, showing the errors produced by automatic switching to achieve direction sensitivity. The error can be reduced, but not eliminated, by careful design.

infancy the results seen so far, albeit with catheters, show tremendous potential. The use of thin film thermal sensors on a needle is still relatively new and the results are good (see Chapter 9); it will be of considerable interest to see a side-by-side comparison with the pulsed ultrasonic device.

Catheter or intraluminal velocity probes of all types suffer from motion artefacts, the thermal and ultrasonic probes probably more so than the electromagnetic, but they can be inserted peripherally and advanced to almost any site within the cardiovascular system. As blood pressure is nearly always also required as well as blood velocity and is easily obtained from the same catheter, catheter probes will still be used for some time to come, especially in clinical applications.

The choice for someone buying a flowmeter today is thus wide. If true flow is of paramount importance, then the electromagnetic method should be used. If velocity profiles or local velocity variations are to be studied, then thermal methods seem at the moment to be best, yet pulsed ultrasound will certainly develop in the near future.

As a clinical tool when surgical exposure of a vessel is to be performed, electromagnetic methods are the choice. For diagnosis, catheter-tip devices utilizing all these methods should be considered, the electromagnetic method perhaps being preferable due to its inherent directional sensitivity and ease of operation. For non-invasive clinical diagnosis, ultrasound is the only method; yet great care must be taken in interpreting the results and it must be remembered it is a velocity device, not a flowmeter.

REFERENCES

Baker, D. W. (1966). Pulsed ultrasonic flowmeter. *In* "Methods in Medical Research" (R. F. Rusher, ed.), Vol. 11, Year Book Medical Publishers Inc., Chicago.

Baker, D. W., Stegall, H. F. and Schlegal, W. A. (1964). A sonic transcutaneous blood flowmeter. *Proc. 17th Ann. Conf. Eng. Med. Biol.* **6**, 76.

Barefoot, C. A. (1970). Electromagnetic catheter blood flow probe. U.S. Patent 3, 487, 826.

Beck, R., Morris, J. A. and Assali, N. S. (1965). Calibration characteristics of the pulsed field electromagnetic flowmeter. *Amer. J. Med. Electron.* **4**, 87–97.

Bellhouse, B. J. and Bellhouse, F. H. (1968). Thin film gauges for the measurement of velocity or skin friction in air, water or blood. *J. Sci. Inst.* **1**, 1211–1213.

Bellhouse, B. J., Bellhouse, F. H. and Gunning, A. J. (1969). A straight needle probe for the measurement of blood velocity. *J. Sci. Inst.* **2**, 936–938.

Bellhouse, B. J., Schultz, D. L., Karatzas, N. B. and Lee, G. de J. (1967). A catheter tip method for the measurement of the pulsatile blood flow velocity in arteries. *In* "Blood Flow Through Organs and Tissues" (W. H. Bain and A. M. Harper, eds), S. Livingstone Ltd., Edinburgh.

Benchimol, A., Stegall, H. F., Maroko, P. R., Brener, L. and Gartlon, J. L. (1969). Aortic flow velocity in man during cardiac arrhythmias measured with the Doppler-catheter flowmeter system. *Amer. Heart J.* **78**, 649–659.

Bergel, D. H. and Gessner, U. (1966). The electromagnetic flowmeter. *In* "Methods in Medical Research" (R. F. Rusher, ed.), Vol. 11, Year Book Medical Publishers Inc., Chicago.

Bergel, D. H. and Makin, G. (1968). Experience with calibration procedures. *In* "New Findings in Blood Flowmetry" (C. Cappelen, ed.), Universitetsforlaget, Oslo.

Bevir, M. (1969). Induced Voltage Electromagnetic Flowmeters. Ph.D. Thesis, University of Warwick.

Bevir, M. (1971). Sensitivity of electromagnetic velocity probes. *Phys. Med. Biol.* **16**, 229–232.

Bond, R. F. (1967). *In vivo* method for calibrating electromagnetic flowmeter probes. *J. Appl. Physiol.* **22,** 358–361.

Bond, R. F. and Barefoot, C. A. (1967). Evaluation of an electromagnetic catheter tip velocity sensitive blood flow probe. *J. Appl. Physiol.* **23,** 403–409.

Brunsting, J. R. and Ten Hoor, F. (1968). Factors preventing accurate *in vitro* calibration of non-cannulating electromagnetic flow transducers. *In* "New Findings in Blood Flowmetry" (C. Cappelen, ed.), Universitetsforlaget, Oslo.

Cappelen, Chr. and Hall, K. V. (1967). Electromagnetic blood flowmetry in clinical surgery. *Acta. Chir. Scand.* Suppl. 368.

Case, R. B., Roselle, H. A. and Nassar, M. E. (1966). Simplified method for calibration of electromagnetic flowmeters. *Med. Res. Eng.* **5,** 38–40.

Chiche, P., Kalmanson, D., Veyrat, L. and Toutain, G. (1968). Enregistrement transcutané du flux artériel par fluxmétre directionnel à effet Doppler. Description d'un appareillage et premiers résultats. *Bull. Mém. Soc. Méd. Hôp. Paris* **119,** 87–97.

Clark, D. M. and Wyatt, D. G. (1968). The effect of magnetic field inhomogeneity on flowmeter sensitivity. *In* "New Findings in Blood Flowmetry" (C. Cappelen, ed.), Universitetsforlaget, Oslo.

Clark, D. M. and Wyatt, D. G. (1969). An improved perivascular electromagnetic flowmeter. *Med. Biol. Eng.* **7,** 185–190.

Dedichen, H. and Schenk, W. G., Jr. (1968). Influence of haematocrit changes in square wave electromagnetic flowmeter calibration. *In* "New Findings in Blood Flowmetry" (C. Cappelen, ed.), Universitetsforlaget, Oslo.

Denison, A. B., Spencer, M. P. and Green, H. D. (1955). A square wave electromagnetic flowmeter for application to intact blood vessels. *Circulation Res.* **3,** 39–46.

Dennis, J. and Wyatt, D. G. (1969). Effects of haematocrit value upon electromagnetic flowmeter. *Circulation Res.* **24,** 875–886.

Ferguson, D. J. and Landahl, H. D. (1966). Magnetic meters: effects of electrical resistance in tissue on flow measurements and on improved calibration for square wave circuits. *Circulation Res.* **19,** 917–929.

Ferguson, D. J. and Wells, H. S. (1959a). Frequencies in pulsatile flow and response of magnetic meter. *Circulation Res.* **7,** 336–341.

Ferguson, D. J. and Wells, H. S. (1959b). Harmonic analysis of frequencies in pulsatile blood flow. *I.R.E. Trans. Med. Elect.* **6,** 291–294.

Flax, S. W., Webster, J. G. and Updike, S. J. (1970). Statistical evaluation of the Doppler ultrasonic blood flowmeter. *Biomed. Sci. Inst.* **7,** 201–222.

Folts, J. D. (1970). Electronic zero for chronic application of electromagnetic flowmeter probes. *J. Appl. Physiol.* **28,** 237–241.

Franklin, D. L., Schlegal, W. A. and Rushmer, R. F. (1961). Blood flow measured by Doppler frequency shift of backscattered ultrasound. *Science, N.Y.* **134,** 564–565.

Franklin, D. L., Baker, D. W. and Rushmer, R. F. (1962). Pulsed ultrasonic transit time flowmeter. *I.R.E. Trans. Bio. Med. Electron.* **9,** 44–49.

Fricke, G., Studer, U. and Scheu, H. (1970). Pulsatile velocity of blood in the pulmonary artery of dogs—measurement by an ultrasound gauge. *Cardiovasc. Res.* **4,** 371–379.

Gessner, U. (1961). Effects of vessel wall on electromagnetic flow measurements. *Biophys. J.* **1,** 627–637.

Gessner, U. (1969). The performance of the ultrasonic flowmeter in complex velocity profiles. *I.E.E.E. Trans. Bio. Med. Eng.* **BME-16,** 139–142.

Goldman, S. C., Marple, N. B. and Scolnik, W. C. (1963). Effects of flow profile on electromagnetic flowmeter accuracy. *J. Appl. Physiol.* **18**, 652–657.

Goodman, A. H. (1968). Low pass filters for electromagnetic flowmeters. *Med. Biol. Eng.* **6**, 477–486.

Goodman, A. H. (1969). A transistorized squarewave electromagnetic flowmeter I. *Med. Biol. Eng.* **7**, 115–132.

Gosling, R. (1970). Personal communication.

Grahn, A. R., Paul, M. H. and Wessel, H. U. (1968). Design and evaluation of a new linear thermistor velocity probe. *J. Appl. Physiol.* **24**, 236–246.

Grahn, A. R., Paul, M. H. and Wessel, H. U. (1969). A new direction sensitive probe for catheter tip thermal velocity measurement. *J. Appl. Physiol.* **27** 407–412.

Guz, A. (1968a). Measurement of cardiac output simultaneously with indicator-dilution technique. *In* "New Findings in Blood Flowmetry" (C. Cappelen, ed.), Universitetsforlaget, Oslo.

Guz, A. (1968b). Analysis of frequency response of a flowmeter—measurements and requirements. *In* "New Findings in Blood Flowmetry "(C. Cappelen, ed.), Universitetsforlaget, Oslo.

Hainsworth, R., Ledsome, J. R. and Snow, H. M. (1968). Dynamic testing of electromagnetic flowmeters by mechanical and electronic methods. *J. Appl. Physiol.* **25**, 469–472.

Hill, W. S. (1960). On the theoretical basis of electromagnetic methods to measure rates of flow. *Bol. Fac. Ing. Agri-Mensura Montevideo.* **7**, 295–324.

Hognestad, H. (1966). Square wave electromagnetic flowmeter with improved baseline stability. *Med. Res. Eng.* **5**, 28–33.

Hutcheon, I. C. and Harrison, D. N. (1960). Transistor quadrature suppression for a.c. servo systems. *Proc. I.E.E.* **107B**, 73–82.

Jochim, K. E. (1962). The development of the electromagnetic flowmeter. *I.R.E. Trans. Med. Electron.* **9**, 228–235.

Kanai, H. (1969). The effects upon electromagnetic flowmeter sensitivity of non-uniform fields and velocity profiles. *Med. Biol Eng.* **7**, 661–676.

Kalmanson, D., Toutain, G., Novikoff, N., Derai, C., Chiche, P. and Cabrol, C. (1969). Le Cathétérisme Velocimétrique du Coeur et des gros vaisseaux par sonde Ultrasonique Directionnelle à effet Doppler. Rapport Préliminaire. *Ann. Médicine Interne.* **11**, 685–700.

Katsura, S. R., Weiss, R., Baker, D. W. and Rushmer, R. F. (1959). Isothermal blood flow velocity probe. *I.R.E. Trans. Med. Elec.* **ME 6**, 283–285.

Kivilis, S. S. and Reshetnikov, V. A. (1965). Effect of a stabilized flow profile on the error of ultrasonic flowmeters. *Measurement Techn.* **3**, 276–278.

Kolin, A. (1936). An electromagnetic flowmeter. Principle of the method and its application to blood flow measurements. *Proc. Soc. Exp. Biol. Med.* **35**, 53–56.

Kolin, A. (1938). Electromagnetic rheometry and its application to blood flow measurements. *Amer. J. Physiol.* **122**, 797–804.

Kolin, A. (1941a). A variable phase transformer and its use as an a.c. interference eliminator. *Rev. Sci. Inst.* **12**, 555.

Kolin, A. (1941b). An a.c. induction flowmeter for measurement of blood flow in intact blood vessels. *Proc. Soc. Exp. Biol. Med.* **46**, 235–239.

Kolin, A. (1944). Electromagnetic velometry, I. A method for the determination of fluid velocity distribution in space and time. *J. Appl. Physics.* **15**, 150–164.

Kolin, A. (1952). A method of adjustment of the zero setting of an electromagnetic flowmeter without interruption of flow. *Rev. Sci. Inst.* **24,** 178–179.

Kolin, A. (1960). Blood flow determination by electromagnetic method. *In* "Medical Physics" (O. Glasser, ed.), Vol. 3, Year Book Medical Publishers Inc., Chicago.

Kolin, A. (1967). An electromagnetic intravascular blood flow sensor. *Proc. Nat Acad. Sci.* **57,** 1331–1337.

Kolin, A. (1969). A new principle for electromagnetic catheter flowmeters. *Proc. Nat. Acad. Sci.* **63,** 357–363.

Kolin, A. (1970a). A new approach to electromagnetic blood flow determination by means of a catheter in an external magnetic field. *Proc. Nat. Acad. Sci.* **65,** 521–527.

Kolin, A. (1970b). An electromagnetic catheter blood flowmeter of minimal lateral dimensions. *Proc. Nat. Acad. Sci.* **66,** 53–56.

Kolin, A., Archer, J. D. and Ross, G. (1967). An electromagnetic catheter flowmeter. *Circulation Res.* **21,** 889–899.

Kolin, A., Ross, G., Grollman, J. H. and Archer, J. D. (1968). An electromagnetic catheter flowmeter for determination of blood flow in major arteries. *Proc. Nat. Acad. Sci.* **59,** 808–815.

Kolin, A. and Vanyo, J. (1967). New design of miniature electromagnetic flow transducers suitable for semi-automatic fabrication. *Cardiovasc. Res.* **1,** 274–286.

Kolin, A. and Wisshaupt. R. (1963). Single coil coreless electromagnetic blood flowmeters. *I.E.E.E. Trans. Bio. Med. Eng.* **BME 10,** 60–67.

Lauridsen, P., Uhrenholdt, A., Engell, H. C. and Lunding, M. (1968). Simultaneous measurements of cardiac output by an electromagnetic flowmeter and dye dilution techniques in calves. *In* "New Findings in Blood Flowmetry" (C. Cappelen, ed.), Universitetsforlaget, Oslo.

Light, H. (1969). Non-injurious ultrasonic technique for observing flow in the human aorta. *Nature, London* **224,** 1119–1121.

Ling, S. C. and Atabek, H. B. (1966). Measurement of aortic blood flow in dogs by a hot film technique. *Proc. 19th Ann. Conf. Eng. Med. Biol.*, p. 212, Institute of Electrical and Electronic Engineers, New York.

Ling, S. C., Atabeck, H. B., Fry, D. L., Patel, D. J. and Janicki, J. S. (1968). Applications of heated film velocity and shear probes to haemodynamic studies. *Circulation Res.* **23,** 789–801.

McDonald, D. A. (1960). "Blood Flow in Arteries", Arnold, London.

McLeod, F. D., Jr. (1967). A directional Doppler flowmeter. Digest 7th Int. Conf. Med. Biol. Eng., p. 213. The Organizing Committee for the 7th International Conference on Medical and Biological Engineering, Stockholm.

Mills, C. J. (1966). A catheter tip electromagnetic velocity probe. *Phys. Med. Biol.* **11,** 323–324.

Mills, C. J. and Shillingford, J. P. (1967). A catheter tip velocity probe and its evaluation. *Cardiovasc. Res.* **1,** 263–273.

Mills, C. J., Gabe, I. T., Gault, J. H., Mason, D. T., Ross, J., Jr., Braunwald, E. and Shillingford, J. P. (1970). Pressure flow relationships in vascular impedance in man. *Cardiovasc. Res.* **4,** 405–417.

Olmsted, F. (1959). Measurement of cardiac output in unrestrained dogs by an implanted electromagnetic meter. *I.R.E. Trans. Med. Elec.* **ME 6,** 210–213.

O'Rourke, M. F. (1967). Pressure and flow waves in systemic arteries and the anatomical design of the arterial system. *J. Appl. Physiol.* **23**, 139–149.

O'Rourke, M. F. (1965). Dynamic accuracy of the electromagnetic flowmeter. *J. Appl. Physiol.* **20**, 142–147.

Peronneau, P., Chevrier, J. L., Bui-Mong-Hung, Leger, F. and Hinglais, J. (1969). Blood flow velocity measurement by ultrasonic Doppler effect velocity profile and velocity–flow rate relation. 4th Congress European Society for Experimental Surgery, Davos, Switzerland.

Peronneau, P., Deloche, A., Bui-Mong-Hung and Hinglais, J. (1969). Débitmétrie Ultrasonore-Développements et applications expérimentales. *Europ. Surg. Res.* **1**, 147–156.

Philips, C. M. and Davila, J. C. (1965). Frequency response of three commercial electromagnetic flowmeters. *Amer. J. Med. Elec.* **4**, 166–169.

Rice, S. O (1944). Mathematical analysis of random noise. *Bell System Tech. Jour.* **23**, 282–332.

Rice, S. O. (1945). Mathematical analysis of random noise. *Bell System Tech. Jour.* **24**, 46–156.

Rummel, T. and Ketelsen, B. (1966). Inhomogenes Magnetfeld ermöglicht Induktive Durchblutmessung bei allen in der Praxis vorkommenden Strömungsprofilen. *Regelungstecknik* **6**, 262–267.

Scheu, H., Sager, O. and Veragut, U. (1965). Eine Neue Methode Zur Intravasalen Messung Von Strömungsgeschwindigkeiten: Die Ultraschallsonde. *Klin. Wschr.* **43**, 608–611.

Schultz, D. L., Tunstall-Pedoe, D. S., Lee, G. de J., Gunning, A. J. and Bellhouse, B. J. (1969). Velocity distributions and transition in the arterial system. *In* "Ciba Foundation Symposium on Circulatory and Respiratory Mass Transport" (G. E. W. Wolstenholme and J. Knight, eds), Churchill, London.

Seed, W. A. and Wood, N. B. (1969). An apparatus for calibrating velocity probes in liquids. *J. Sci. Inst.* **2**, 896–898.

Seed, W. A. and Wood, N. B. (1970). Development and evaluation of a hot film velocity probe for cardiovascular studies. *Cardiovasc. Res.* **4**, 253–263.

Shercliff, J. A. (1962). "The Theory of Electromagnetic Flow Measurement". Cambridge University Press.

Shercliff, J. A. (1968). The effects of non-uniform magnetic fields and variations of the velocity distribution in electromagnetic flowmeters. *In* "New Findings in Blood Flowmetry" (C. Cappelen, ed.), Universitetsforlaget, Oslo.

Spencer, M. P. and Barefoot, C. A. (1968). Sensor design for electromagnetic blood flowmeters. *In* "New Findings in Blood Flowmetry" (C. Cappelen, ed.), Universitetsforlaget, Oslo.

Spencer, M. P. and Denison, A. B. (1959). The square wave electromagnetic flowmeter for surgical and experimental application. *In* "Methods in Medical Research" (G. D. Bruner, ed.), Vol. II, Year Book Medical Publishers, Chicago.

Stegall, H. F., Rushmer, R. F. and Baker, D. W. (1966). A transcutaneous ultrasonic blood velocity meter. *J. Appl. Physiol.* **21**, 707–711.

Stein, P. D. and Schuette, H. (1969). New Catheter tip flowmeter with velocity flow and volume flow capabilities. *J. Appl. Physiol.* **26**, 851–856.

Stone, H. L., Stegall, H. F., Bishop, V. S. and Laenger, C. (1967). Continuous measurement of blood flow velocity with an intravascular Doppler flowmeter. Digest 7th Int. Conf. Med. Biol. Eng., p. 215. The Organizing Committee for the 7th International Conference on Medical and Biological Engineering, Stockholm.

Studer, U., Fricke, G. and Scheu, H. (1970). Testing of an improved ultrasound flowmeter technical description and results of testing *in vitro*. *Cardiovasc. Res.* **4**, 380–387.

Warbasse, J. R., Hellman, B. H., Gillilon, R. E., Hawley, R. R. and Babitt, H. I. (1969). Physiologic evaluation of a catheter tip electromagnetic velocity probe. *Amer. J. Cardiol.* **23**, 424–433.

Weber, K. C., Engle, J. C., Lyons, G. W., Madsen, A. J. and Fox, I. J. (1968). *In vivo* calibration of electromagnetic flowmeter probes on pulmonary artery and aorta. *J. Appl. Physiol.* **25**, 455–460.

Wells, P. N. T. (1969). "Physical Principles of Ultrasonic Diagnosis". Academic Press, London and New York.

Wetterer, E. (1937). Eine neue methode zur Registrierung der Blutströmungs-geschwindigkeit am uneröffneten Gefass. *Z. Biol.* **98**, 26–36.

Wetterer, E. (1963). Flowmeters: their theory, construction and operation. *In* "Handbook of Physiology" (W. F. Hamilton and P. Dow, eds), Section II, Vol. 2, American Physiological Society, Washington, D.C.

Wyatt, D. G. (1960). A simple wave filter. *Electron. Eng.* **32**, 155–157.

Wyatt, D. G. (1961a). A 50 c/s cannulated electromagnetic flowmeter. *Electron. Eng.* **33**, 650–655.

Wyatt, D. G. (1961b). Problems in the measurement of blood flow by magnetic induction. *Phys. Med. Biol.* **5**, 289–352.

Wyatt, D. G. (1964). Electromagnetic flowmeter for use with intact vessels. *J. Physiol.* **173**, 8P.

Wyatt, D. G. (1965). An input transformer with low earth leakage currents. *Electron. Eng.* **37**, 16–19.

Wyatt, D. G. (1966a). Base line errors in cuff electromagnetic flowmeters. *Med. Biol. Eng.* **4**, 17–45.

Wyatt, D. G. (1966b). Noise in electromagnetic flowmeters. *Med. Biol. Eng.* **4**, 333–347.

Wyatt, D. G. (1968a). Dependence of electromagnetic flowmeter sensitivity upon encircled media. *Phys. Med. Biol.* **13**, 529–534.

Wyatt, D. G. (1968b). The electromagnetic blood flowmeter. *J. Sci. Inst.* 2, **7**, 1146–1152.

Yanof, H. M. (1961). A trapezoidal wave electromagnetic blood flowmeter. *J. Appl. Physiol.* **16**, 566–570.

Yanof, H. M., Rosen, A. L. and Shoemaker, W. C. (1963). Design of an implantable flowmeter transducer based on the Helmholtz coil. *J. Appl. Physiol.* **18**, 227–230.

Chapter 4

The Measurement of Lengths and Dimensions

D. H. BERGEL

Fellow of St. Catherine's College, Oxford:
University Laboratory of Physiology, Oxford, England

1. INTRODUCTION

Generally speaking, in studying the circulation one needs to measure pressures, flows and dimensions. The first two of these are discussed elsewhere in this volume, the third type of measurement merits brief discussion. The dimensions are such measurements as the diameters of a blood vessel, the volume and shape of a cardiac chamber or the wall thickness of the left ventricle. At first sight it might be thought that these are rather trivial compared with the measurement of phasic blood flow through an unopened artery but in fact the methods available are generally rather clumsy, inaccurate and not readily applicable to the human subject. It is not uncommon to find that the velocity of blood flow may be measured rather accurately, and that to estimate volume flow use is made of a very crude estimate of luminal cross-sectional area based on external diameter measurements.

It is not intended to mention here all the methods that have been employed at one time or another to measure dimensions of some sort. Attention will be given to those techniques which seem to hold the greatest promise, and especially those which have a frequency response which allows measurement of changes occurring in the time of a heart beat. Good general discussions of transducer design principles may be found in Lion (1959) and Neubert (1963).

2. General Principles

A. linearity

It is preferable that the output of any measuring device, whatever its form, be linearly related to its input, the variable to be detected. This means that proportional changes in the one must produce proportional changes in the other, though it will nearly always be the case that linearity applies only over some limited range. Thus before choosing any technique one needs some idea of the likely range in which one is to work. This can generally be known from the literature but sometimes a pilot study will be necessary.

Strictly speaking, true linearity applies when the input/output relationships of the system plot as a straight line through the origin, e.g. measurement of length from a photograph of known magnification. Where some form of transducer is used there is generally no unique significance attached to zero output and a working definition of linearity would be one in which the relationship plots as a straight line in the region of interest. Once linearity has been verified within a known error subsequent two-point calibrations will be sufficient, but in order to reduce the effects of random errors more points will generally be needed. From this one can define both the sensitivity of the device and the baseline (output for zero input, or conversely). It is perfectly possible to make measurements with a non-linear device provided the form of the non-linearity is known (the cross-sectional area of a regular cylinder can be "measured" with a ruler), if the device is sufficiently stable and the form of the input–output function known either from first principles or empirically. Generally the practical difficulties with a non-linear system are great. Calibration may be very tedious, small changes in baseline may produce large errors and visual monitoring of the output for general quality may be misleading. Nevertheless, non-linearity of a system is not of itself an absolute bar to its use which may be greatly simplified by the increasing availability of analogue or digital computing devices.

B. UNIQUENESS OF THE RESPONSE

Ideally a system should respond to changes in the measured variable and to none other. If we include time as a variable then this includes stability as it is generally understood. In practice the requirement for a unique response means that the effects of alterations of irrelevant variables should be either negligible or known. It is necessary to know in advance the differences of environment and delays in time to be expected between the calibration procedure and the actual measurement. Only very rarely can one forecast these with accuracy. Those most likely to cause trouble are time and temperature, but it should never be assumed that the performance of any system will not be affected by such diverse influences as acidity, gravity, mains voltage fluctuations, radiation or whatever. The cardinal principle is to attempt to calibrate against some reference standard during the experiment, and if this is impossible, to match the calibration conditions as closely as possible to the experimental conditions with the minimum delay possible.

C. ACCURACY

This is a much abused word. To specify the accuracy of an instrument is to make a statistical statement about the likely value of the measured variable which corresponds to a certain output measurement. Often a partly subjective judgment must be made as to an acceptable degree of accuracy in a given situation. One will need to know the amount of "noise" present at the input (this word is used to mean a purely random variation, but in biological work at least it often means unaccountable variation). The input noise may be considered to be partly due to biological variation; there is no point at present in measuring cardiac output to the last cubic millimetre nor in measuring the weight of an animal to the last milligram. To the input noise is added noise generated in the whole system; this can be estimated and need not be much smaller than the unaccountable biological variation.

Thus the requirements for accuracy stem partly from the degree of accountability present in the system and they thus increase as understanding increases. It is very tempting to pursue accuracy for its own sake, but more often realistic to trade this against the cost and complexity of the system and choose an instrument suited to the present problem. The accuracy of a system can only be stated within the range covered by the calibration procedure.

D. CALIBRATION

Calibration must be carried out over the range of input amplitudes and frequencies to be expected in use. Calibration involves determination of the response of the entire system including the recording apparatus and any devices that may be introduced when the instrument is applied to the tissue.

The conditions must be as similar as possible to the experimental situation. Thus it has recently been shown (Patel *et al.*, 1969) that the output of a transducer for measuring arterial diameter was detectably different when attached to a vessel than when tested with a micrometer *in vitro*.

Before determining the frequency response some knowledge is required of the frequency content of the input and the range in which one is interested. Again it is essential to test the entire system. For devices designed to follow changes with each cardiac cycle it is considered desirable (McDonald, 1960) to determine the frequency response to the tenth harmonic. This can be done either by subjecting the system to sinusoidal input variations over this frequency range or by applying a step function. In the latter case one may merely verify that the response time is at least an order of magnitude smaller than the time of any changes to be detected, or one may, if the system is adequately known, compute the response for the frequencies of interest (see Chapter 2).

It must be remembered that the method of calibration should be suitable for the experiment planned. To illustrate the point consider a report (Parrish *et al.*, 1964) on the frequency response of a mercury-in-rubber strain-gauge used to measure pulsatile arterial expansion. The device is used when tied around the vessel and was tested by attaching it to an instrument which stretched it at various frequencies. While this would test part of the response characteristics it would be equally important to know how the mechanical impedance of the gauge altered with frequency. This would not be measured unless the source impedance of the stretcher was comparable to that of the pulsating artery.

E. LONG-TERM IMPLANTATION OF DEVICES

It is becoming increasingly clear that the acute effects of surgery and anaesthesia on the cardiovascular system can be very great. While a great deal of fundamental information has been gained in these studies, knowledge of performance of the whole system in the healthy unanaesthetized animal is the ultimate goal. This can be achieved by preparing the animal for measuring at a preliminary operation. At a later date the attached wires, cannulae, etc., can be reached with little further disturbance. This technique introduces serious restrictions on the materials suitable for transducers which must have no biological effect and be unaffected by prolonged immersion in physiological fluids with continual mechanical disturbance. Generally speaking the solution has been to encase the transducer and associated equipment in epoxy resins and/or silicone rubbers, but meticulous attention to the details of the embedding process is essential if the device is to have a reasonably long useful life. Wire connections are subject to repeated flexural strain and are often the first part to fail. Unless the output can be telemetered from within the animal, which will generally exclude all systems with an appreciable (i.e. more than a few mW) power consumption, considerable difficulties will arise at the point where the leads penetrate the skin. The site is very liable to become infected and the cables will be chewed through unless placed in a very inaccessible area, e.g. between the shoulder blades.

F. PHYSICAL EFFECTS

Most biological materials are highly extensible and compliant when compared to metals. In order to determine, say, some length and to follow its alterations accurately it is essential that the device does not restrict the movement or otherwise distort the specimen. Instruments used for measuring displacements of stiff structures, e.g. resistance strain gauges, will follow infinitesimal strains without impeding them noticeably, but in biology these strain gauges are most commonly used as stress gauges in manometers and force transducers. The mechanical compliance of the system used must be matched to that of the materials under study, and this necessity is one of the major difficulties in this field.

The Young's modulus of soft body tissues such as the arterial wall is of order 10^6 dynes cm^{-2} and strains of 1 or more may occur. This is also true for unvulcanized rubber. If one desires to measure arterial circumference and its changes with a rubber strain gauge the only satisfactory solution will be to choose the most compliant material possible and to reduce its cross-sectional area to the minimum. Reduction in size will be effective, since the longitudinal coupling in the arterial wall itself will spread the load due to the transducer across an (unknown) length of vessel. Since the effectiveness of this load-spreading cannot be easily determined it is wise to use a material whose elasticity is as low as possible and to use as small a tube as is practicable. The Silastic tubes used by Parrish et al. (1964) had an outer diameter of 0·38 mm and bore of 0·17 mm. Assuming a Young's modulus of 10^7 dynes cm^2 and that the gauge would be stretched by 10 per cent in application, the force produced would be about 3×10^2 dynes, whereas the hydrostatic force acting on an arterial wall segment 1 mm long is normally about 10^5 dynes. It would seem that these very thin gauges would not produce significant distortion of an artery, but in the case of a vein which is thinner and generally more distensible its suitability would need to be directly verified. The problem of measuring ventricular dimensions is rather different, the myocardium may be considered stiff during systole when it is also shortening, but it is very compliant in diastole when a very small pressure head suffices to refill it. In addition a device attached to the surface of the ventricle will, unless care is taken to couple it to deep muscle, only load the superficial fibres. Thus the movement of the myocardium under the gauge may be considerably impeded and it is by no means certain that measurements with rubber gauges are satisfactory here. Recent work by Wilson (unpublished) shows considerable variation in the measured changes of diastolic ventricular dimensions, when using mercury-in-rubber transducers. A source of some of this variation is almost certainly the loading produced by the device.

Other devices which develop no restoring forces have been used to follow ventricular dimensions. In this case the inertial and viscous loading must be determined and shown to be low. The exact nature of the load imposed and the amount of muscle so loaded are very difficult to measure and the only truly satisfactory answer, often very hard in practice, is to measure directly the effect of the device on the tissue studied.

G. BIOLOGICAL EFFECTS

Any dissection necessary to prepare the site of measurement may alter the behaviour of the tissue. It has been suggested (Arndt et al., 1968) that the clearing of an arterial segment may increase the elasticity of an artery, but this has not been directly demonstrated. There will inevitably be some local damage if the device must be sutured in place; this will both alter the properties of the specimen and introduce additional uncertainty into the coupling between tissue and device. It has even been shown (Furchgott, 1955) that smooth muscle reacts to light.

Where a device is to be implanted the effects of dissection and attachment will be very noticeable if fibrosis occurs. The use of tissue adhesives (e.g. Eastman 410) has been recommended but in at least one such study (Aars, 1969) it appears that the tissue reaction to the glue may greatly increase the stiffness of the tissue (Aars, 1971). Although many commercial plastics and polymers appear to be biologically inert in themselves, they frequently contain residual amounts of catalysts, curing agents, mould release agents, etc., and these are often very reactive.

H. TYPES OF SYSTEMS

The systems to be described will be classified as continuous, semi-continuous and discontinuous. Continuous methods are those in which the output at all times represents the instantaneous value of the measure; this definition neglects the necessarily finite frequency response of the system. Semi-continuous methods include those in which repeated measurements are made automatically at some rate which is reasonably fast compared to the heart rate. The output has the form of a series of plateaux (generally of voltage) each of which represents the value of the measure at some earlier time. Nevertheless the output is a recordable analogue representation of the biological event. In discontinuous methods the data are recorded once or at intervals for later analysis. Such methods include all photographic and radiographic techniques; although exposures can readily be made quite rapidly subsequent analysis may be extremely time-consuming. Another method involves measurements made on fixed tissues post mortem. A very great deal of information can be obtained by such methods such as the careful measurement of fixed and sectioned tissues (Curtis, 1960; Weibel, 1963; Glazier *et al.*, 1967) though such studies have to date been almost entirely confined to the lung. A further application is the measurement of casts and contrast angiograms of vascular systems (e.g. Reid, 1968). There is still very great need for representative values for such relatively mundane measurements as area ratios at vascular branches, lengths of vascular segments, capillary network morphology, etc., and their lack is a real impediment to progress in many areas (see, for example, Chapter 19). It is not proposed to deal further with these post-mortem measurements here for the principles of the techniques are relatively straightforward.

3. CONTINUOUS METHODS

A. VARIABLE RESISTANCE TRANSDUCERS

(1) *Low compliance strain gauges*

When a metal is stretched its electrical resistance (R) changes because of the length change, the change in cross-sectional area and a change in the resistivity of the material. These three effects are seen in the three terms of the expression

$$\frac{\Delta R}{R} = \frac{\Delta L}{L} + 2\sigma \frac{\Delta L}{L} + \frac{\Delta \rho}{\rho} \tag{3.1}$$

where L is length, σ is Poisson's ratio and ρ is resistivity. The strain sensitivity S of the material can then be expressed as

$$S = \frac{\Delta R/R}{\Delta L/L} = 1 + 2\sigma + \frac{\Delta \rho/\rho}{\Delta L/L} \tag{3.2}$$

Most metals have $\sigma = 0\cdot3$ and thus the sensitivity or gauge factor will be at least $1\cdot6$. In fact, for the materials in common use, $S = 2$–5. It should be remembered that if a metal is overstrained it will undergo a plastic deformation; in this event, which generally occurs with strains $> 0\cdot2$–$0\cdot6$ per cent, the gauge factor falls and some degree of irreversible change will have occurred. More recently semi-conductor materials have been used as strain sensitive elements. For these materials the resistivity change is very much greater than for metals and strain sensitivity may be an order of magnitude higher.

The chief disadvantages of stiff strain gauges in the measurement of physiological strains are that the gauge is many times stiffer than the tissue.

Thus complex and bulky impedance matching devices have to be employed. Two versions are discussed below. In addition all strain gauges show temperature sensitivity which will produce zero drift and also sensitivity changes. This effect is generally reduced by the use of a two or four active-arm bridge circuit in which all elements are exposed to the same thermal environment. If this is impracticable compensating resistors can be used.

(2) *Metallic foil transducers*

Printed foil units (Mallos, 1962), which are relatively cheap and small, and can be readily attached to any surface, are used. In Mallos' design the gauges are attached to a piece of shimstock which is arched between the two arms of a calliper. The output is nearly linear, though detailed calibration reveals the necessity for non-linear corrections (Patel *et al.*, 1969), and it is simple to manufacture units suitable for application to a variety of vessels down to the 3–4 mm diameter range. The manner of attachment to the vessel is critical, and ideally, calibration should be performed *in situ*. The frequency response is inherently good. Great care must be taken in designing for a suitable mechanical impedance. In Mallos' original device an elastic load of about 0·7 g was present and an additional inertial loading of 0·3 g was estimated (inertial effects might be relatively greater for small callipers). The effect of this loading on an aortic specimen was estimated to be a reduction in diameter of about 0·5 per cent (the restriction of pulsatile changes due to inertial effects might be 3 4 times as great, still acceptably low). This instrument has been extensively used by the Bethesda group (see Chapter 11) and has proved reliable, provided extremely careful *in situ* calibration is undertaken. Bonded foil strain gauges have also been used to measure the thickness of the ventricular wall (Feigl, 1966). In principle these devices could be adapted for use in almost any circumstance, but the mechanism used to match the impedances of tissue and gauge are generally bulky which severely limits their applicability.

(3) *Semi-conductor strain gauges*

Although these devices, which are more expensive than foil gauges, could well be attached to the Mallos calliper, they have so far been used on strained beams. The deflection (x) of a cantilever beam (length, L, width, w, thickness, h, and elasticity, E) is given by

$$x = \frac{FL^3}{3EI} \tag{3.3}$$

where F is the normal force applied to the free end of the cantilever. I is the moment of inertia of the beam, for a rectangular cross-section $I = wh^3/12$.

The material on the surfaces of the beam will be either compressed or expanded and two strain gauges applied here and connected as a bridge will give increased sensitivity and temperature compensation. If the sensing element is placed at a distance x from the free end the longitudinal strains (ε) at that point will be

$$\varepsilon = \pm Fxh/2IE. \tag{3.4}$$

A device of this sort using two calliper arms of spring steel has been described by Peterson (1966). Peterson has also described a modification for intravascular use in which the two beams may be protruded from the end of a catheter to make contact with the internal wall of the vessel. The frequency response is good, and the impedance of the device has been calculated to produce less than 1 per cent change in arterial radius. It would, however, be desirable to have more details of their actual behaviour before concluding that all technical problems have been solved.†

(4) Highly compliant strain gauges

The first instrument of this sort was designed by Whitney (1953) for measuring the circumference of the human forearm as an alternative to volume plethysmography. It consists of a fine tube of rubber containing mercury. Connections are made at either end by means of metal plugs. The change in resistance is due to the elongation and narrowing of the mercury column ($\sigma = 0.5$) and thus the gauge factor is 2. The instrument has been used to measure aortic and ventricular circumferences and its development for these purposes is described by Baker et al. (1960). These devices are relatively simple to make, can be attached with relatively little interference and are suitable for long-term implantation. One major defect is that the resistance of the mercury column is very low ($< 10 \, \Omega$) which makes accurate measurements difficult. Attempts to overcome this by the use of other fluids have not been very successful. Rubber can be made conductive when heavily loaded with graphite but this material is electrically noisy and relatively stiff. The thermal coefficient of resistivity of mercury is $0.0009/°C$ and Whitney's original design incorporated a compensating element of copper; most later workers have dispensed with this. When used internally the temperature should be constant enough to allow use provided calibration is carried out at the same temperature. The mechanical effect of a rubber tube tied to an organ is hard to access because of difficulties in determining the exact conditions of contact and uncertainties as to the dynamic impedance of the gauge. The rough calculations shown earlier suggest that little interference would be produced with the motion of an artery. Unless extremely fine gauges can be produced, which would be possible, their use on veins

† Such a device has been shown to have good characteristics by Murgo et al. (1971).

would not be satisfactory. Several reports exist on their use for measuring cardiac dimensions (see Peterson, 1966) but it is not clear that relaxation in diastole would not be significantly impeded.

The use of mercury in rubber strain gauges in limb plethysmography has been generally accepted and shown to compare well with direct measurements of volume (Burger et al., 1959).

(5) Potentiometers

Where relatively forceful movements are to be measured a sliding or rotating potentiometer can be used. In this case sensitivity and stability can be very great but resolution may be limited if wound-wire potentiometers are used. A rotating potentiometer specially selected for its low impedance has been used in acute measurements of left-ventricular segment length (Mitchell et al., 1960). Clearly these instruments are bulky and not suitable for implantation. They do not appear to have found other applications, chiefly on account of high mechanical impedance.

(6) Tissue impedance

The resistance between two electrodes placed on some tissue will clearly vary with their separation. This principle has been used but there are many difficulties due to electrode polarization, resistivity changes of the tissue, and non-uniform electric fields between electrodes. Such effects can be overcome to some extent (Geddes and Hoff, 1964) but the principle can at present only be considered semi-quantitative.

B. INDUCTIVE TRANSDUCERS

The inductance of a coil is

$$L = n^2 G \mu \mu_0 \tag{3.5}$$

where n is the number of turns, G is a geometric form factor and $\mu\mu_0$ the effective permeability of the medium. All these can be altered mechanically. A transducer can employ a single coil (self-induction) or can use two coils and vary the magnetic coupling between them (mutual inductance); see Fig. 1. Changes of inductance can be measured relatively easily and with high accuracy, generally employing a bridge circuit. These devices have been used in many situations and the most useful will be mentioned. Measurement involves the use of a.c. circuits which will generally make it necessary to compensate for capacitative and resistive changes. All such devices will be affected by external magnetic fields due to the proximity of any magnetic material. This will generally be less severe with iron cored devices ($\mu = $ ca. 200). In general these devices will be non-linear. The use of two inductances back to back (differential transformer) improves the situation.

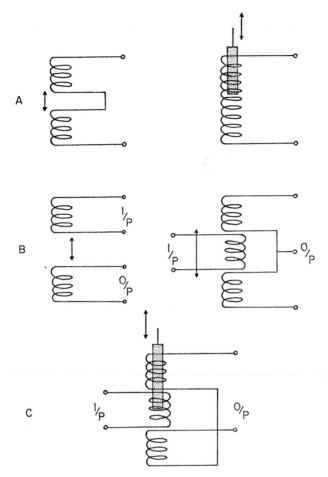

FIG. 1. Inductive transducers: A. Self-inductance; B. Mutual inductance C. Differential transformer.

It is usually necessary to limit the measurement range to some quasi-linear portion.

(1) *The differential transformer*

This is possibly the most successfully used variable inductance device. The coupling between two coils is altered by the motion of a high permeability slug between them. Two or three coils may be used, the principle is the same for both but the more complex device (Fig. 1c) uses two secondary coils connected in opposite sense to permit a greater region of linearity. Some non-linearity has to be tolerated but Neubert (1963) discusses the construction of optimal devices.

These devices can be made extremely small thus achieving low inertia (Gerova and Gero, 1969; Dobrin and Rovick, 1969). Sensitivity is high and can be adjusted to some extent by choice of operating frequency. It is necessary to ensure that the slug moves freely along the coil axis and the construction of small differential transformers calls for a high degree of skill. There appears to be only one application (Rushmer, 1954) where they have been implanted but the device can be used intravascularly and is not affected by immersion in electrolyte solutions.

In Rushmer's application the transducer was in the form of a piston in a cylinder and the two halves were attached to opposite walls of the left ventricular cavity. This device functioned well after implantation, but it is difficult to achieve smooth and frictionless travel and its performance was occasionally affected by blood clotting. A good description of the construction and calibration of a differential transformer calliper for measuring vessel diameter has been given by Gow (1966); see also Chapter 12. Gow's device uses a tiny differential transformer mounted on one calliper arm, the other carries a ferrite slug ($\mu = $ ca. 1000) which is moved within the secondary coils. Good performance will only be attained when the slug is moving across the boundary of the two secondary coils, consequently a range of transducers must be employed to suit different vessels. In addition Gow incorporated an adjustable knee joint on one calliper arm allowing for final adjustment in situ. The device was shown to have a flat frequency response to 20 Hz and, to impose no detectable mechanical load on a model arterial segment.

Differential transformers are robust and can be made small enough to be mounted on the tip of a catheter for intravascular use where they have been used to measure pressure and flow velocity. Pieper and Paul (1968) have described a development in which two transducers are mounted on a catheter of about 3 mm diameter. One system is used to measure vessel diameter by means of three jointed arms which contact the internal surface. The motion of the arms is sensed by the displacement of a ferromagnetic sleeve acting as the core of a differential transformer. These instruments can only be used in large (> 10 mm diameter) vessels and it is doubtful if they are intrinsically safe enough to use in humans. The force exerted by each arm is given as 9000 dynes and it was stated that no distortion of the vessel was observed. Nevertheless, the force exerted by the three arms, $2 \cdot 7 \times 10^4$ dynes, is only one-fifth of the hydrostatic force per mm length of vessel (ca. $1 \cdot 5 \times 10^5$ dynes) which suggests the need for caution. A modified device with greater compliance has been used in large veins (Yates, 1969) but its use in this situation needs more evaluation.

(2) Mutual inductance transducers

A good description of mutual inductance transducers is given by Van Citters (1966). The great advantage is that measurement is made with simple hand wound coils which are attached to either side of a blood vessel or other organ. Alternating current is passed through one and the magnitude of the current induced in the other is measured with conventional demodulator and amplifier circuits. The best frequency to use is that at which the secondary circuit is in resonance; this is generally determined empirically. The great simplicity of this device has led to its widespread use in a number of applications, especially those involving implantation. The assumption is made that the variations in induced current are due to changes in separation of the coils. The relation between separation and induced current is non-linear, for two plane coaxial coils with radii R_1, R_2 and number of turns n_1, n_2 at a separation x, the mutual induction (M) is

$$M = \frac{\mu\mu_0 R_1^2 R_2^2 n_1 n_2}{2x^3} \qquad (3.6)$$

where the term $\mu\mu_0$ is the magnetic permeability of the medium. Unless the working range can be kept small the non-linearity of the relationship must be taken into account.

Equation (3.6) is true where $x \gg R$ which is not generally the case in practice. However, the inverse cube relationship has been verified empirically for the coils used in measuring vessel diameter (Van Citters, 1966). A potentially serious error will result if the relative movement of the coils is not limited to displacement along the mutual axis. If one coil is allowed to rotate through an angle θ, the current induced in the other will be reduced in proportion to $\sin \theta$, but when the coils are very close together (and even bent into a saddle shape), the errors may be much greater. No systematic study of these effects has been reported and the performance of these devices in situ has not been compared with any acceptable standard. It is possible that the measurement of vessel diameter could be adequate if the coils were placed with great care and the vessel was truly cylindrical and elastically symmetrical. It is uncertain that satisfactory performance would result with other organs such as the application described by Hinds et al. (1969).

(3) Self-inductive transducers

The self-induction principle has not been greatly used for the measurement of lengths and displacements. The alternations in self-inductance of a coil produced by movement of a magnetic body in the vicinity will not be linearly related to displacement; the differential transformer is a better device. The one advantage of the self-induction transducer is its low power requirement, a variable inductance incorporated in a resonant circuit will produce large signal variations in a form suitable for radiotelemetry.

C. CAPACITANCE TRANSDUCERS

The capacity (C, farads) between two conducting plates each of area A and separation t (metres) is given by

$$C = \varepsilon\varepsilon_0 A/t \tag{3.7}$$

where ε_0 is the dielectric constant of free space, $(36\pi.10^9)^{-1}$, and ε is the relative dielectric constant of the medium ($= 1$ for vacuum and air). It will be noted that the capacitance of a simple air dielectric system will generally be extremely low. A simple formula gives C in $\mu\mu$F where A and t are measured in centimetres.

$$C = 0.0885A(N-1)/t \tag{3.8}$$

where N is the number of plates.

The most successful use of the capacitance transducer has been in pressure measurement where one plate of the capacitor is moved by the applied pressure and it is possible to make t very small. The advantages of capacitance transducers are that they are relatively simple to construct and can have an excellent frequency response. There are, however, formidable difficulties, the circuitry is relatively complex, the cables to the transducer are prone to introduce errors and temperature stability is generally poor. Capacitance displacement transducers for use *in vivo* will be very adversely affected by the conducting fluids generally present. Attempts to measure capacitance changes between a fixed electrode and a piece of tissue have not been successful, but the principle has been employed with good results in volume plethysmography (Fewings and Whelan, 1966).

D. PHOTO-ELECTRIC DEVICES

The effects of light on matter are many. In this context the effects of greatest potential usefulness are the photo-conductive effect (the change, generally an increase, in conductivity of certain crystals exposed to light), the photo-emissive effect (the emission of electrons from a surface when light falls on it) and the photo-voltaic effect (the generation of an e.m.f. when radiant energy falls on a junction of two dissimilar materials). By a suitable choice of materials the spectral sensitivity can be chosen to cover almost any application. The photo-conductive and photo-emissive effects have found the widest application.

In one common type of application the amount of light falling on a device is altered by the movement of the material under study. This may be accomplished by the motion of an opaque vane interposed between the light source and photo cell, but unless the vane is carefully shaped and the response of the cell uniform over its whole surface, linearity will be hard to obtain. A better principle is to use a moving wedge or other device with variable optical density, or to make arrangements to destroy the image of the vane with a diffuser. Commercial devices of this sort are readily available.

Thus there is little difficulty in simple photo-electric transducers provided the tissue can be coupled satisfactorily to the moving part of the instrument. An ingenious refinement of the photo-conductor device is the "photo-pot", (Ross and Brust, 1966). Here the photo-conductive material is laid down as a strip between two linear resistive elements. If arrangements are made to allow a light spot to move along the central strip the effect is that of a moving slider connecting the two resistance strips. This device will give large outputs with excellent linearity. In all of these applications the frequency response and mechanical characteristics will be governed by the mechanical components.

In another application the structure being studied is made to vary the amount of light falling on the detector. Such a device, incorporating a photo-multiplier was used (Bergel, 1961) to measure diameter changes of blood vessels *in vitro*. Providing a diffuser was used to integrate the total light passing the specimen, linearity was excellent over a wide range, coupled with great sensitivity. It is necessary to have unobstructed access to the specimen, which is unlikely to be possible *in vivo* and that the tissue be optically opaque (the use of coloured filters may be helpful here).

A very refined use of optical techniques has been described by Gordon *et al.* (1966). The device was used to measure the length changes of the central portion of a single muscle fibre to which were attached two tiny opaque markers. The light from the two spots of a twin-beam cathode ray oscilloscope was made to pass the markers and fall on a pair of photo-transistors. Feedback circuits were used to control the spot positions so that at all times they were semi-occluded by the markers; the deflection voltages generated were proportional to the position of each marker.

Rather similar principles are employed in commercial optical trackers. These are highly sophisticated and expensive devices which allow the automatic tracking of the position of a suitable target in space. In one physiological application (Moritz, 1969) two units were used to follow the motion of the arterial wall. The targets used were small pieces of card displaying a single black–white interface. By these means the torsional, radial and axial motion of an artery were recorded.

The major disadvantage of these optical methods is that they are generally not suitable for use *in vivo*, and where they are to be so used considerable dissection is necessary to ensure a clear view. With this important reservation these methods do have the advantages of great sensitivity, good linearity and there is no mechanical restraint of the specimen. In addition, some such devices may often be constructed in any normal laboratory. The greatest single advantage, however, is that, through the use of conventional optical systems, the methods can be applied to very small structures. It is this fact that has led to the development of the scanning devices to be described in the following section.

4. SEMI-CONTINUOUS METHODS

A. ULTRASONIC TECHNIQUES

In recent years there has been a rapid development in the medical applications of ultrasonics. This stemmed largely from the need to devise alternative techniques for radiography in situations where the possibility of radiation damage existed. It is now clear that ultrasonic techniques possess other advantages and many new applications have been found. Of particular relevance here is the use of the Doppler principle in blood flow studies (see Chapter 3). It will not be possible to cover all applications but those in search of further details are referred to the monograph by Wells (1969).

In the applications to be discussed here use is made of the fact that sound waves propogate through materials at a determinable velocity and distance measurements become time measurements. When the wavelength of the sound waves is very small compared to the diameter of the source a well-defined sound beam can be generated. Sound waves will be reflected at tissue discontinuities and objects whose size is of the same order as the wavelength can be "seen". Although the term ultrasound generally refers to waves whose frequency is above 20 kHz the above facts mean that practical systems involve much higher frequencies in the range 1–10 MHz.

The velocity of sound waves (c) in a fluid is given by $c^2 = K_a/\rho$, where K_a is the adiabatic bulk (compressional) modulus of elasticity and ρ is fluid density. In a fluid the only waves propagated are pressure waves and the particle displacement is along the axis of wave propagation. The adiabatic bulk modulus is not very frequency dependent for high frequencies and thus ultrasonic waves in water are only mildly dispersive with a velocity of 1525 m s^{-1}. The temperature coefficient of the velocity is about 0·03%/°C. At 1 MHz the wavelength (λ) is about 1·5 mm and thus such waves travelling in blood within a large artery will behave as though they were in an infinite medium with a velocity of about 1570 m s^{-1} rather than at the Moens–Korteweg velocity at which the long wavelength disturbances of the arterial pulse wave travel.

Wave propagation in solids is more complex because of the existence of shear waves but the velocity of high frequency sound in soft tissues is about the same as in water (Wells, 1969). At any junction where the wave velocity changes a proportion of the energy will be reflected according to the relation where the reflection coefficient (R) is $(Za-Zb)/(Za+Zb)$, where Za and Zb are the acoustic impedances of the two media. Now the acoustic impedance is proportional to the characteristic wave velocity and the differences between the velocity in most soft tissues is only about 2·5 per cent. Thus the proportion of ultrasound reflected at most tissue interfaces (excluding bone surfaces) will be of the order of 1 per cent.

Ultrasonic waves are also attenuated as they travel and in most tissues the attenuation per wavelength is not greatly altered by frequency, thus attenuation is roughly proportional to frequency. Typical attenuation values show that 5 MHz $(\lambda = 0\cdot3$ mm) waves will travel about 1 cm in muscle before being attenuated to 10 per cent (for blood the distance is ten times greater). The use of echolocation techniques to detect tissue interfaces within the body is relatively new and has much to offer but it is as well to remember that small signals are being detected and much attention to details will be required if the results are to be satisfactory. Ultrasonic beams can cause tissue damage, and are used in therapy for this purpose, but the energy used in echolocation and similar techniques is much lower than the damage threshold (a sound intensity of about $0\cdot1$ W cm^{-2}).

For echolocation purposes one requires an ultrasonic generator which can be coupled to the body, and a detector, generally but not necessarily the same unit as the generator. The elapsed time between the impulse and its echo yields the distance to the reflector if the velocity is known. Ultrasound is generated by the excitation of piezo-electric materials, the most commonly used materials are quartz, which has to be accurately cut along the appropriate crystal axis, and the polarized polycrystalline ferro-electric materials such as barium titanate and its derivatives. These materials can be formed in a suitable shape and subsequently polarized by the application of a strong electric field while cooling from above the Curie temperature, around 350 °C. They are excited by applying an electric field across two electrodes which are generally electroplated on to the transducer. If the material is in the form of a disc (thickness ≪ diameter) it will be found to resonate when excited at a frequency such that the thickness is an odd integral number of half wavelengths. The wave velocity in these materials is of order 4×10^3 m s^{-1} and thus a disc 2 mm thick will resonate at about 1 MHz. To generate a single short pulse a single high voltage impulse is used and the material will produce a damped train of waves at resonant frequency. It is very important in echolocation techniques to produce a short clean pulse to achieve this; meticulous attention to the mechanical arrangement of the transducer is called for (Wells, 1969). If a narrow beam is not required the diameter of the crystal may be reduced or curved lenses may be employed.

These details are mentioned to illustrate the fact that it is very hard to produce a single pulse of ultrasound so that there is inevitably some uncertainty as to when the pulse actually occurred. A similar difficulty arises in the accurate detection of the time of arrival of a pulse. The waveform will have altered spread while travelling because the high frequency components are more strongly attenuated. If an echo is being detected the amplitude will have been further reduced by incomplete reflection. The attenuation is so great that most systems used employ "swept gain" techniques whereby the gain of the receiver is continually increased (by up to 50 dB) following the generation of each spike. The echo will be detected when the sound pressure amplitude has risen to some value. The range resolution will thus be determined by many factors. These are discussed in detail by Wells (1969, Section 4.1b) but it is roughly the case that resolution is limited to at least one wavelength under the most favourable conditions; this is 0·3 mm at 5 MHz, a significant distance when, for example, measuring blood vessel dimensions. It is not possible to increase the frequency without limit on account of the direct relationship between attenuation and frequency. If two crystals are employed on either side of the object being measured the difficulties due to attenuation are somewhat reduced.

There are thus considerable technical problems to be overcome before using ultrasound for distance measurements either by echolocation or with transmitter–receiver pairs. Meticulous attention to engineering details will be required. The advantages of these methods make them well worth the trouble; the systems are inherently linear and performance is rather stable. The transducers can be made quite small and are eminently suitable for implantation. The cardinal advantage, however, is that ultrasound can be used transcutaneously in many applications. The output is semi-continuous but since pulse trains may be repeated at very high rates the system can be regarded as one with continuous output. Ultrasonic methods have been used in the measurement of cardiac dimensions (Baker, 1966) and for the measurement of vessel diameter in the experimental animal (Aars, 1969; Lie et al., 1970) and in man (Arndt et al., 1968). In clinical medicine ultrasonics have chiefly been used in neurosurgery for the detection of cerebral shifts (White, 1967) and in obstetrics (Donald, 1968), but there are numerous other applications which are discussed by Wells (1969). Other applications of interest here are the measurement of the velocity of the anterior cusp of the mitral valve (Joyner et al., 1963) and the measurement of aortic diameter (Evans et al., 1967).

It is noticeable, however, that there is little direct evidence that could indicate the accuracy of ultrasonic measurements in vivo. Although it appears that the estimation of gross vascular dimensions (Evans et al., 1967) is at least as good as that given by other techniques, the accuracy with which pulsatile changes can be measured is not established. Pulsations at the heart rate can readily be seen in ultrasonic scan displays of vascular tissues but the changes are predominantly in the amplitude of the echoes, presumably due to small changes in the orientation of reflecting surfaces. It is important that amplitude changes should not produce output signals representing range shifts. The best data on pulsatile arterial changes are found in Arndt *et al.* (1968) but the pulsations measured are greater than those expected on the grounds of earlier estimations of pulse-wave velocity. There is a great need for a careful study of these techniques by means of simultaneous wave velocity and pulsatile expansion measurements.

B. SCANNING PHOTOELECTRIC METHODS

These methods depend on the detection of optical density or reflectance changes at some interface; this is generally the margin of the specimen studied but may be a specially placed marker. Frequency response and linearity are inherently good and conventional optical systems allow studies on very small specimens. The main disadvantage is that the apparatus is generally complex and needs to be physically massive to maintain optical alignment and stability. The conventional optical systems have been developed to allow studies *in vivo*, but the situations in which they may be applied are rather limited.

The flying spot angiometer of Johnson and Greatbatch (1966) may be taken as the simplest example. A conventional, but highly accurate, saw-tooth voltage is used to produce a spot on an oscilloscope face moving at constant velocity. The tube faces a microscope eyepiece and a focused and reduced image of the spot (5–10 μm diameter) is projected on the specimen, typically a piece of mesentery, containing a blood vessel, spread across the microscope stage. Below the stage a condenser lens collects the light and focuses it on a detector; because of the small size of the object field a high sensitivity device of the photo-multiplier type must be used. Thus light-transmission is reduced as the spot traverses the vessel.

The resulting output signal ideally has the form of a rectangular dark-pulse repeated at the scan-rate (ca. 30 s^{-1} in this instance). Because of the finite spot-size and variations in density of object and background, together with the finite response-time of the photo-multiplier and its circuits, the rectangular waveform is somewhat degraded, but this is restored by using the signal to trigger a flip/flop circuit at a predetermined light level. The width of the resulting pulses is proportional to the width of the object. A voltage proportional to object size is generated by starting and stopping a ramp-voltage generator and recording the final voltage with a synchronized sample-hold device.

Devices of this sort give a semi-continuous output delayed in time by the interval between scans. If N scans are made every second the highest frequency at which measurements may theoretically be made is $1/(2N-1)$ Hz with a phase lag of order $2\pi/N$ rad/Hz, but it may be necessary to add a low pass output filter with cut-off frequency somewhat below $1/N$ Hz, which will introduce further errors. However, the frequency response will be fixed and determinable so that corrections may be made if required.

The device described by Johnson and Greatbatch gave linear outputs over the range 20–200 μm with errors of order 1–2 per cent.

A similar instrument was devised by Wiederhielm (1963). In this case the scanning is performed by the electron beam of a commercial vidicon television camera tube. The output video output signal is gated so that only a selected portion of a single line scan is used. Thus the exact portion of the simultaneously displayed television image to be observed can be selected and this portion is displayed on the monitor screen by a white marker. The instrument was developed for studies on small vessels and the camera is coupled to a microscope. Calibration of the flying spot angiometer was achieved by focusing on a set of standard wires or engraved lines. In the gated television system a stage micrometer is used, the sampling marker being adjusted to fit this; the resulting calibration was found to be linear within ± 2 per cent over the range 15–150 μm with a standard error of $\pm 3 \cdot 7$ μm.

In the original gated television system the commercial field repetition rate (60 Hz in U.S.A., 50 Hz in U.K.) dictated the measuring frequency. Since the gate opens for less than the time of one line scan the whole measurement was performed within about 5 μs and high frequency techniques were necessary. It is possible to operate a commercial vidicon to be at considerably lower scan rates and thus allow more time for each measurement. One such system is under development in Oxford. In this instrument the normal scan is interrupted when recording; the horizontal deflection system is disconnected and a 100 Hz triangular wave applied to the vertical deflection amplifiers. The amplifiers will function perfectly well at this frequency and thus the scanning spot moves steadily up and down the vidicon face, taking 5 ms for each traverse. Every other sweep is sampled giving a sampling rate of 100 Hz with no requirements for high frequency equipment.

Although scanning devices are expensive and cumbersome they are capable of making measurements on very small vessels.† The range is easily altered by changing the optical system. The object is entirely unloaded, but must be prepared so that a clear view is obtained. Much difficult development work is avoided by making use of readily available and relatively cheap commercial systems.

† The quite different system, using an image splitter (Baez, 1968) should be mentioned in this context.

5. Discontinuous Measurements

Techniques in this category are predominantly those in which the object is photographed, generally by visible light or by X-rays, for subsequent analysis. Other applications include histological preparation and observation, and the preparation of solid casts of hollow organs. The latter will not be mentioned further save to mention that this sort of measurement is frequently invaluable for an *in situ* calibration of some other system (see for example Patel *et al.*, 1969).

Where study of the living tissue is required, photography offers advantages of simplicity. No tissue restraints are involved and a series of photographs before and during the application of some other device will often be the best way of determining its effects on the organ. For most studies X-rays will be required with some technique to improve contrast. Such techniques include radio-opaque material painted on the organ before the study (see Chapter 13), the implantation of two or more metallic markers (Noble *et al.*, 1969), the use of non-implanted intravascular markers (Neufeld *et al.*, 1965) or fluid contrast media (Caro, 1965). All these techniques carry some risk of altering the behaviour of the system; there is no evidence to suggest that the changes are large, but conventional contrast media produce large changes in the peripheral bed. Calibration is simple though often tedious since it involves precise measurement of tube–object and tube–film distances. Resolution is limited to the extent that the object–film distance cannot generally be made very small. It is also governed by the effective diameter of the source; modern fine-focus tubes allow the resolution of distances down to about 150–200 µm.

The most severe practical difficulty arises in studies in which the movement of an object is followed by conventional or high speed cinematography. Such methods are currently often employed in the measurement of ventricular volume (see Hawthorne, 1969). Several hundred frames per second may be necessary, often taken simultaneously in two planes. Very many pictures must be analysed, and even with electronic coordinate reading systems and digital computation, the process is extremely tedious with a rather small output for a great deal of effort. The only reason for using such methods is that there are currently no other entirely acceptable methods for the estimation of ventricular volumes and dimensions. Measurement difficulties are one of the major limitations on progress in this field.

References

Aars, H. (1969). Relationship between blood pressure and diameter of ascending aorta in normal and hypertensive rabbits. *Acta Physiol. Scand.* **75**, 397–405.

Aars, H. (1971). Diameter and elasticity of the ascending aorta during infusion of noradrenaline. *Acta Physiol. Scand.* **83**, 133–138.

Arndt, J. O., Klauske, J. and Mersch, F. (1968). The diameter of the intact carotid artery in man and its change with pulse pressure. *Pflüger's Arch.* **301**, 230–240.

Baez, S. (1968). Vascular smooth muscle: quantification of cell thickness in the wall of arterioles in the living animal *in situ*. *Science, N.Y.* **159**, 536–538.

Baker, D. W. (1966). Sonocardiometer. *In* "Methods in Medical Research" (R. F. Rushmer, ed.), Vol. 11, pp. 31–34, Year Book Medical Publishers Inc., Chicago.

Baker, D. W., Franklin, D. F. and Ellis, R. M. (1960). Miniature electronic instruments for medical research. *Research* **13**, 275–280.

Bergel, D. H. (1961). The static elastic properties of the arterial wall. *J. Physiol.* **156**, 445–457.

Burger, H. C., Horreman, H. W. and Brakkee, A. J. M. (1959). Comparison of some methods for measuring peripheral blood flow. *Phys. Med. Biol.* **4**, 168–175.

Caro, C. G. (1965). Extensibility of blood vessels in isolated rabbit lungs (see appendix by Saffman, P. G.). *J. Physiol.* **178**, 193–210.

Curtis, A. S. G. (1960). Area and volume measurement by random sampling. *Biol. Med. Illustr.* **10**, 261–266.

Dobrin, P. B. and Rovick, A. A. (1969). Influence of vascular smooth muscle on the contractile mechanics and elasticity of arteries. *Am. J. Physiol.* **217**, 1644–1651.

Donald, I. (1968). Ultrasonics in obstetrics. *Brit. Med. Bull.* **24**, 71–75.

Evans, G. C., Lehman, J. S., Segal, B. L., Likoff, W., Ziskin, M. and Kingsley, G. B. (1967). Echoaortography. *Am. J. Cardiol.* **19**, 91–96.

Feigl, E. O. (1966). Transducer for measuring myocardial wall thickness. *In* "Methods in Medical Research" (R. F. Rushmer, ed.), Vol. 11, pp. 24–25, Year Book Medical Publishers Inc., Chicago.

Fewings, J. D. and Whelan, R. F. (1966). Difference in forearm blood flow measured by capacitance and volume plethysmography. *J. Appl. Physiol.* **21**, 334–340.

Furchgott, R. F. (1955). The pharmacology of vascular smooth muscle. *Pharm. Rev.* **7**, 183–265.

Geddes, L. A. and Hoff, H. E. (1964). The measurement of physiological events by electrical impedance. *Am. J. Med. Electronics* **3**, 16–27.

Gerova, M. and Gero, J. (1969). Range of the sympathetic control of the dog's femoral artery. *Circulation Res.* **24**, 349–359.

Glazier, J. B., Hughes, J. M. B., Maloney, J. E. and West, J. B. (1967). Vertical gradient of alveolar size in lungs of dogs frozen intact. *J. Appl. Physiol.* **23**, 694–705.

Gordon, A. M., Huxley, A. F. and Julian, F. J. (1966). Tension development in highly stretched vertebrate muscle fibres. *J. Physiol.* **184**, 143–169.

Gow, B. S. (1966). An electrical caliper for measurement of pulsatile arterial diameter changes *in vivo*. *J. Appl. Physiol.* **21**, 1122–1126.

Hawthorne, E. W. (ed.) (1969). Dynamic geometry of the left ventricle. *Fed. Proc.* **28**, 1323–1367.

Hinds, J. E., Hawthorne, E. W., Mullins, C. B. and Mitchell, J. W. (1969). Instantaneous changes in the left ventricle lengths occurring in dogs during the cardiac cycle. *Fed. Proc.* **28**, 1351–1357.

Johnson, P. C. and Greatbatch, W. H. (1966). The angiometer: a flying spot microscope for measuring blood vessel diameter. *In* "Methods in Medical

Research" (R. F. Rushmer, ed.), Vol. 11, pp. 220–227, Year Book Medical Publishers Inc., Chicago.

Joyner, C. R., Reid, J. M. and Bond, J. P. (1963). Reflected ultrasound in the assessment of mitral disease. *Circulation* **27**, 503–511.

Lie, M., Sejersted, D. M. and Kiil, F. (1970). Local regulation of vascular cross section during changes in femoral arterial blood flow in dogs. *Circulation Res.* **27**, 727–737.

Lion, K. S. (1959). "Instrumentation in Scientific Research", McGraw-Hill, New York.

McDonald, D. A. (1960). "Blood Flow in Arteries", Arnold, London.

Mallos, A. J. (1962). Electrical calliper for continuous measurement of relative displacement. *J. Appl. Physiol.* **17**, 131–134.

Mitchell, J. H., Linden, R. J. and Sarnoff, S. J. (1960). Influence of cardiac sympathetic and vagal nerve stimulation on the relation between left ventricular diastolic pressure and myocardial segment length. *Circulation Res.* **8**, 1100–1107.

Moritz, W. E. (1969). Transmission characteristics of distension, torsion and axial waves in arteries. SUDAAR report 373, Stanford University.

Murgo, J. P., Cox, R. H. and Peterson, L. H. (1971). Cantilever transducer for continuous measurement of arterial diameter *in vivo. J. Appl. Physiol.* **31**, 948–953.

Neubert, H. K. P. (1963). "Instrument Transducers", Clarendon Press, Oxford.

Neufeld, H. H., Leibinsohn, S. H., Goor, D. and Nathan, D. (1965). A new method of measuring the diameter of blood vessels *in situ. Lancet*, 1965 (i), 1002–1003.

Noble, M. I. M., Milne, E. N. C., Goerke, R. J., Carlsson, E., Domenich, R. J., Saunders, K. B. and Hoffman, J. I. E. (1969). Left ventricular filling and diastolic pressure–volume relations in the conscious dog. *Circulation Res.* **24**, 269–284.

Parrish, D., Strandness, D. E. and Bell, J. W. (1964). Dynamic response characteristics of a mercury-in-silastic strain gauge. *J. Appl. Physiol.* **19**, 363–365.

Patel, D. J., Janicki, J. S. and Carew, T. E. (1969). Static anistropic elastic properties of the aorta in living dogs. *Circulation Res.* **25**, 769–779.

Peterson, L. H. (1966). General types of dimensional transducer. *In* "Methods in Medical Research" (R. F. Rushmer, ed.), Vol. 11, pp. 5–23, Year Book Medical Publishers Inc., Chicago.

Pieper, H. T. and Paul, L. T. (1968). Catheter-tip gauge for measuring blood flow velocity and vessel diameter in dogs. *J. Appl. Physiol.* **24**, 259–261.

Reid, L. (1968). Structural and functional reappraisal of the pulmonary artery system. *In* "Scientific Basis of Medicine Annual Reviews", 1968, 289–301, Athlone Press, London.

Ross, S. M. and Brust, M. (1966). Photopot isotonic myogram. *J. Appl. Physiol.* **21**, 293–294.

Rushmer, R. F. (1954). Continuous measurements of left ventricular dimensions in intact, unanaesthetized dogs. *Circulation Res.* **2**, 14–27.

Van Citters, R. L. (1966). Mutual inductance transducers. *In* "Methods in Medical Research" (R. F. Rushmer, ed.), Vol. 11, pp. 26–30, Year Book Medical Publishers Inc., Chicago.

Wells, P. N. T. (1969). "Physical Principles of Ultrasonic Diagnosis", Academic Press, London and New York.

Weibel, E. R. (1963). "Morphometry of the Human Lung", Springer-Verlag, Berlin.

114 D. H. BERGEL

White, D. N. (1967). The limitations of echo-encephalography. *Ultrasonics* **5,** 88–90.

Whitney, R. J. (1953). The measurement of volume changes in human limbs. *J. Physiol.* **121,** 1–27.

Wiederhielm, C. A. (1963). Continuous recording of arteriolar dimensions with a television microscope. *J. Appl. Physiol.* **18,** 1041–1042.

Yates, W. G. (1969). Experimental studies of the variations in the mechanical properties of the canine abdominal vena cava. SUDAAR report 393, Stanford University.

Chapter 5

The Use of Control Theory and Systems Analysis in Cardiovascular Dynamics

K. SAGAWA

Department of Biomedical Engineering,
Johns Hopkins University School of Medicine,
Baltimore, Maryland, U.S.A.

In this chapter, the author intends to present both a brief historical account of control theory and systems analysis, and a review of examples of its application to cardiovascular system analysis.

Elementary knowledge of classical control theory based on transfer function representation is assumed as well as some knowledge of the neural control of the cardiovascular system. Because of the nature of this book, discussion is limited to the hemodynamic aspects of the basic cardiovascular system though this limit is passed where considered necessary. Throughout the emphasis is on the understanding of the interactions between the system components in overall circulatory dynamics and the methodology used. When dynamic aspects are discussed the frequency range of interest is confined to below 0·1 Hz since it is the range which has been most neglected and which is important from the control viewpoint.

1. CONTROL THEORY AND SYSTEMS ANALYSIS

Control theory and system analysis are fields of engineering primarily concerned with analysis and synthesis of a "system" with the object of improving its performance. The system in question may be given or arbitrarily conceived, but it must be clearly defined as to its boundary, environment, input and output variables of interest, time or frequency range of interest, and above all, its ultimate goal. A clear-cut definition of the goal (or goals) of a given system is prerequisite even for analysis by the systems approach. In this respect, these engineering disciplines differ radically from classical biology or physiology where the purpose has been to understand with or without the intent of improvement. Historically, biologists have positively rejected such a teleological approach to life processes in order to safeguard modern physiology from medieval contamination by Aristotelian philosophy. Though this attitude greatly contributed to establishing physiology, biophysics, and biochemistry as modern sciences, a trend toward another direction is being felt today. Many contemporary biologists, and medical investigators in particular, emphasize the need for a teleological interpretation of biological mechanisms because it gives direction to research areas, sheds new light over the ever increasing mass of factual and fractional knowledge and stimulates new working hypotheses. Since medicine is clearly a humanity oriented science this trend is natural and perhaps should be encouraged.

Early control theory evolved from the design of speed controllers for steam engines and developed into systematized knowledge of techniques to control position, pressure, fluid level, temperature, etc. of technological systems. The systems to be analyzed were usually simple enough to be conceived as consisting of two major sub-systems, a controller and a plant (Fig. 1(a)). The variable to be controlled was usually singular and the principle of negative feedback control was invariably used by providing a single (major) feedback path which sensed the controlled variable and conveyed the feedback signal to the controller via a comparator. Most components in each sub-system were linear or approximated as linear and had time-invariant parameters. A major concern of control engineers in those days was "stability" and "optimization" of the dynamic performance of a system with such a feedback control.

The mathematical technique for dealing with relatively simple problems is characterized by applying Laplace transforms to time variables in the system and representing appropriately lumped system components in terms of the transfer function; a form of operator to relate an input to an output across the component. Expressing the property of the open-loop system or lumped elements in the frequency domain, predictions of the oscillatory nature of the performance of the closed-loop system were easily made by inspecting the frequency response plotted in a Bode or Nyquist diagram. Shortly thereafter the root locus method was applied to the design of airplanes and then to more complex systems such as distributed parameter systems or random signal systems. Boolean algebra and other mathematical logic were also used.

Before large-scale digital computers were available and engineers had to depend on manual computation or graphical analysis, the above methods provided powerful tools to predict the closed-loop behavior of those systems. With the Laplace operator, the complex procedure of solving high-order differential equations is reduced to a simple algebraic calculation. This is the essential feature of classical control theory.

With the rapid advance of computer technology and the ever-increasing demand from industry, engineers expanded their technique to a new field which may be called "vector control theory". In this new class of control theories, such as Lyapunov's theorem on stability and Pontryagin's maximum principle in optimal control, nth-order differential equations which describe the system are replaced with a set of n first-order differential equations in which the variables $\dot{x}$, $\ddot{x}$, $\dddot{x}$, etc., are collectively termed a "state vector". The state vector is an n-dimensional vector and the set of equations is a vector differential equation which represents the internal state of a given system in the time domain. Correspondingly, both the input and output variables are represented by single or m-dimensional vectors. Vector representation in the time domain facilitated a more direct connection of the system's state with its digital computer model than that with classical control theory. Some important rules which determine whether an input to a system governs all the internal states and whether a system output reflects all the internal states (Kalman's conditions for controllability and observability) could be reached only by this vector representation. The design of multi-variate control systems, for which the older approach was inherently powerless, was also aided.

In principle, a technological adaptive control system is endowed with the following capabilities (see Fig. 1(b)):

(i) *Identification of plant dynamics.* There is a specially developed sensor part which identifies plant dynamics. When the changes in environment are drastic, the properties of the controlled (plant) system will vary to such an extent that a set of controller signals may result in

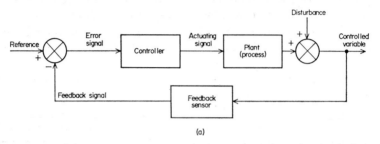

(a)

Fig. 1(a). Structure of a typical feedback control system in classical control engineering. It is characterized by a single input and output variable, single feedback path, a simple (arithmetic) comparator, and a simple mode of introducing disturbances into the system.

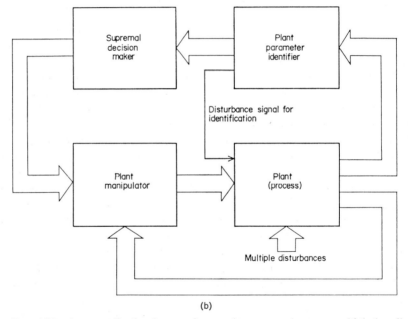

(b)

Fig. 1(b). A generalized scheme of a modern control system which handles multiple input-output variables (denoted by the open arrows), identifies the plant state, decides multiple references based on the identified state, and thus adapts to given environments which disturb at multiple sites. Note the much closer similarity of this type of structure to biological control systems.

an entirely different performance from that expected in ordinary conditions. Therefore, it becomes necessary to re-identify the plant performance as precisely as possible. The identification is achieved by feeding a set of test perturbation signals into the plant (often superimposed on normal control signals), and studying the plant responses. The information on identified plant dynamics is then passed to the decision maker.

(ii) *Deciding the proper control strategy.* Due to the changing environments, the performance-index optimum is slowly changing its position in the state space. The adaptive controller must contain some logic to evaluate the present position of the index with reference to the optimum and then take action to drive the system toward the optimum through the next process.

(iii) *Modification of controller parameters.* Signals based on the decision of the decision maker are passed to the controller which changes the parameters in its network. In practice, the modification is achieved by altering resistances via servo-motors.

All these elements in the adaptive process involve such complex and precise calculations that the identification block and decision maker in Fig. 1(b) are in essence special purpose computers, handling multiple inputs and outputs and solving an nth-order vector equation. Because the adaptation process is provided by a feedback loop in addition to the fast inner feedback loop, the system is called a closed-loop adaptive control system.

Whether the functional structure of biological adaptations resembles that of a technological adaptive system is a stimulating question. It is likely that the brain is capable of such a job, and yet no one has been able to show definite evidence for the presence of a reference signal, decision-making process or a plant identification mechanism. At best, we know that the baroreceptor reflex, for example, is quite strongly modified by stimulating some portions of the cerebral cortex or hypothalamus (Gebber and Snyder, 1970; Hilton, 1966; Hockman *et al.*, 1969; Smith *et al.*, 1968; Weiss and Crill, 1969). Insight into the role of the higher levels of the brain in the control of the circulatory system may be gained by extensive neurophysiological studies together with some imagination and some understanding of technological adaptive control systems. At any rate, modern control theory has proved a powerful aid in the design of complex adaptive control systems. However, it must be mentioned here that the newer theory is by no means unconditionally superior to the older. For example, when one is concerned with the input impedance of a network, the older technique is the more convenient because of the frequency domain in which it operates. The same is true if one's interest is in analysis of noise in a system. On the other hand, if the investigator's concern extends to the identification of system parameters in the network of elements, vector representation is superior due to its immediate access to these parameters. The new theory is essential for a sophisticated control system with adaptive control, which requires automatic (on-line) computer identification of system parameters and instant decision making based on the observed internal state. The older approach tends to lump these parameters in black boxes.

Nevertheless, both techniques supplement each other and are of course interrelated fundamentally. Engineers use either technique depending on the nature of the problems, and practical application is still mostly limited to linear systems with time-invariable constants. In this chapter all examples pertain to the use of transfer functions to represent circulatory black boxes. This is simply because the new approach has not yet permeated into circulatory systems analysis, due partly to its novelty but also due to its demand for explicit formulations of involved elements. Some models of vascular impedance are directly translatable to vector state representation.

Under socioeconomical pressures further expansion of the systems approach has taken place to analyze problems involving large-scale systems with many unidentifiable factors. New general and abstract theories are emerging continually. Particularly interesting to the biologist is a class of theories concerning multi-level and multi-goal hierarchical systems. Physiological regulation operating at the levels of individuals and of organ systems is obviously of such a nature. Therefore, development of large-scale system theories is highly desirable for the understanding of physiological regulations. Unfortunately, they are still in their infancy and most discussion deals with the definition of hierarchy and the mathematical formulation of problems in a very general form. Therefore, no reference can be made in this chapter to their future role in cardiovascular physiology.

The monographs listed in the references may be helpful in understanding control theory and systems analysis and their application to biological systems. In addition, there are extensive areas of engineering techniques (e.g. signal analysis, network analysis, etc.) which can greatly help biologists to formulate the problem and find techniques to solve it. For this purpose the text books of biomedical engineering listed in the references should be consulted.

2. Mechanical Analysis of the Circulatory System: General Considerations

A. the cardiovascular system as a "plant"

It was pointed out in the previous section that the control theory approach presupposes a clearly defined goal or goals of the system to be analyzed. The circulatory system transports blood throughout the body around a closed system. Through its transport function, it serves to transfer nutrients, waste products, heat and chemical signals. By changing either the total flow (cardiac output) or the distribution of flow among various parts of the body, it serves the homeostasis of the whole body. This is achieved at the expense of temporary metabolic imbalances in certain areas of the body. There is sufficient physiological reserve both in the circulatory system and in the tissue metabolic system to tolerate moderate degrees of stress; however, at times of extreme stress, the circulation to some tissue may be maintained at the expense of another. For example, exercise in a normal environment results in such increases of blood flow in both the exercising muscles and the skin that neither core temperature nor metabolite concentrations in the muscle become abnormal. However, in a hot and humid environment, the homeostatic decision maker appears to weigh temperature regulation more heavily than metabolic balance in the muscle and flow is diverted from muscles to skin.

It is obvious that the circulatory system serves many goals related to various facets of homeostasis (e.g. temperature, pH, osmolarity, tissue metabolism, etc.). It is also clear that the circulatory system is not the only supporter of homeostasis; it is merely one of many subsystems of the homeostatic control system (Fig. 2). This suggests that the sub-goal assigned to the circulatory system cannot be defined without specifying the situation of the whole body, and that the circulatory sub-goal varies dynamically depending upon the decisions made by the hierarchical homeostatic controllers. We must therefore confine the mechanical studies on the circulatory system to that of "plant identification" in control theory (Fig. 2). The identification of plant performance is nevertheless very important in systems analysis. It is the first step in modeling a system for the purpose of designing or analyzing the controller.

Unfortunately, experimental identification of the cardiovascular plant is not so easy as in most engineering systems. Surgical or pharmacological elimination of the neural and humoral controllers immediately throws the cardiovascular plant in such a collapsed state that the information obtained is almost useless, unless the large shifts in the operating points of components are somehow compensated. The only practical method to bring the plant operation back to a nearly normal range is the infusion of norepinephrine and the injection of other important hormones (such as ACTH). Ideally, the neural and hormonal signals should be present at their steady resting level, without responding to any changes in hemodynamic variables. A very incomplete imitation of such a state may be attained by cutting the aortic baroreceptor afferent nerves in the vagi and maintaining the isolated carotid sinus pressure at a constant level, but hormonal control signals will still be operative in such preparations.

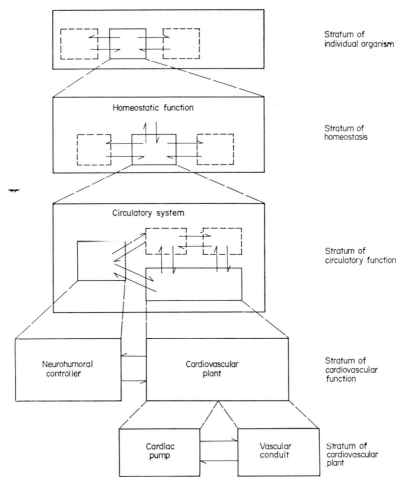

FIG. 2. Levels of understanding of circulatory function. One can start either at the level of the individual organism or at the plant level, or anywhere in between. From the system's viewpoint, understanding is gained by going up or down the levels. However, for this vertical move to be complete, interactions between blocks within the same stratum must be identified.

B. THE CARDIOVASCULAR SYSTEM AS A CLOSED HYDRAULIC LOOP

The fundamental feature of the cardiovascular plant is that it constitutes a closed-loop hydraulic system. Unless special stresses are imposed over a prolonged period of time (e.g. hemorrhage or severe cardiac failure), the blood volume within the system remains fairly constant. Since this constant amount of blood is forced to flow by the cardiac pump from the veins to the arteries, and since the vascular compliance is not infinitely large, mechanical signals propagate in both directions through the system with each heart beat, with respiratory fluctuations of stroke volume associated with intra-thoracic and abdominal pressure changes, and with any other reasonably quick changes in some system parameters (e.g. rhythmic contraction of the spleen). Thus, it becomes clear that any change in pressure or flow in one part of the loop is bound to influence the rest of the loop with signals flowing with and against blood flow. These two flows of mechanical signals eventually return to their origin. It follows that study of an isolated portion of the circulatory loop is incomplete for the understanding of the mechanical events in that portion within the normal closed-loop system. The general axiom that the whole is not a mere sum of parts is particularly true in the circulatory system. Analysis of arbitrarily segmented components is liable to omit information, particularly on the shifts of blood from one part of the system to another and the pressure or flow variations associated with this.

C. ANALYSIS OF THE CIRCULATION AS A CHAIN OF TWO-PORT ELEMENTS

The above warning may become more explicit by applying the concept of two-port analysis to the cardiovascular loop. When a part of the circulatory system is isolated from the rest (either surgically or conceptually), the portion of interest generally has at least two junctions: the inflow port and outflow port. At each of these a direct mechanical interaction takes place with the adjacent parts of the original loop, resulting in the passage of energy through them (Fig. 3(a)). Strictly speaking, the cardiovascular loop should be treated as a network of at least three energy port elements

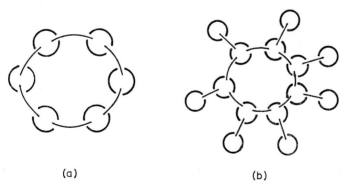

(a)   (b)

FIG. 3(a). The circulatory loop as a chain of two-port elements.
FIG. 3(b). The loop as a network of three-port elements. The interrupted circles represent the components and the bars connecting them the exchange of energy between the components.

since both heart and vessels are surrounded by physiological spaces of finite compliance (Fig. 3(b)).

The pressure-flow relationship across a linear two-port element is generally represented by a set of equations which deal with two pairs of pressure and flow variables at both ends. For convenience, let us represent the time-dependent component of these four variables by Fourier or Laplace transform, p_1^*, q_1^*, p_2^*, and q_2^*. In Fig. 4, note that the directions of a pair of

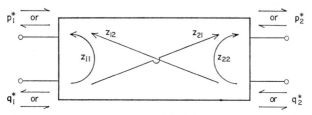

FIG. 4. A hydraulic two-port system or black box. Z_{ij} represent the impedance parameters of the system seen from inflow and outflow ports.

arrows denoting pressure and flow at one port are always opposite. This means that one cannot arbitrarily assign both pressure and flow at each port; one is always dependent on the other and on the property of the system. From the interrelationships among these four variables, we can define the system in the following manner:

(1) Impedance $[Z_{ij}]$:

$$p_1^* = q_1^* Z_{11} + q_2^* Z_{12}$$
$$p_2^* = q_1^* Z_{21} + q_2^* Z_{22} \tag{2.1}$$

(2) Admittance $[Y_{ij}]$:

$$q_1^* = Y_{11} p_1^* + Y_{12} p_2^*$$
$$q_2^* = Y_{21} p_1^* + Y_{22} p_2^* \tag{2.2}$$

where Z_{11} is "input driving-point impedance with constant outflow" or,

$$Z_{11} = \left. \frac{p_1^*}{q_1^*} \right|_{q_2^* = 0} \tag{2.3}$$

Similarly, Z_{22} is "output driving-point impedance with constant inflow" or,

$$Z_{22} = \left. \frac{p_2^*}{q_2^*} \right|_{q_1^* = 0} \tag{2.4}$$

Z_{21} is "inflow to outflow transfer impedance with constant outflow" or,

$$Z_{21} = \left. \frac{p_2^*}{q_1^*} \right|_{q_2^* = 0} \tag{2.5}$$

and Z_{12} is "reverse transfer impedance with constant inflow" or,

$$Z_{12} = \left. \frac{p_1^*}{q_2^*} \right|_{q_1^* = 0} \tag{2.6}$$

The system property may also be expressed in matrix form using Z_{ij} or Y_{ij} as defined above:

$$\begin{vmatrix} p_1^* \\ p_2^* \end{vmatrix} = \begin{vmatrix} Z_{11} & Z_{12} \\ Z_{21} & Z_{22} \end{vmatrix} \begin{vmatrix} q_1^* \\ q_2^* \end{vmatrix} \tag{2.7}$$

or

$$\begin{vmatrix} q_1^* \\ q_2^* \end{vmatrix} = \begin{vmatrix} Y_{11} & Y_{12} \\ Y_{21} & Y_{22} \end{vmatrix} \begin{vmatrix} p_1^* \\ p_2^* \end{vmatrix} \tag{2.8}$$

The transmission parameter is represented by:

$$\begin{vmatrix} p_1^* \\ q_1^* \end{vmatrix} = \begin{vmatrix} A & B \\ C & D \end{vmatrix} \begin{vmatrix} p_2^* \\ -q_2^* \end{vmatrix} \tag{2.9}$$

and the reverse transmission parameter is:

$$\begin{vmatrix} p_2^* \\ q_2^* \end{vmatrix} = \begin{vmatrix} A & B \\ C & D \end{vmatrix} \begin{vmatrix} p_1^* \\ -q_1^* \end{vmatrix} \tag{2.10}$$

Assuming linearity in the frequency and magnitude ranges of interest, the following relationships exist among the above parameters:

$$\begin{aligned} Z_{11} &= A/C, & Z_{12} &= (AD-BC)/C \\ Z_{21} &= 1/C, & Z_{22} &= D/C \end{aligned} \tag{2.11}$$

and

$$\begin{aligned} Y_{11} &= D/B, & Y_{12} &= (-AD+BC)/B \\ Y_{21} &= -1/B, & Y_{22} &= A/B \end{aligned} \tag{2.12}$$

The purpose of stating these comprehensive representations of a two-port system is to recognize that most conventional studies on pressure-flow relationships in the vascular system have concentrated heavily on the arterial-end driving point impedance, with no specification of the venous end. To understand thoroughly an element in the circulatory loop, more comprehensive studies from both arterial and venous ends are necessary. Without such efforts, the information on components will never lead to the synthesis of the whole chain of two-port elements.[†] A recent study by Sato et al. (1971) is a good example of two-port analysis of an isolated vascular bed.

[†] On this subject, the reader may find the following citation from Folkow and Mellander (1964) interesting. "The cardiovascular system has many facets, each of which may spellbind an investigator. Thus, to a cardiologist it consists of the heart, to which there happens to be connected a system of tubes, justified mainly because it allows the output to return to the heart. To the expert on peripheral circulation it consists of a fascinating system of tubes for flow studies, wherein, incidentally, the pressure head is said to have something to do with the heart. Again, to the investigator who is biophysically minded it is an inexhaustable source for the creation of stunning formulae of profound beauty and doubtful applicability. Lastly to the expert on capillaries it is a vast and delicate exchange membrane, which unfortunately has to be connected to other, far duller cardiovascular sections for providing the flow needed to put the all-important exchange into action. The only common denominator of these superspecialists would probably be their raised eyebrows if someone dared to suggest that the veins might be important, too."

In the following sections, progressive openings in the circulatory loop will be discussed to illustrate a class of systems approach to cardiovascular plant identification. The central idea is to reverse the conventional direction of approach from the components toward synthesis into that from the total toward the components, so as not to lose the vital information on interactions among the divided plant components.

3. OPENINGS IN THE CIRCULATORY LOOP

A. SINGLE OPENING

As a first step, let us assume that we open the circulatory loop at a single point where the flow is physiologically lumped. The appropriate sites are the right ventricular-pulmonary arterial junction, pulmonary vein-left atrial junction and left ventricular-ascending aortic junction, proximal to the coronary ostia. From an experimental viewpoint, the easier site is either the venae caval–right atrial junction or the ascending aorta distal to the coronary ostia. Let us discuss a case in which the right atrium is uncoupled from the venae cavae.

The opened circulatory loop can be analyzed as a four-terminal black-box analogous to the two-port element discussed in Section 2 C. However, at the very beginning of the analysis of this opened system, we encounter a basic constraint which is inherent to the system but often neglected; this is the constancy of total blood volume in the natural circulatory system. A properly designed open-loop experiment should also ensure constancy of total blood volume, and this constraint limits the choice of input and output variables in the open-loop study. If we assign $\bar{q}_1$ and $q_1(t)$ (mean and time-varying components of atrial inflow) differently from $\bar{q}_2$ and $q_2(t)$ (mean and time-varying components of venous return), the blood volume in the system will change, violating the natural constraint. Hence $\bar{q}_1 = \bar{q}_2$ and $q_1(t) = q_2(t)$ must hold. These conditions will never be met if one chooses $\bar{p}_1$, $p_1(t)$, $\bar{p}_2$ and $p_2(t)$ as the input variables, unless one is lucky enough to assign such a unique set of pressure values that the blood volume happens to remain constant. Such extreme luck cannot be expected. The constraint of constant blood volume makes it inevitable that we choose a single flow variable $\bar{q}$ and q^* as the input forcing in the analysis of the system, and then p_1^* and p_2^* become the output variables of the black-box. The previously described four impedance parameters reduce therefore to the following simple set.

$$Z_{11} = Z_{12} = p_{ra}^*/q^*$$
$$Z_{22} = Z_{21} = p_{cv}^*/q^* \qquad (3.1)$$

where p_{ra}^* indicates time-dependent component of right atrial pressure and p_{vc}^* that of vena caval pressure.

(1) *Static analysis*

Although the above discussion dealt with the dynamics of the opened system, the same constraints hold for the static case. Static analysis is indispensable in giving the approximate performance of the system over a wide range of input and output signals. Quite often it reveals key basic properties of the system which cannot be understood by dynamic performance analysis. Systematic static analysis of the opened circulatory loop had not been performed until Guyton (1955) and his associates initiated a series of studies on venous return in open-chest dogs whose central nervous system was rendered inoperative by spinal anesthesia and the cardiovascular tone was maintained by norepinephrine infusion.

This group stated their concept of input and output variables differently from the above discussion. In fact, they by-passed the right ventricle by a perfusion pump which drained the blood from the right atrium via a collapsible tube. The pump speed was continuously adjusted so that it was always equal to the venous return attained at the right atrial pressure set by the hydrostatic level of the collapsible tube. Guyton's group first set the level of the collapsible tube and then adjusted the perfusion pump, and on this basis, they state that atrial pressure was the input and the venous return was the output. However, because of the reciprocity law, it really does not matter whether one changes right atrial pressure or the flow through the pump first.

The curve labeled $VR-P_{cv}$ in Fig. 5 represents the relationship between venous return and central venous pressure. As the latter was elevated to 7 mmHg, venous return ceased, or, in accordance with our previous discussion, when the input flow was made zero, systemic venous pressure rose to 7 mmHg. Since there is no flow in the system where the same pressure exists throughout the systemic vascular bed, Guyton (1955) called this pressure "mean systemic filling pressure" (MSP). The slope of the $VR-P_{cv}$ curve represents the d.c. resistance of the systemic vascular bed seen from the venous end; Guyton (1955) termed it "resistance for venous return". When central venous pressure was lowered below atmospheric partial collapse occurred centrally and spread gradually to the distal veins. Venous return could not increase further due to the increased resistance of the collapsed portion of the vein ("vascular waterfall"). This plateau is extremely important because it limits the maximum cardiac output (and venous return) attainable simply by providing an active flow source at the opened ends of the circulatory loop.

On the same diagram, a curve is plotted which illustrates the property of the cardiac pump, that is, the relationship between cardiac output and mean right atrial pressure ($CO-P_{ra}$ curve in Fig. 5). This is equivalent to the Frank–Starling cardiac output curve; it represents the resistance or con-

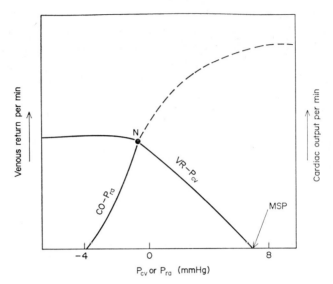

FIG. 5. An equilibrium diagram for the circulatory loop uncoupled at the vena cava–right atrial junction. (Modified from Guyton, 1955.)

ductance seen from the right atrial end of the opened circulatory loop. This curve also has a ceiling which is however much higher than that of the $VR-P_{cv}$ curve. Part of the $CO-P_{ra}$ curve is indicated by a broken line because that portion of the curve cannot be seen unless an excessive amount of blood is added to the system, or the property of the vascular system is varied by some means. In fact, Guyton *et al.* (1958) obtained the $CO-P_{ra}$ relationship curve from a separate group of dogs in which the constancy of total blood volume was disregarded.

The intersection (N) of these two curves represents graphically the equilibrium at which the circulatory system arrives when the loop is closed. A few important points become apparent from this equilibrium diagram:

(a) The closed system is stable since the two open-loop curves intersect with opposite slopes.

(b) Near the equilibrium point, the $CO-P_{ra}$ curve is somewhat steeper than the $VR-P_{cv}$ curve, indicating that the static overall gain of the loop is more than unity with negative sign (see discussion on dynamic performance).

(c) The fact that the equilibrium point is very close to the ceiling of the $VR-P_{cv}$ curve indicates that cardiac output cannot increase much above normal however hard we push the cardiac (or perfusion) pump, unless the $VR-P_{cv}$ curve shifts to the right or increases in slope.

The last point was shown to be the case in patients with artificial pace-makers as well as in animals (Ross *et al.*, 1965); by increasing heart rate to 120–150/min no substantial increase of cardiac output occurred.

To explain the physiological meaning of the VR–P_{cv} curve, Guyton developed the model of the circulatory system shown in Fig. 6. Although greatly simplified, it is very useful for understanding the importance of blood

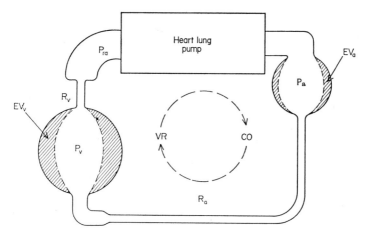

FIG. 6. Guyton's simplified model of the circulatory loop. EV_a or EV_v represents the volume of blood in the lumped systemic arteries or veins in excess of their unstressed volume. (Modified from Guyton, 1963a, b.)

volume and vascular tone in the dynamics of the whole system. In this model, if the heart–lung pump ceases to transfer blood from the vein to artery ($q = 0$), the pressures in all the segments of the systemic vascular bed will equalize. Therefore,

$$P_a = P_v = P_{ra} = \text{MSP} \equiv \frac{EV_s}{C_s} \quad (q = 0) \qquad (3.2)$$

where EV_s is the blood volume in excess of the unstressed systemic vascular volume V_o (i.e. EV_s = total systemic volume − $V_o = EV_a + EV_v$), and C_s is the sum of arterial and venous compliances defined as $C = \Delta EV/\Delta P$ (i.e. $C_s = C_a + C_v$). Thus, MSP is a function of the blood volume, compliance and unstressed volume of the systemic vessels.

If the pump generates a steady flow ($\bar{q} > 0$), then the mean arterial and venous pressures will be:

$$P_a = \bar{q}(R_v + R_a) + P_{ra} \qquad (3.3)$$

$$P_v = -\bar{q} \cdot R_v + P_{ra} \qquad (3.4)$$

where R_v and R_a are venous and arterial resistances, respectively. Note that the model lumps the venous resistance proximal to the lumped venous capacitance, which therefore corresponds to the site of the small veins and venules in the real system. For simplicity the compliance of the heart-lung section is disregarded.

From (3.3) and (3.4) and the definition of MSP given by (3.2), the arterial and venous pressures generated in the vascular bed in response to a given flow $\bar{q}$ can be given as functions of the vascular parameters and MSP.

$$P_a = \text{MSP} + \bar{q}.R_a$$

$$P_{ra}(= P_{cv}) = \text{MSP} - \left[\frac{R_v C_v + (R_v + R_a)C_a}{C_v + C_a}\right] \times \bar{q} \qquad (3.5)$$

Note that the above equations hold for the vascular bed as a passive circuit and have nothing to do with the property of the cardiac pump. Since C_v is roughly 20 times as large as C_a, (3.5) can be approximated as:

$$P_{ra} = \text{MSP} - \left(R_v + \frac{R_a}{20}\right)\bar{q} \qquad (3.6)$$

This states that right atrial pressure (= central venous pressure) is given as the difference between mean systemic filling pressure and a pressure which is related to the existing flow (forced by the pump) and the sum of venous resistance and the arterial resistance weighted by the ratio of venous to arterial compliance. An important implication of this is that a change of venous resistance is 20 times as effective as one of arterial resistance in changing right atrial pressure. Since the steady-state output of the cardiac pump is extremely sensitive to its input filling pressure (P_{ra}), but almost insensitive to arterial pressure load (Herndon and Sagawa, 1969), a change in venous pressure has a much greater effect on cardiac output than an equal change in arterial resistance. For this reason, an increase in venous resistance decreases cardiac output far more than a similar increase in arterial resistance. That this is in fact the case was shown in the dog's closed-loop circulation (Guyton et al., 1959).

Another important implication of this equation is that either variation of blood volume or alteration of vascular compliance affects P_{ra} through a change in MSP, and thereby affects cardiac output. The equilibrium diagram in Fig. 7 illustrates the effect of such parameter changes. The VR curve, indicated by a broken line, shows the $VR-P_{cv}$ relationship obtained in a group of reflexless dogs which were bled about 12 per cent of total blood volume. The intersection with the normal cardiac output curve correspondingly shifts, to N_1, indicating that cardiac output should decrease to approximately 420 ml/min or about 50 per cent of control (Guyton et al., 1958). On the other hand, transfusion of about 10 per cent of total blood volume caused the $VR-P_{cv}$ relationship to shift upwards and to the right (dotted line),

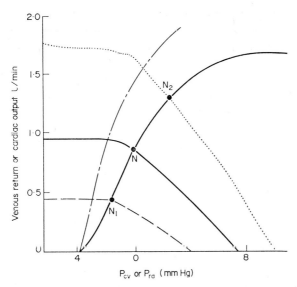

FIG. 7. The effect of hemorrhage or transfusion on the equilibrium between cardiac output, venous return and central systemic venous pressure (= right atrial pressure). (Modified from Guyton, 1955.)

resulting in an intersection N_2 which indicates an equilibrium cardiac output of 1400 ml/min or 40 per cent above the control. The high sensitivity of the MSP and of the equilibrated flow to blood volume changes derives from the relatively small compliance of the systemic vascular bed.

From the relationship between variations in mean systemic filling pressure and changes in (total) blood volume observed in a separate group of reflexless dogs, Richardson *et al.* (1961) concluded that the acutely measured compliance is in the order of 0·6 ml/mmHg in a 10-kg dog. However, the compliance recently measured in the author's laboratory by a different method taking two minutes gave a value 3 to 4 times greater than this (Shoukas and Sagawa, 1970), and with such a compliance value the variation of cardiac output after alteration of blood volume should be more moderate. Note that these studies, which dealt only with static pressure flow relationships, led to a quantitative estimate of the importance of blood volume and capacitive property of the vascular bed in regulating cardiac output.

Many other implications of the equilibrium diagram have been explored with reference to various situations such as the opening of an arterio-venous fistula, infusion of vasoconstrictor agents, body tilting, muscular exercise, compensated and decompensated heart failure and hypoxia (Guyton, 1963a).

An obvious but often forgotten virtue of the model approach to a system is simplification of the complex reality for specific problems or purposes. Guyton's approach to the understanding of overall circulatory regulation in terms of a simplified model such as the one shown in Fig. 4 has been greatly appreciated by clinical investigators. Graphical analysis by the venous return–cardiac output equilibrium diagram is useful and accurate. One can incorporate any observed shifts of the non-linear relationships with time and other variables and can predict the equilibrium under closed-loop conditions. This is often done by systems engineers and should not be underestimated even when computers are available.

As stated before, one may cut the loop of the circulation at several alternative sites where the flow is conveniently lumped. This will give equilibrium diagrams concerning flows and pressures at different sites and reveal the interactions in the overall system at different energy ports.

(2) Dynamic performance

Sagawa (unpublished observations) studied the dynamic performance of the circulatory loop, opened between venae cavae and the heart, with a method using sinusoidally varying flow forcing. A constant flow perfusion pump with little compliance was inserted between the venae cavae and right atrium, and its mean flow rate was adjusted so that P_{ra} and P_{cv} were equal. The frequency range of interest was limited to beteeen $\frac{1}{4}$ and 8 cycles/ min. The amplitude of the flow variation was confined to about $+30$ per cent the control. Figure 8 illustrates an example of frequency-dependent changes in the moduli of impedance seen from atrial and vena caval ends of the opened circulatory loop. The modulus seen from the atrial end ($|RAP_{(j\omega)}/F_{(j\omega)}|$) remained fairly constant within the investigated range of frequency, whereas that seen from the vena caval end ($|SVP_{(j\omega)}/F_{(j\omega)}|$) began to attenuate above 1 cycle/min. These characteristics obviously reflect both a quick response of the right heart which may be regarded as zero-order proportional element within the frequency range, and also the relatively large compliance of the central systemic veins. The absolute value of the ratio $|SVP_{(j\omega)}/RAP_{(j\omega)}|$ (amplitude ratio of vena caval pressure waves over right atrial pressure waves) indicated an attenuation of roughly -20 dB/decade over the frequency range above 2 cycles/min (0·033 Hz) in this and other examples. Below this frequency, the ratio was found to be approximately unity (or greater in some dogs). In this lower frequency range, $SVP_{(j\omega)}$ and $RAP_{(j\omega)}$ are shifted in phase by approximately $180°$.

The fact that the above modulus ratio is unity or greater in the low frequency region suggests a good dynamic stability of the closed circulatory loop in this frequency range. The ratio reflects the relative magnitudes of the two opposing forces that the system generates at the right atrial–venae

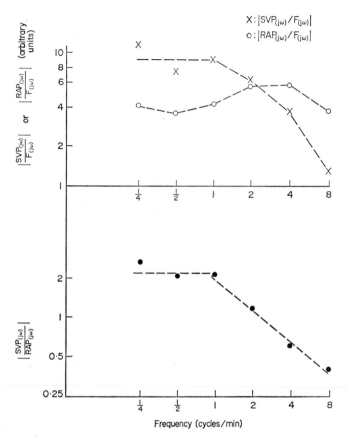

Fig. 8. "Ultra-low" frequency responses of the circulatory loop with a single opening, seen simultaneously at the right atrial and vena caval ports. The opened loop was forced by a sinusoidally varying flow with a fixed flow amplitude and frequencies from ¼ to 8 cycles/min. The upper panel shows the moduli of impedance at the two ports, the lower panel indicates their ratio. An example from a dog.

caval junction in response to a given disturbance in P_{ra} or flow; it is equivalent to the gain of a negative feedback control system in this sense.

With an increase in forcing frequency, however, the amplitude ratio became smaller while the phase shift increased; this means that the mechanical circulatory loop is less stable for a disturbance with higher frequency components. At the frequency of respiration (15 cycles/min) the negative feedback gain is about one quarter of the plateau value. If respiration is slower with an identical depth, the closed-loop system will attenuate the respiratory change in cardiac output to a greater degree. However, a sign of instability, i.e. a gain near unity with a phase lag of 360° was absent in all the dogs studied (negative feedback is equivalent to 180° phase shift, and 360° lag is a further shift of 180°). Thus it is highly improbable that the closed circulatory system goes into an oscillation through the mechanical feedback loop.

Spontaneous waves with a period of 15–30 sec often appear in the mean arterial pressure in man or animal. It is clear in reference to the above finding that these waves are neither produced nor amplified by the closed-loop structure of the circulation. The cause might be instability in the arterial baro- and chemoreceptor reflexes, since the slow oscillation was observed even when the heart was driven by a constant flow pump, but was greatly attenuated after sectioning the sino-aortic nerves.

B. DOUBLE OPENING

The next step in the analysis of the circulation is to open it at two appropriate sites. Sagawa's group studied the basic behavior of the circulatory system by opening the venae cavae–right atrial junction and the left ventricular–ascending aortic junction (Fig. 9), thus dividing the loop into two major sections, the heart–lung and the systemic vascular bed. As indicated by the arrows in Fig. 9, the input variables to the heart–lung are the outputs from the vascular bed, whereas the input to the latter is the cardiac output (= venous return) of the heart–lung section. In studying the flow generating capacity of the heart–lung section, its compliance was disregarded. That is, the blood volume changes needed to fill the heart and lungs so as to cause different flows was not measured. For the heart–lung section to alter its flow by the Frank–Starling mechanism, some blood must shift to or from the vascular bed. For this reason, the compliance of the heart–lung is an important system parameter. Roughly speaking, the compliance is estimated as about ⅛ that of the systemic vascular bed (Guyton, 1963b). If this is true, only small amounts of blood will have to shift from or to the systemic vascular bed in order to vary the performance of the heart.

(i) The heart–lung

a. *Static response.* The three-dimensional graph in Fig. 10 represents cardiac output (strictly speaking, ascending aortic flow less coronary flow), as a function of mean right atrial pressure and mean aortic pressure under steady-state conditions (about 2 minutes after changing these pressure loads), (Herndon and Sagawa, 1969). There were no reflex effects on the heart from the sino-aortic baroreceptors because the vagi were cut and the carotid sinuses and brain were perfused at constant pressure. The cardiac output surface was constructed from (i), a family of curves relating cardiac output to mean aortic pressure with mean right atrial pressure held at various levels, and (ii), a family of mean right atrial pressure–cardiac output curves

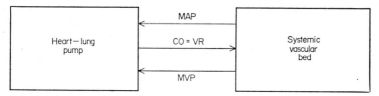

FIG. 9. Diagrammatic representation of a double opening in the circulatory loop at the venae cavae-right atrial junction and at the left heart (including the coronary ostia)–ascending aortic junction.

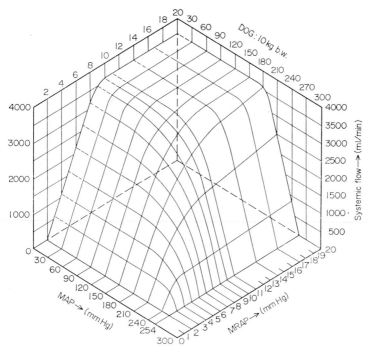

FIG. 10. Three-dimensional plot of the steady-state (2 min) flow output of the heart-lung in response to inflow and outflow pressure loads. (From Herndon and Sagawa, 1969).

(Starling cardiac output curves) at various mean aortic pressures. The important feature of the surface is that within the physiological pressure range cardiac output is highly dependent on inflow (venous) pressure, but almost independent of the outflow (arterial) pressure load.

It must be emphasized that the relatively constant outflow from the left heart over a wide range of aortic pressures was observed only when a steady state was reached after a sudden change in aortic pressure. Sarnoff *et al.*

(1960) observed a similar adaptive recovery of cardiac output with time following elevation of aortic pressure in the isolated left heart preparation perfused at constant coronary pressure. Since the end-diastolic pressure in this preparation was found to return to the control level as the cardiac output recovered to its control value, they assumed that the adapted heart was pumping a similar flow from an identical end-diastolic volume despite the greater pressure afterload. For this reason, they called this intrinsic adaptive mechanism "homeometric autoregulation" in contrast to the Starling mechanism which results from a change in end-diastolic volume and is therefore "heterometric". Recently, however, Clancy *et al.* (1968) re-investigated homeometric autoregulation in a similar left heart preparation and found that creep or stress relaxation occurred in the left ventricle during the transient period of increased residual volume and elevated end-diastolic pressure after a sudden increase in aortic pressure. Clancy and his associates consider this creep the major source of the apparently homeometric autoregulatory adaptation. That is, although the end-diastolic pressure returned to the same level as the control, the end-diastolic volume was actually greater than before; since the heart is extremely sensitive to changes in end-diastolic volume they feel that heterometric autoregulation caused by the creep phenomenon is far more important than homeometric autoregulation in the recovery of cardiac output after increasing aortic pressure.

In the heart–lung preparation, it is obvious that the Starling mechanism operates in the left heart as the aortic pressure load is altered, and the residual volume in the left heart increases or decreases. When mean left atrial pressure is controlled (instead of right atrial pressure), the role of the Starling mechanism will be greatly minimized. This difference is illustrated by the two sets of curves in Fig. 11. The solid curves, obtained from the left heart while maintaining mean left atrial pressure at a constant level, indicate a greater decrease in output with increase in aortic pressure above 120 mmHg, compared with the broken-line which represents the outflow from the heart–lung over the same range of aortic pressure.

To achieve greater outflow against the high pressure afterload, the heart–lung section must be filled with a greater amount of blood. How much this extra amount will be depends upon the compliance of the heart–lung section and the sensitivity of the Starling mechanism in the left heart, and the extra blood volume must come from the systemic bed.

Figure 12 shows the left heart outflow surface (A) and external work output per minute, calculated as $\bar{p}_{ao} \times \bar{q}_{ao}$ (B). The surfaces were calculated for a 10-kg dog based on the data from another group of dogs under open-chest reflexless conditions (Sagawa, 1967). Compared with that of Fig. 10, the surface in Fig. 12A is more sensitive to changes in mean aortic pressure, particularly when the atrial pressure is high and therefore when there is a

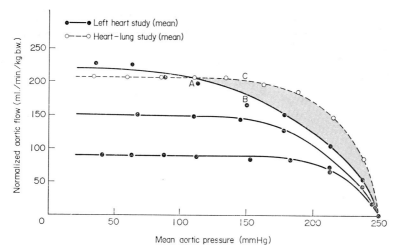

FIG. 11. Comparison of the static mean arterial pressure (MAP)–Cardiac output (CO) curves, one obtained with fixed mean right atrial pressures (solid circles) and the other with a fixed mean left atrial pressure. The shaded area reflects the difference in cardiac output between the characteristics of the heart–lung (MRAP fixed) and that of the left cardiac pump alone (MLAP fixed). (From Herndon, 1969.)

large flow output at a relatively low arterial pressure. An empirical description of the relationship between the three variables appears as follows:

$$\bar{q}_{ao} = K(\bar{p}_{la} - \bar{p}_{la,0}) \left\{ 1 - \exp\left[-100 \left(1 - \frac{\bar{p}_{ao}}{\bar{p}_{ao,\max}} \right) \middle/ A \times K(\bar{p}_{la} - \bar{p}_{la,0}) \right] \right\} \times \text{B.W.}$$

(3.7)

$\bar{p}_{la,0}$ is the lowest left atrial pressure at which the left heart can pump blood. K is a linear slope constant which relates the effective mean left atrial pressure $(\bar{p}_{la} - \bar{p}_{la,0})$ to the greatest aortic flow, $\bar{q}_{ao,\max}$, which the left heart can pump against a low aortic pressure (approximately 50 mmHg). $\bar{p}_{ao,\max}$ is the maximum mean aortic pressure at which the left heart can pump blood (apart from coronary flow). A is an empirical constant which was obtained in the following manner. When the data on mean aortic flow, normalized for body weight, were plotted against mean aortic pressure relative to $\bar{p}_{ao,\max}$ as 100 per cent, the observations lay around exponential curves which intersected with the P_{ao} axis at $P_{ao,\max}$ and tended towards one of three values of q_{ao} determined by $K(\bar{p}_{la} - \bar{p}_{la,0})$ for the three different $\bar{p}_{la}$'s tested. Thus the $\bar{q}_{ao} - \bar{p}_{ao}$ curves could be fitted with an exponential formula,

$$\bar{q}_{ao} = \bar{q}_{ao,\max}\{1 - \exp\left[-100(1 - \bar{p}_{ao}/p_{ao,\max})/\alpha \right]\}$$

(3.8)

The slope constant α was found to be proportional to $\bar{q}_{ao,\max}$ and this, in its turn, was related to $\bar{p}_{la}$ by $K(\bar{p}_{la} - \bar{p}_{la,0})$. The constant relating α and

$\bar{q}_{ao, \max}$ is termed A. The maximum value of the aortic pressure against which the heart could pump, $\bar{p}_{ao, \max}$, did not vary significantly with the left atrial pressure, $\bar{p}_{la}$; it was about 250 mmHg after sino-aortic denervation and 180 mmHg when the baroreceptor reflexes were intact. B.W. is the body weight of the dog in kg.

Because of this interdependence of the effects of preload and afterload on cardiac output, the peak of the work-output surface is also a function of both pressure loads (Fig. 12B). The higher the preload, the lower was the optimum afterload pressure at which the peak external work was achieved.

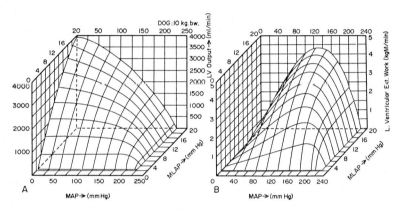

FIG. 12. Static characteristics of flow output (A) and the external mechanical work output (B) at left heart as a function of mean left atrial pressure (MLAP) and mean aortic pressure (MAP). The work was calculated as [CO/min] × [MAP]. Compare A with the cardiac output surface in Fig. 10. Note in B that the MAP at which the work output is maximum shifts with changes in MLAP. The values of the co-ordinates are for a 10-kg dog, calculated from (3.7), see text. (From Sagawa, 1967.)

b. *Dynamic analysis*. Dynamic properties of a system can be analyzed by forcing the system with waves of various forms. Herndon (1969) forced the heart–lung preparation with sinusoidally varying aortic pressure. The mean aortic pressure, $\bar{p}_{ao}$, was set at either 60 or 120 mmHg and sinusoids, p^{*}_{ao}, with a small fixed amplitude (30 mmHg) and at frequencies from $\frac{1}{2}$ to 16 cycles/min were superimposed on the former (Fig. 13).

The mean right atrial pressure was controlled (at one of two levels) so that the mean aortic flow $\bar{q}_{ao}$ was 60 or 150 ml/min/kg. The control of atrial pressure was somewhat imperfect in the higher frequency range. The aortic flow responses, q^{*}_{ao}, to these arterial pressure waves were determined in terms of an amplitude ratio and phase lag and plotted as a function of the input frequency (Fig. 14).

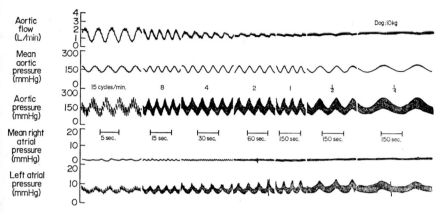

FIG. 13. Part of an experimental record showing the frequency response of the heart–lung output to imposed sinusoidal variations of constant amplitude (± 30 mmHg) in mean aortic pressure; the mean right atrial pressure was held as constant as possible. Notice the diminishing fluctuations of aortic flow as the frequency of the aortic pressure variations was reduced from 15 to $\frac{1}{4}$ cycles/min. (From Herndon, 1969.)

With respect to the amplitude ratios, it was found that the ratio of the decrease or increase in aortic flow to the rise or fall in aortic pressure became greater with frequency, the slope being roughly $+20$ dB/decade between 1 and 15 cycles/min. Below 1 cycle/min, the curve appeared to level off. Above 7·5 cycles/min, another plateau was noted in some experiments though this is not seen in the averages in Fig. 14. The phase curve indicated an increasing lead as the frequency was increased up to 4 cycles/min but thereafter the lead diminished, which again suggests that there might be another break point at a frequency between 0·5–1 Hz. The suspected plateau was clear in experiments where the dynamic response of the left heart to sinusoidal changes of aortic pressure was studied (Sagawa, 1967). Combining these results the following transfer function approximately describes the dynamic response of the heart–lung section in the range from $\frac{1}{2}$ to 15 cycles/min:

$$\frac{q_{ao}^*}{p_{ao}^*} = \frac{k(1+\tau_2 s)}{(1+\tau_1 s)} \tag{3.9}$$

where q_{ao}^* and p_{ao}^* represent Laplace transforms of the sinusoidally changing components of aortic flow and pressure, s the Laplace operator, k a negative constant, and τ_1 and τ_2 time constants. The values of k, τ_1 and τ_2 are function of mean atrial and aortic pressures. The constant k is different from K in (3.7); k represents the piece-wise linearized slope at various points on the curves in Fig. 10 projected on the $\bar{q}_{ao} - \bar{p}_{ao}$ plane. The value ranged

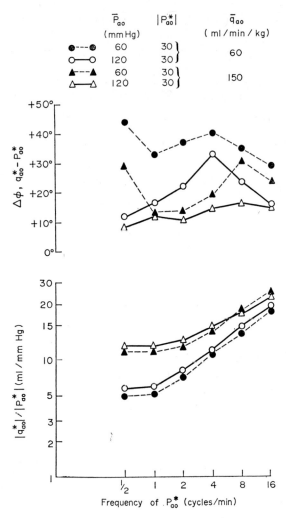

FIG. 14. Bode plots of the averaged frequency responses of the heart-lung output, q_{ao}^*, with sinusoidally varied aortic pressure, p_{ao}^*, ± 30 mmHg (in 5 dogs) studied at two different levels of mean right artrial pressure (MRAP) (and therefore of flow) and two different mean levels of $\bar{p}_{ao}$. Notice the elevation of the plateau levels at low input frequencies and diminishing slopes of the amplitude ratio curves with higher mean flows. The fall in the amplitude ratio curves, as the frequency of the imposed sinusoidal variations in mean aortic pressure (MAP) was reduced, corresponds to the diminished aortic flow (AF) fluctuations seen in Fig. 13. (Redrawn from Herndon, 1969.)

from about zero to 5 ml/mmHg. The values of τ_1 and τ_2 were approximately 1 sec and 10 sec respectively in these experiments.

The above description in the frequency domain (3.9) represents the dynamic performance of a first-order derivative element. The $\bar{q}_{ao}$ response in the time domain to step changes in aortic pressure is shown in Fig. 15. The relationship between the constants in (3.9) and the parameters of the response of aortic flow ($\bar{q}_{ao}$) is illustrated in the figure.

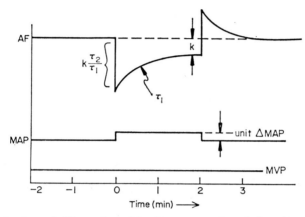

FIG. 15. A schematic illustration of the time course of aortic flow (AF) in response to unit step changes in aortic pressure (MAP). The coefficients in (3.9) are related to the characteristic features of the aortic flow curve.

Those who have only studied the instantaneous effect of step changes in arterial impedance on left ventricular output (Wilcken et al., 1963) observed the initial large change shown in Fig. 15. Consequently they concluded that the heart is a flow source with relatively small internal resistance. Those who extended observation to the static relationship established some minutes after the change in aortic pressure load found only a small change in flow and maintained that the cardiac pump behaves like a constant flow generator with a large source resistance. Either statement is true and incomplete. The linear equation (3.9) includes both properties over a small range of aortic pressure changes and frequency.

Scher et al. (1968) approached the problem by multiple regression analysis between stroke volume and its determinants such as filling pressure, afterload systolic pressure and filling time of the left ventricle in unanesthetized dogs. The effect of respiratory changes in arterial pressure on stroke volume, independent of other factors, was found to be in the order of 0·04 ml/mmHg change in aortic pressure. Converting this into ml/min, we obtain about 40 ml/mmHg in a 13-kg dog. Since the respiratory frequency is close to the upper limit of the range covered in Sagawa's and Herndon's experiments, the result of Scher's study appear to agree reasonably well with those of the latter experiments. However, this apparent agreement may be coincidental because regression analysis deals with the instantaneous input–output relationship, whereas frequency response analysis separates the amplitude from the phase relationship. Additionally in Scher's experiments the baroreceptor reflex and other neural controls were participating while these were eliminated in the experiments of Sagawa and Herndon.

(ii) *The systemic vascular bed*

a. *Static analysis.* The static pressure-flow relationship of the whole systemic vascular bed is a subject of controversy. Yet it is becoming increasingly important to understand it for surgical procedures involving whole body perfusion. Here again, perfusion experiments on individual vascular beds does not help in the synthesis of the overall pressure-flow relationship, just as the overall information cannot contribute much to the knowledge on the former. We need to know both far better than we do now, particularly with regard to the resistance (and impedance) seen from the venous outflow end. The experimental analyses by Guyton (1963a) are still the best example of the systems approach to static equilibrium conditions in this vascular bed.

The curves in Fig. 16 reflect the degree of discrepancy on the total systemic pressure-flow relationship seen from the arterial end. There are many differences in the experimental details including the animal species, the time allowed for measurement after changing pressure or flow, the constancy of blood volume in the system, and the intensity of nervous control of vasomotor tone. Consequently, the curves vary from linear (Grodins *et al.*, 1960) to a power function, $F = kp^n$, the exponent, n, of which varies from 0·75 (Folkow, 1952) to a value larger than 1 (Read *et al.*, 1957).

It is important to note that, as far as the physiological range of pressure and flow is concerned, the non-linearity if any is rather insignificant. The linearized curves of Levy *et al.* (1954) as well as Herndon's (1969) extrapolate toward a large negative pressure (−40 mmHg) at zero flow. From extensive experience of isolated cat's limb perfusion experiments, Folkow (1952) asserted that the exponent is less than unity as long as the preparation possesses active vasomotor tone. This is also true for the total vascular bed at very low pressures and flows, but does not seem to be so in a narrow range near the physiological pressure level. The well-known autoregulation of flow in many individual vascular beds (kidney, brain, heart, and skeletal muscle) appears insignificant when the total systemic resistance is investigated by short-term whole body perfusion experiments. The reason for this is not known. However, there is recent evidence (Granger and Guyton,

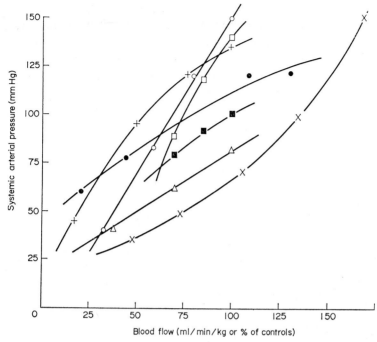

FIG. 16. Aortic pressure-flow relationships reported by various investigators. Note the wide discrepancies seen.

+, Read, Kuida and Johnson (1957); ○ and ●, Levy *et al.* (1954); ×, Folkow (1952); △, Grodins *et al.* (1960); ■ and □, Herndon (1969). The flows in Levy's and Grodins' reports were given neither relative to control nor body weight. Therefore these were estimated from the average weight of the animals used. ●, Pressure in the isolated carotid sinuses held at 210 mmHg. ○, both sinus nerves and vagi cut, ■, sinoarotic nerves left intact, □, both nerves cut.

1969) that, if one extends observation to some hours after the change of pressure or flow in decapitated dogs, autoregulation of flow may also become prominent in the whole bed. Further experimental studies are badly needed in which the damage to perfused blood and vessels is minimized and the period of observation is extended to a reasonably long period.

b. *Dynamic analysis.* Herndon (1969) perfused the vascular bed with sinusoidally varying flow, using the experimental dog's own heart as the perfusion pump and controlling aortic flow by an implanted pericardial balloon. The balloon compressed the right atrium so that the desired aortic flow ($\bar{q}_{ao} + q_{ao}^*$) was maintained by a servo-mechanism. The frequency ranged from $\frac{1}{4}$ to 8 cycles/min. The amplitude of the flow sinusoid ($|q_{ao}^*|$) was fixed at about ± 10 per cent of the control aortic flow while the mean level of flow $\bar{q}_{ao}$ was set at 85 and 70 per cent of the control cardiac output (Fig. 17). Thus the total blood volume remained constant despite the sinusoidal change in cardiac output. Figure 18 shows the frequency response of systemic arterial pressure p_{ao}^*, Fig. 19 shows that of systemic venous pressure p_v^*, and Fig. 20 that of the arterial-venous pressure difference p_{a-v}^*, with and without arterial baroreceptor reflexes.

Only two major conclusions will be mentioned here. One is that the arterial impedance curve, which indicated a slope of -6 dB/decade, cannot be modeled by a simple network consisting of arterial capacitance, total peripheral resistance and venous capacitance, as used in several models of the whole circulatory system (see Chapter 6). A model with many series and parallel CR network elements, as used by Beneken (Beneken and DeWit, 1967) and Rideout (Synder and Rideout, 1969) is needed. Another implication is that baroreceptor reflex control caused a resonance phenomenon in the frequency range near 4 cycles/min (Fig. 18), whereas the venous pressure response did not indicate any significant difference whether the reflex was intact or not. The so-called spontaneous vasomotor waves in arterial pressure are perhaps related to this resonance phenomenon since both frequencies fall in the same range.

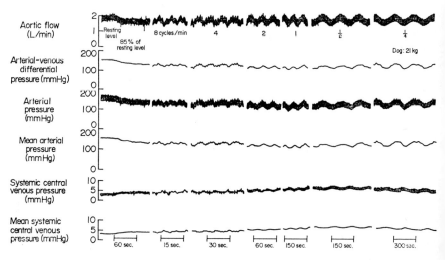

FIG. 17. Recording of an experiment in which the dynamic responses of arterial, venous, and arterial-venous pressure differences to variations of aortic flow were studied. The dynamic response of the system was determined by imposing sinusoidal variations in aortic flow with a constant amplitude ($\pm$ 10 per cent of control) over a frequency range of 8 to $\frac{1}{4}$ cycles/minute. (From Herndon, 1969, see text for details.)

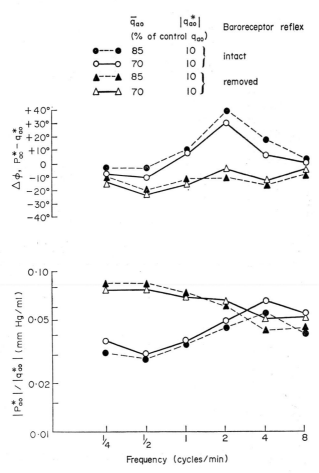

FIG. 18. (see legend under Fig. 20.)

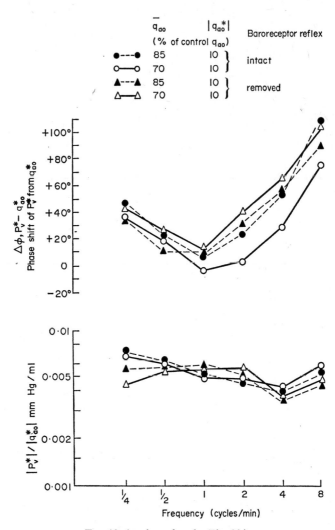

FIG. 19. (see legend under Fig. 20.)

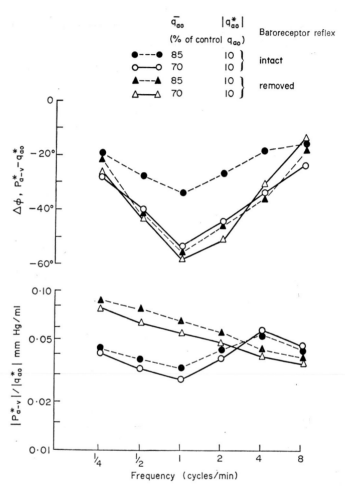

FIG. 20. Figs. 18–20 are Bode plots of the average results from experiments in which the frequency responses of arterial pressure, P_{ao}^* (Fig. 18), venous pressure, P_v^* (Fig. 19) and arterial-venous differential pressure, P_{a-v}^* (Fig. 20), to imposed sinusoidal variations in aortic flow, q_{ao}^*, of constant amplitude, were examined at two mean flow levels with and without the influence of the carotid and aortic baroreceptor reflexes. Note the resonance phenomenon (peaking of the amplitude ratio curve) seen in the frequency range of 1–8 cycles/min when the reflexes were intact, in Figs. 18 and 20, and its absence in Fig. 19. The mean control flow was $98 \cdot 5 \pm 1 \cdot 7$ ml/min/kg body weight.

The variation in aortic flow was $\pm$ 10 per cent of the control value, superimposed on a mean flow of 85 per cent of control ($\blacktriangle$) and of 75 per cent of control ($\triangle$). $\bigcirc$ and $\bullet$, baroreceptor reflexes intact; $\triangle$ and $\blacktriangle$, baroreceptor reflexes removed. (Redrawn from Herndon, 1969.)

Taylor (1966) investigated the arterial impedance in dogs in a similar very low frequency range. He used vagal stimulation with random bursts of stimulation to produce varying periods of reduced aortic flow. The resulting arterial pressure-flow relationship was analyzed by spectral density methods (see Chapter 10) to yield the frequency response curve shown in Fig. 21. It is strikingly similar to that in Fig. 18, both in the shape of the basic (reflexless) impedance curve and its modification by the autonomic nervous system.

Most previous studies on arterial impedance have not paid much attention to the ultra-low frequency range discussed above. However, this range is

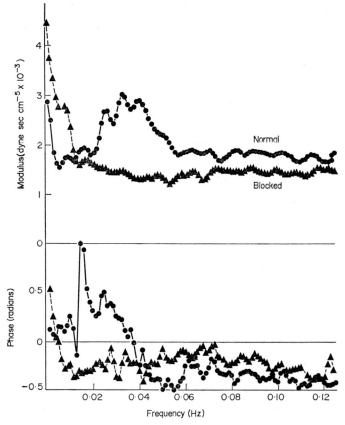

FIG. 21. Aortic impedance in the ultra-low frequency range before and after ganglionic blockade, studied in a dog. The heart rate was altered for random periods and the resulting changes in aortic flow and pressure analyzed. Note the similarity of both modulus and phase curves to those in Fig. 18, including the effect of eliminating the reflex control. (From Taylor, 1966.)

importantly related to the dynamic performances of many neural and some humoral reflex control systems, e.g., many analyses of the carotid sinus reflex (Scher and Young 1963) or aorticarch baroreceptor reflex (Allison *et al.*, 1969) indicate that the time course of vasomotor control in response to step forcing is about 20 to 30 sec. Therefore, for an accurate estimation of the reflex modification of vascular impedance we need to know the basic vascular impedance in this frequency range. Reflex control of vascular impedance can be accurately appreciated only when we know the dynamic characteristics of arterial impedance of the vascular bed in the absence of reflex responses.

(iii) *Coupling of the heart–lung pump and the systemic bed*

This subject is discussed on a beat-to-beat basis elsewhere (Chapter 7). Here, we concern ourselves with the static equilibrium between those two components of the cardiovascular plant. This can be done by solving simultaneously the equations which describe the interrelations between cardiac output, arterial pressure, and venous pressure. However the same can be achieved graphically, as was demonstrated by Guyton (1963b). Figure 22 shows such an equilibrium diagram, which deals with the shift of

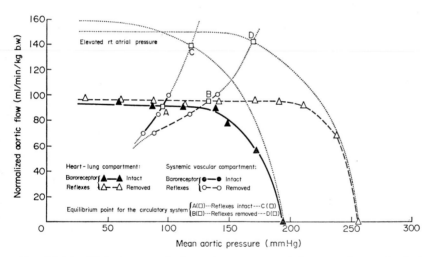

FIG. 22. Equilibria between the heart–lung pump and the systemic vascular bed seen at the left heart-ascending aortic junction. A and B represent equilibrium points for the cardiovascular system with a flow level of about 95 ml/min/kg body weight with and without the arterial baroreceptor reflexes, respectively. C and F represent equilibrium points for the system operating at a flow of about 140 ml/min/kg body weight with and without the arterial baroreceptor reflexes, respectively. (From Herndon, 1969.)

arterial pressure associated with an increase in blood volume. The inter-section A represents the normal equilibrium in a dog whereas the inter-section B is that which was seen when the arterial baroreceptor reflexes were removed from the experimental animal.

As the blood volume is expanded and the filling pressure of the heart–lung pump increased, the relationship between the cardiac output and arterial pressure shifts from the solid curve to the dotted curve which starts at a higher cardiac output level but intersects the arterial pressure axis at the same point as before. The new equilibrium is represented by the inter-section C which indicates an elevation of about 20 mmHg in arterial pressure and an increase of approximately 40 per cent in cardiac output. When the animal's barostatic reflex was removed, the control arterial pressure was higher due to the different systemic resistance (dashed curve) and after blood volume expansion, an approximately equal increase in cardiac output (point D) occurred. Note that the shifts of equilibrium from A to C with the reflex and B to D without the reflex cannot be understood without full knowledge of the non-linear performances of both system components in those pressure and flow ranges.

Figure 23 represents a similar shift of the equilibrium in a three-dimensional form, which enables one to see the change in central venous pressure as well. With computer aided devices, such complex interrelationships among three variables can readily be displayed. This type of information represented could be of great clinical value. For this to be possible, much more knowledge must be collected on the interactions of these major variables.

C. MULTIPLE OPENINGS IN THE CIRCULATORY LOOP

Further opening of the circulatory loop has been studied in models, for example, Grodins (1963) defined four segments: the right heart, the pulmonary circuit, the left heart and the systemic vascular bed. Defares *et al.* (1963) used a similar model. Both studies dealt with the basic mechanical system without any neural and humoral controls. Beneken and DeWit (1967) and Snyder and Rideout (1969) divided their models further, including decoupling of the parallel and series elements in the systemic vascular beds. All these will be discussed elsewhere (see Chapter 6).

The major use of such large models lies in predicting the quantitative role of a mechanism found experimentally in isolated portions of the circu-latory system (e.g. the effect of vascular flow-autoregulation on the total system) and then testing the prediction against experimental results. Such an interaction between the model and the experimental study has been limited thus far. To improve the situation arrangements are needed to aid the interchange of information between experimental physiologists and modellers. The physiologist could request specific information on the

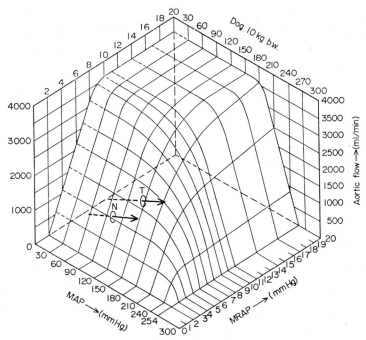

FIG. 23. A schematic three-dimensional equilibrium diagram for the heart–lung pump and the systemic circuit. Two arrows, which are superimposed on the cardiac output surface shown in Fig. 10, represent the static pressure-flow relationships in the systemic circuit, seen at both arterial and venous ports. The arrow, which intersects the cardiac output surface at point N, represents the normal total peripheral resistance, whereas the arrow, intersecting at point T, indicates the changes in vascular parameters (mean systemic pressure and resistance) after a large transfusion. Theoretical prediction for a dog without nervous control.

predicted properties of some real system and provide reference data, while the model predictions could be used to suggest crucial experiments. At the moment such collaboration is arranged on a personal basis and there is no doubt that the potential of the large computer model has not been fully exploited.

4. APPLICATION TO THE NEURAL CONTROL OF THE CIRCULATION

In this section, a few examples will be discussed in which control theory has been applied to the neural control of the circulation without much concern over the relation to the rest of the system.

A. BARORECEPTOR REFLEX CONTROL OF MEAN ARTERIAL PRESSURE

Because of its similarity to process control devices, the carotid sinus baroreceptor reflex control of mean arterial pressure has attracted investigators who were interested in applying control theory to biological mechanisms.

Koch (1931) pioneered open-loop analysis of the carotid sinus reflex and used the term "Selbststeuerung" (automatic control) before the engineers. Although his analysis was confined to the static performance of the open-loop system with a non-pulsatile pressure input to the isolated sinuses, the results of his study are still valid today. Recently, Scher and Young (1963) approximated the static non-linearity of this reflex system by the following equation:

$$\Delta P_o = -[G_m - K_o(P_i - P_m)^n](\Delta P_i) \tag{4.1}$$

where ΔP_o and ΔP_i are changes in output and input mean pressures respectively, G_m is maximal gain ($\Delta P_o/\Delta P_i$), P_m is the input pressure at which G_m is obtained, k_o is a positive constant and n is an even number.

The necessity for dealing with multiple input factors became clear when Ead et al. (1952) drew attention to the depressor effects of pulsations superimposed on a static sinus pressure. It was shown that this derived from an asymmetric rate sensitivity, which may be largely due to the properties of the baroreceptors themselves. Disregarding this dynamic non-linearity, the dynamic performance of the system can be approximated by the following description (Scher et al., 1967).

(i) Time domain expression:

$$k_2(dP_o/dt) + k_3(d^2P_o/dt^2) = k_1(dP_i/dt)(t - t_o) \tag{4.2}$$

(ii) Frequency domain expression:

$$\frac{P_{o(s)}}{P_{i(s)}} = \frac{k_4\, e^{-sL}}{(1 + \tau_1 S)^2} \tag{4.3}$$

where $t - t_o = L =$ transportation lag (or latency) of the reflex system, the observed value being about 1 to 2 sec, and τ_1 is a time constant of 4 to 10 sec. The Bode plots in Fig. 24 show the data from several studies in which the isolated sinus pressure was varied sinusoidally with a fixed small amplitude and over a frequency range from 0·5 to 10 cycles/min.

Scher and Young (1963) termed the depressor effect mentioned which was caused by superposition of high frequency sinusoids (up to 2 Hz) on the steady sinus pressure, "frequency dependent rectification"; and gave the following expression:

$$\Delta P_o = -G_R(P_i + dP_i/dt - K)\frac{[\text{Sgn}\,(P_i + dP_i/dt - K) + 1]}{2} \tag{4.4}$$

where ΔP_o is the change in mean arterial pressure due to the pulsatile com-

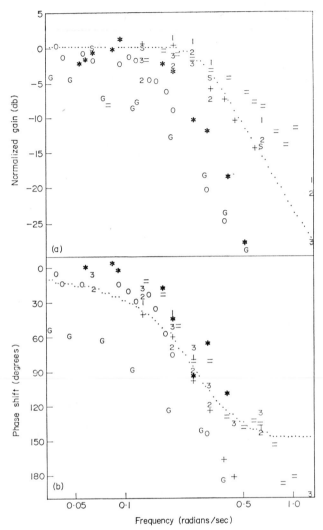

FIG. 24. Bode plots of the open-loop dynamic performance of the carotid sinus reflex system (intrasinus pressure as the input and mean arterial pressure as the output). Data from various authors are superimposed in this plot, and theoretical curves (dotted line). The upper half shows normalized gain against frequency and the lower half shows phase lag between changes in arterial pressure and changes in intrasinus pressure against frequency. Points labelled (1), (2) and (3) are from Levison et al. (1966); (G) Grodins (1963); (S) Scher and Young (1963). Symbols $(+)$, $(=)$, $(*)$ and $(\bigcirc)$ are from Ito (in Scher et al., 1967). The dotted curves were obtained by Scher et al. (1967) by solving the transfer function $k_2 (s + 2\cdot77)/(s + 55\cdot5) (s^2 + 1\cdot15s + 0\cdot255^2)$. The theoretical linear curves appear to account satisfactorily for the Bode plots of the frequency response data.

ponent of the input pressure, G_R is the amplification factor for the rectification effect, P_i is the amplitude of the superimposed sinusoids, K is a constant and Sgn is a function which has a value of $+ 1$ when the content of the bracket is positive and $- 1$ when the content is negative.

Levison *et al.* (1966) demonstrated further non-linear features of the dynamic behavior of the system. For example, a positive impulse with a short duration caused a depressor response whereas a negative impulse with a similar duration also caused a depressor response. A similar paradoxical response was found by Scher and Young (1963) (Fig. 25). Levison *et al.* (1966) also demonstrated that superposition of high frequency sinusoids on a slower sinusoidal pressure in the carotid sinuses diminished the amplitude of the reflex response of mean arterial pressure to the slow pressure waves

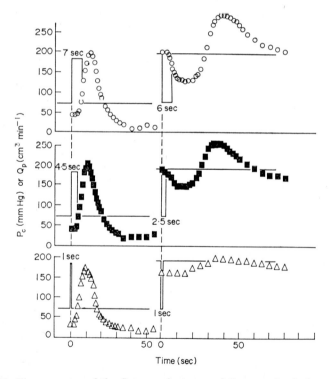

FIG. 25. The response of the flow conductance of the vascular bed to a square pressure pulse input into the isolated carotid sinuses shown by the lines. Note that with a short positive pulse, the conductance showed a marked increase, whereas no decrease but a slight increase was observed in response to a negative input pulse of similar duration (bottom panel). (From Scher *et al.*, 1967.)

(Fig. 26). This was confirmed by other investigators. Many textbooks state the baroreceptors respond "more effectively" to a pulsatile than to a non-pulsatile input. The overall reflex gain, however, attenuates if the input sinus pressure is pulsatile. Only if the amplitude of the pulsation diminishes simultaneously with the fall of the mean sinus pressure, may the overall reflex gain remain the same as (or be greater than) that obtained with a non-pulsatile input. Such a mechanism has been suspected in hemorrhage where both mean arterial pressure and pulse pressure decrease (Neil, 1952). Kumada et al. (1970) studied mild hemorrhage but failed to find evidence for the importance of the pulsatile signal in the reflex compensation of arterial pressure.

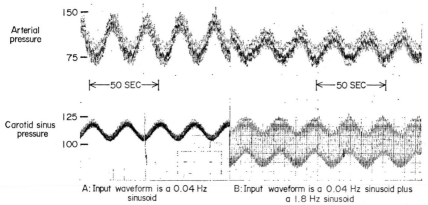

FIG. 26. Frequency responses to forcing of the opened carotid sinus reflex system at 0·04 Hz. A: input pressure in the carotid sinuses with pulsation at 0·04 Hz. B: a sinusoid of 1·8 Hz with a fixed amplitude of 25 mmHg was superimposed on the input pressure. Notice the drastic attenuation of the systemic arterial pressure response produced by the pulsation. (From Levison et al., 1966.)

Stegeman and Tibes (1969) demonstrated another important non-linearity which depends on the mean level of carotid sinus pressure. They showed that the frequency-dependent rectification reversed its polarity of rectification when the mean sinus pressure was above 180 mmHg. Fortunately, in the pressure range up to 150 mmHg, such a reversal has not been seen, and mean arterial pressure seldom rises above this level in response to ordinary acute stresses. This non-linearity appears to derive, at least in part, from a property of the receptor, since early work by Landgren (1952) and other recent studies on the receptor (Christensen et al., 1967; Koushanpour and McGee, 1968) indicate that the receptor fires more frequently in response to an identical step or pulsatile input when this is superimposed on a low initial or mean pressure than on a higher pressure.

The so-called vasomotor waves (Traube-Hering waves, Mayer waves, etc.) have been postulated to be positive feedback oscillations elicited via the baroreceptor reflex system (Guyton and Harris, 1951). Definite evidence for this has never been presented. The reported gain or phase margin of the open-loop carotid sinus reflex system (after vagotomy) is large enough to indicate a fair stability of this system (see Fig. 24). The stability of the aortic (and subclavian) baroreceptor reflex system also appears to be sufficient (Allison et al., 1969). However, no one has succeeded in driving both reflex systems in an open-loop condition to find the stability of the two baroreceptor reflex systems operating simultaneously in parallel, nor is the summation law of these parallel feedback loops in the center known.

    Those who have opened the carotid sinus loop after vagotomy and then closed it with an artificial external loop have often seen oscillations of arterial pressure due to slight delays in the artificial loop. This suggests that the closed-loop behavior of the reflex system might differ from that expected from the open-loop analysis due to some non-linearity. Therefore, it is possible that a slight change in some part of the sino-aortic feedback control system might alter it from a stable negative feedback mechanism into a hunting, or under-damped control system. Exactly what is or are those slight changes which elicit the instability remains to be known. The presence of multiple input factors and of many parallel reflex loops makes accurate appreciation of the baroreceptor reflex performance in natural closed-loop conditions extremely difficult.

B. CEREBRAL ISCHEMIC PRESSOR RESPONSE

This is an example of positive feedback oscillations which has been shown to result from a negative feedback mechanism in the cerebral control of the circulation. When the brain is rendered severely ischemic, the medullary center maximally excites both cardiac and vasoconstrictor centers for a few minutes. The result is an acute and drastic elevation of systemic arterial pressure which in turn improves the cerebral circulation. It may be regarded as an emergency type of negative feedback control of cerebral blood flow. Sagawa and Guyton (1961) opened this loop by isolating the cerebral perfusion pressure and lowering it in steps toward a level as low as 10 to 20 mmHg. The static relationship between cerebral perfusion pressure and systemic arterial pressure was found to be hyperbolic (Sagawa et al., 1961). In the low perfusion range, the performance of the system indicated a large overall open-loop gain (7·0 on average) with a long transportation lag (10 sec) and with a first- or second-order delay. The Nyquist diagram in Fig. 27 is an example of the open-loop performance of the cerebral ischemic pressor response. Notice that the vector locus crosses the instability point of

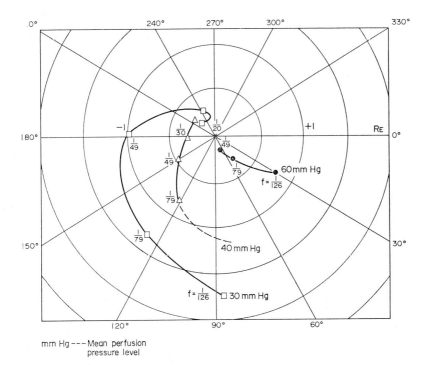

mm Hg – – – Mean perfusion
                pressure level

FIG. 27. Nyquist diagrams obtained from open-loop analysis of the cerebral
ischemic pressor response in the dog. Notice the strong influence of the d.c. voltage
level of input pressure (mean cerebral perfusion pressure) on the paths of the
vector loci, mainly in the gain parameter. Since the locus obtained at a mean
pressure of 30 mmHg crossed the —1 point, instability of the system under closed-
loop conditions was predicted. (From Sagawa, *et al.*, 1961.)

— 1 when the mean perfusion pressure was 30 mmHg. Therefore the closed-
loop behavior is expected to be unstable provided that the cerebral arterial
perfusion pressure is biased from the systemic arterial pressure to an appropriate degree (Sagawa *et al.*, 1961). The prediction from the open-loop
analysis was further verified by a closed-loop experiment in which the
isolated cerebral perfusion pressure was biased from systemic arterial pressure
by a constant amount, using a pressure bias device (Sagawa *et al.*, 1962). The
predicted oscillations did occur at the expected level of pressure bias and
at predicted frequencies (Fig. 28(a)). The oscillation is obviously similar
to that elicited by acutely elevating the intracranial pressure to near or
above the animal's arterial pressure (Fig. 28(b)). At the turn of the century,
Cushing (1901) described this phenomenon and explained it as a feedback
oscillation, though in medical terms. Guyton and Satterfield (1952) expanded
the idea of feedback oscillation as the basic mechanism of this effect. The

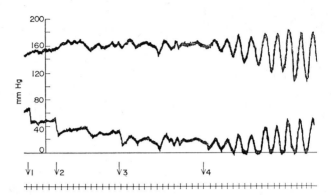

FIG. 28(a). A positive feedback oscillation in the dog's arterial pressure when the instability condition predicted from open-loop analysis of the cerebral ischemic pressor response was fulfilled. This was that the mean cerebral perfusion pressure be lowered to 15–30 mmHg while changes in mean arterial pressure are transmitted directly to the cerebral perfusion pressure. This was achieved by a servo-controlled perfusion of the brain. At the arrows the mean cerebral pressure (lower curve) was biased away from the systemic pressure (upper curve) by introducing a greater biasing d.c. voltage between the feedback (cerebral pressure) signal and the reference (systemic pressure) signal in the servo system. When the cerebral perfusion pressure was sufficiently reduced a sustained oscillation of mean arterial pressure occurred with amplitudes of 40–70 mmHg. Time intervals, 15 sec. Compare with Fig. 28(b). (From Sagawa *et al.*, 1962.)

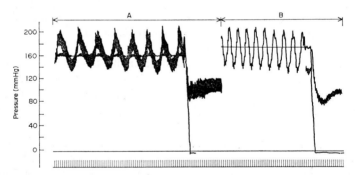

FIG. 28(b). The Cushing wave. The intra-cranial pressure of a dog was raised to the animal's mean arterial pressure, which then went into sustained oscillation. The horizontal line shows the intra-cranial pressure. The left half of the recording was obtained with the sino-aortic nerves intact and the right half after denervation. Time intervals, 5 sec. (From Guyton and Satterfield, 1952.)

open-loop analysis followed by the closed-loop verification by Sagawa *et al.* (1961, 1962) finally presented definite evidence that Cushing's waves are indeed feedback oscillations of the cerebral ischemic response.

C. NEURAL CONTROL OF RESISTANCE AND CAPACITANCE VESSELS

The dynamic aspects of neural control of the vessels can be studied by stimulating the vasomotor nerve innervating a vascular bed with sinusoidally modulated stimulus frequencies and relating the observed changes in resistance or capacitance to the frequency used. The normal nervous control of vasomotor tone acts through both frequency modulation of the impulse train in individual fibers and recruitment of different fibers. The above method involves only the former mechanism. However, the stimulus input to the nervous system can be controlled by holding the intensity at a supramaximal level and modulating the frequency around the mean or center frequency (e.g. about 4 Hz).

Using this method, Peňáz and his associates studied the dynamic characteristics of the nervous control of various resistance vessels (Peňáz and Buriánek, 1963; Peňáz *et al.*, 1966) and of the capacitance vessels in rabbit's ears (Peňáz, 1963). The frequency responses of the resistance of the carotid bed was studied by perfusing one carotid artery at a constant pressure and measuring the changes in blood flow in response to sinusoidal changes in stimulus frequency given to the ipsilateral cervical sympathetic nerve. The Bode plot in Fig. 29 shows the amplitude ratio (in arbitrary units) and phase shift in 24 experiments. The averaged flow amplitude curve showed a constant value from about 1 to 3 cycles/min and an attenuation of about 20 dB/decade in the range above the corner frequency (0·062 Hz). The phase lag reached −180° at 0·192 Hz, i.e. at this frequency the blood flow increased as the stimulus frequency increased. The broken line in the phase plot shows the system delay corrected for the transportation lag (or response latency) which was about 1·5 sec. The maximum delay of the system was then found to plateau at −90°, suggesting that the vasomotor response can be described approximately as a first-order delay system with a time constant of 2·5 sec and a transportation lag of 1·5 sec.

In many instances, the amplitude ratio curve showed a peak at an average frequency of 0·04 Hz; this is close to the resonance frequency observed in the systemic arterial impedance (Fig. 21). Peňáz's group (1963, 1966) also tested the system's response to step changes in stimulus frequency and found there was often an over- or under-shoot of flow, particularly when the stimulus frequency was decreased. The response subsided in a damped oscillatory fashion and the frequency of this damped oscillation was approximately 0·05 Hz. For the mechanism(s) underlying this resonance, the authors postulate competition between the nervous control and local auto-

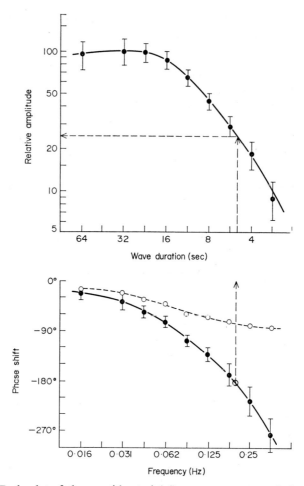

FIG. 29. Bode plot of the carotid arterial flow response to cervical sympathetic stimulation in the rabbit. The stimulus frequency was modulated sinusoidally at various frequencies (abscissa). The amplitude and phase lag of the flow variations are plotted after normalization of amplitude, as the means and standard deviations, from 24 experiments. The broken line in the phase plot shows the system delay after correcting for transportation lag. (From Peňáz and Buriánek, 1963.)

regulation of flow. Whatever the cause, these properties of the peripheral vasomotor control system explain some features of the baroreceptor reflex system such as the latency, delay and attenuation of reflex gain with increase in input frequency, and the asymmetric rate sensitivity to rising and falling input pressure.

Essentially the same frequency characteristics of nervous vasomotor control have been observed by the same group in the femoral arterial and the superior mesenteric arterial bed (Peňáz et al., 1966). Both showed an even more prominent peak at about 0·04–0·05 Hz, with comparable corner frequencies. The Bode plot in Fig. 30 represents data obtained in the femoral arterial bed.

Peňáz (1963) studied the dynamic response of the capacitance vessels of the ear to a similar frequency-modulated stimulation of the cervical sympathetic nerve. The changes in the volume of one ear were recorded by plethysmography and related to the frequency. The results of this study differ from those on the resistance vessel in the following respects (compare Fig. 31 with Figs. 29 and 30):

a. The latency of the venous response is longer (3 sec) than that of the resistance vessels.

b. The frequency characteristics of the venous response appear to reflect a second-order delay system rather than a first-order system, as indicated by the greater attenuation of approximately 30 dB/decade.

c. However, the measured phase lag of the capacitance vessels was not so large as that expected from the amplitude ratio curve.

d. No clearcut corner frequency was seen within the frequency range covered; this suggests that the system has a much slower response than the resistance control system.

Strictly speaking, the volume changes must lag behind the changes in capacitance (or compliance) because of the flow limitation due to the resistances distal to many capacitance vessels, and further analysis of vascular capacitance and its control is urgently needed for the better understanding of the circulation, however difficult this may be. The work by Peňáz (1963) certainly represents a step towards the quantitative analysis of the hitherto neglected venous segments.

D. DYNAMIC ANALYSIS OF THE DENERVATED VASCULAR BED

In the foregoing section, it was mentioned that the innervated vascular bed often responded with a damped oscillation of conductance to step changes in the frequency of vasomotor nerve stimulation. A similar oscilla-

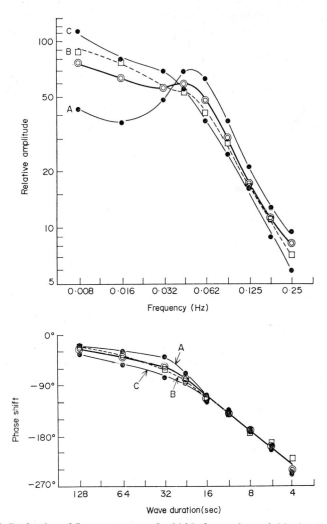

Fig. 30. Bode plot of flow responses of rabbit's femoral arterial bed to frequency-modulated stimulation of the lumbar sympathetic chain. The method and plot are similar to the experiment in Fig. 29. The heavy lines represent the average response from 20 experiments. Roughly one third of the group (A) showed a prominent peaking in the amplitude curve; this was less clear in another third (B) and absent in the remaining third (C). (From Peňáz *et al.*, 1966.)

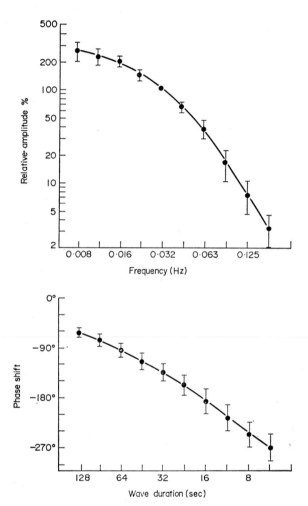

FIG. 31. Bode plot of the response of rabbit's ear capacitance vessels (measured as volume change) to frequency-modulated stimulation of the cervical sympathetic nerve. When compared with the frequency response of the resistance vessels, this system indicates greater attenuation of amplitude and larger increase in phase lag with frequency. Means and standard deviations from 20 experiments. (From Peñáz, 1963.)

tory response has also been noted in denervated vascular beds such as the kidney. Therefore, Başar and Weiss (1968) analyzed the frequency characteristics of conductance in the isolated rat's kidney. The perfusion pressure was elevated by steps from low to high levels. The flow responses were Fourier-analyzed and the results plotted in a Bode diagram as in Fig. 32. This figure shows the frequency responses to different step changes of pressure. Note that when the step was from 60 to 90 mmHg, the amplitude curve (broken line) is that of a simple second or higher order element. In contrast, when the pressure was raised to as high as 180 mmHg, the frequency characteristic curves indicated an irregular peaking in the range between 0·05 and 1 Hz and an irregular concavity in the neighborhood of 0·01 Hz, and similarly, the phase curve showed either a lead or lag at the corresponding frequencies. This peculiarity of the dynamic response of conductance was obviously correlated with flow-autoregulation, for when the step change covered the pressure range where flow autoregulation was operative, the characteristic distortion of the frequency curve was seen. That this was related to active vasomotor tone was demonstrated by another experiment in which the addition of papaverin to the perfusate resulted in the disappearance of the peaks and troughs in the amplitude curve.

The same group of investigators (Başar et al., 1968) used the same approach to the coronary bed of the isolated rat's heart. The heart was either relaxed or in flutter during the test. The frequency characteristic curves obtained (Fig. 33) were almost identical to those from the kidney, and again perfusion with papaverin removed the peaks and troughs.

On the basis of these results, Başar and co-workers contend that both vascular beds possess the same basic mechanical property, and that the dynamic characteristics derive from the myogenic response of the vascular bed to altered distending pressure. The latter contention, however, needs further investigation in view of a number of other findings for other theories on flow-autoregulation in those vascular beds. The major contribution of this study is that it provided an accurate description of vascular conductance in the low frequency range, which has been generally neglected. The identification of the different frequency characteristics for different input steps is particularly important. Thus, their data are useful as test material against which the outputs of various models of vascular autoregulation of conductance may be tested. Similar quantitative descriptions of these and other vascular beds, with the nervous control held at a normal level, and forced with pressure or flow inputs at both the arterial and venous ends will provide an even better description of the subsystems of the circulatory system. Unless such analytical data accumulate to some extent no detailed and reasonably isomorphic mechanical model of the entire cardiovascular system will be attained.

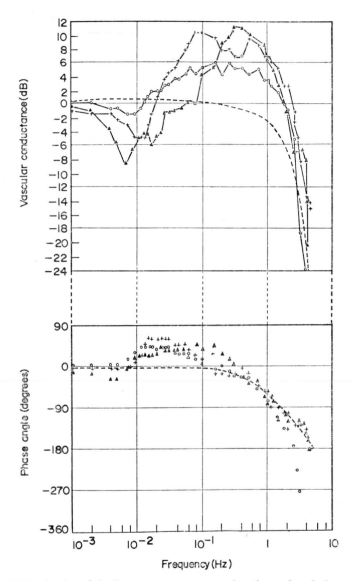

Fig. 32. Bode plot of the flow responses to step elevations of perfusion pressure in the isolated rat's kidney. The pressure steps were from 150 to 180 mmHg (▲), from 90 to 180 mmHg (+), 40 to 180 mmHg (○), and from 60 to 90 mmHg (– – –). Note that, in the last case (– – –) there was no peak in the amplitude ratio curve and no lead in the phase shift curve. The static ratios ($\Delta q/\Delta P$) were different for different steps but were normalized to 0 dB for comparison. Injection of papaverin produced responses lying around the dashed line. (From Başar and Weiss, 1968.)

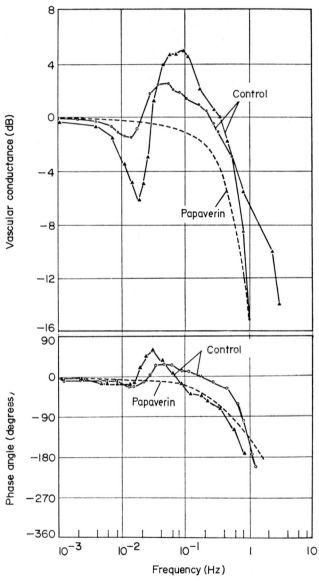

FIG. 33. Bode plots of the coronary flow responses to step increases in perfusion pressure in the isolated rat's heart. ▲, heart in flutter; ○, inactive heart. The broken line is the response after papaverin infusion. Note the similarity of these curves to those in Fig. 32. (From Başar *et al.*, 1968.)

5. CONCLUDING REMARKS

This review of control theory studies may be rather disappointing to some readers. For a fluid dynamicist whose interest is the biophysics of the circulatory system there will be no depth or mathematical rigor. The black-box description is phenomenological, revealing little about underlying mechanisms. To a clinician, the lack of clear integration between the pieces of information at the level of the individual will make the material seem fragmentary. What then are these studies for?

The answer is two-fold. They provide the basic knowledge for the understanding of overall circulatory mechanics, in which the concern lies in the interactions between the major components of the circulatory and other systems (e.g. the kidney as a component of body fluid regulation). For some time to come we cannot hope that such complex problems can be modelled (that is, explained) in terms of cellular or molecular physiology. The sort of description of the behavior of the circulatory system given here is the only feasible path leading to an approximate but reasonably accurate understanding of homeostasis in its broadest context.

Another purpose of the black-box type studies described above is to serve as a convenient set of experimental data to compare with the outputs of models comprising components of the box itself. For systems analysis of complex biological controls it is necessary to define the assumptions, input–output variables, system parameters, constraints and boundaries, etc. Consequently, the design of methods and the presentation of results have to be very well defined. This greatly aids in testing proposed models, without which modelling is a useless game.

For the above reasons, this class of experimental studies is an important bridge between in-depth investigation and integrative understanding. Erroneously, many of them are considered "descriptive" models; there is no such thing as a descriptive model since a model represents understanding in terms of elements and interactive forces. Otherwise, there will be as many models as the number of regression analyses ever performed. Therefore, these black-box descriptions ought rather to be looked upon as the building blocks for a model of larger systems yet to come.

ACKNOWLEDGEMENTS

Grateful thanks are extended to all the authors for their generous offer of permission to reproduce those figures cited in this chapter. Thanks are also due to the publishers of those figures. Figures 21 and 26 were reproduced by permission of The American Heart Association; figures 10, 27, 28(a), (b) by permission of the American Physiological Society; figures 12, 24 and 25 by permission of W. B. Saunders Co.; figure 29 by permission of Pergamon Press; figure 30 by permission of H. Vaillant-Carmanne, S.A., and figures 31, 32 and 33 by permission of Springer-Verlag New York Inc.

REFERENCES

TEXTBOOKS ON CONTROL THEORY

A. *Application of control theory to biological systems*

Grodins, F. S. (1963). "Control Theory and Biological Systems", Columbia University Press, New York.

Milhorn, H. T. (1966). "Application of Control Theory to Physiological Systems", W. B. Saunders, Philadelphia.

Milsum, J. H. (1966). "Biological Control Systems Analysis", McGraw-Hill, New York.

Riggs, D. S. (1970). "Control Theory and Physiological Feedback Mechanisms", Williams and Wilkins, Baltimore.

B. *Introduction to vectorial presentation*

Schultz, D. G. and Melsa, J. L. (1967). "State Functions and Linear Control Systems", McGraw-Hill, New York.

Elgard, O. I. (1967). "Control Systems Theory", McGraw-Hill, New York.

C. *Systems theories of hierarchical systems*

Whyte, L. L., Wilson, A. G. and Wilson, D. (1969). "Hierarchical Structures", Elsevier, New York.

Mesarvoic, M. D., Macko, D. and Takahara, Y. (1970). "Theory of Hierarchical, Multilevel Systems", Academic Press, New York and London.

ORIGINAL REPORTS

Allison, J. L., Sagawa, K. and Kumada, M. (1969). An open-loop analysis of the aortic arch barostatic reflex. *Am. J. Physiol.* **217**, 1576–1584.

Başar, E. and Weiss, C. (1968). Analyse des Frequenzganges druckinduzierter Änderungen des Strömungswiederstandes isolierter Rattennieren. *Pflügers Arch.* **304**, 121–135.

Başar, E., Ruedas, G., Schwarzkopf, H. J. and Weiss, C. (1968). Untersuchungen des zeitlichen Verhaltens druckabhängiger Änderungen des Strömungswiederstandes in Coronargefäss-system des Rattenherzens. *Pflügers Arch.* **304**, 189–202.

Beneken, J. E. W. and DeWit, B. (1967). A physical approach to hemodynamic aspects of the human cardiovascular system. *In* "Physical Basis of Circulatory Transport: Regulation and Exchange" (E. B. Reeve and A. C. Guyton, eds.), pp. 1–45, W. B. Saunders, Philadelphia.

Christensen, B. N., Warner, H. R. and Pryor, T. A. (1967). A technique for the quantitative study of carotid sinus behavior. *In* "Baroreceptors and Hypertension" (P. Kezdi, ed.), pp. 41–50, Pergamon Press, Oxford.

Clancy, R. L., Graham, T. P., Jr., Ross, J., Jr., Sonnenblick, E. H. and Braunwald, E. (1968). Influence of aortic pressure-induced homeometric autoregulation on myocardial performance. *Am. J. Physiol.* **214**, 1186–1192.

Cushing, H. (1901). Concerning a definite regulatory mechanism of the vasomotor center which controls blood pressure during cerebral compression. *Bull. Johns Hopkins Hosp.* **12**, 290–292.

Defares, J. G., Osborn, J. J. and Hara, H. H. (1963). Theoretical synthesis of the cardiovascular system: Study I, The controlled system. *Acta Physiol. Pharmacol. Neerl.* **12**, 189–265.

Ead, H. W., Green, J. H. and Neil, E. (1952). A comparison of the effects of pulsatile and non-pulsatile blood flow through the carotid sinus on the reflexogenic activity of the sinus baroreceptors in the cat. *J. Physiol.* **118**, 509–519.

Folkow, B. (1952). A study of the factors influencing the tone of denervated blood vessels perfused at various pressures. *Acta Physiol. Scand.* **27**, 99–117.

Folkow, B. and Mellander, S. (1964). Veins and venous tone. *Am. Heart J.* **68**, 397–408.

Gebber, G. L. and Snyder, D. W. (1970). Hypothalamic control of baroreceptor reflexes. *Am. J. Physiol.* **218**, 124–131.

Granger, H. J. and Guyton, A. C. (1969). Autoregulation of the total systemic circulation following destruction of the central nervous system in the dog. *Circulation Res.* **25**, 379–388.

Grodins, F. S., Stuart, W. H. and Veenstra, R. L. (1960). Performance characteristics of the right heart bypass preparation. *Am. J. Physiol.* **198**, 552–560.

Grodins, F. S. (1963). "Control Theory and Biological Systems", Columbia University Press, New York.

Guyton, A. C. and Harris, J. W. (1951). Pressoreceptor-autonomic oscillation: A probable cause of vasomotor waves. *Am. J. Physiol.* **165**, 158–160.

Guyton, A. C. and Satterfield, J. H. (1952). Vasomotor waves possibly resulting from CNS ischemic reflex oscillation. *Am. J. Physiol.* **170**, 601–605.

Guyton, A. C. (1955). Determination of cardiac output by equating venous return curves with cardiac response curves. *Physiol. Rev.* **35**, 123–129.

Guyton, A. C., Abernathy, J. B., Langston, J. B., Kaufmann, B. N. and Fairchild, H. M. (1955). Relative importance of venous and arterial resistances in controlling venous return and cardiac output. *Am. J. Physiol.* **196**, 1008–1014.

Guyton, A. C., Lindsey, A. W., Kaufmann, B. N. and Abernathy, J. B. (1958). Effect of blood transfusion and hemorrhage on cardiac output and on the venous return curve. *Am. J. Physiol.* **194**, 263–267.

Guyton, A. C. (1963a). Venous return. *In* "Handbook of Physiology. Section 2", Vol. II, pp. 1099–1133, American Physiological Society, Washington.

Guyton, A. C. (1963b). "Circulatory Physiology: Cardiac Output and Its Regulation", W. B. Saunders, Philadelphia.

Herndon, C. W. and Sagawa, K. (1969). Combined effects of aortic and right atrial pressures on aortic flow. *Am. J. Physiol.* **217**, 65–72.

Herndon, C. W. (1969). Servoanalysis of the cardiovascular system. Ph.D. Thesis: University of Mississippi.

Hilton, S. M. (1966). Hypothalamic regulation of the cardiovascular system. *Brit. med. Bull.* **22**, 243–248.

Hockman, C. H., Talesnik, J. and Livingston, K. E. (1969). Central nervous system modulation of baroreceptor reflexes. *Am. J. Physiol.* **217**, 1681–1689.

Koch, E. (1931). "Die reflektorisch Selbststeuerung des Kreislaufes", Steinkopf, Dresden and Leipzig.

Koushanpour, E. and McGee, J. P. (1968). Demodulation of electrical activity in the carotid sinus baroreceptor nerve. *J. Appl. Physiol.* **24**, 262–266.

Kumada, M., Schmidt, R. M., Sagawa, K. and Tan, K. S. (1970). The carotid sinus reflex in response to hemorrhage. *Am. J. Physiol.* **219**, 1373–1379.

Landgren, S. (1952). On the excitation mechanism of the carotid sinus baroreceptors. *Acta Physiol. Scand.* **26**, 1–34.

Levison, W. H., Barnett, G. O. and Jackson, W. D. (1966). Non-linear analysis of the baroreceptor reflex system. *Circulation Res.* **18**, 673–682.

Levy, M. N., Brind, S. H., Brandlin, F. R. and Philips, F. A. (1954). The relation-ship between pressure and flow in the systemic circulation of the dog. *Circu-lation Res.* **11**, 372–380.

Neil, E. (1952). The carotid and aortic vasosensory areas. *Arch. Middlesex Hospital*, **4**, 16–27.

Peňáz, J. (1963). Frequenzgang der vasomotorischen Reaktionen der kapazitiven Gefässe des Kaninchenohres; ein Beitrag zur Deutung des Plethysmogrammes. *Pflügers. Arch.* **276**, 636–651.

Peňáz, J. and Buriánek, P. (1963). Dynamic performance of vasomotor responses of the resistance vessels of the carotid vascular bed in the rabbit. *Arch. Internat. Physiol. Biochemie*, **71**, 499–517.

Peňáz, J., Buriánek, P. and Semrad, B. (1966). Dynamic aspects of vasomotor and autoregulatory control of blood flow. *In* "Circulation in Skeletal Muscle" (O. Hudlicka, ed.), pp. 255–269, Pergamon Press, Oxford.

Read, R. C., Kuida, H. and Johnson, J. A. (1957). Effect of alterations in vasomotor tone on pressure-flow relationships in the totally perfused dog. *Circulation Res.* **5**, 676–682.

Richardson, T., Stallings, J. O. and Guyton, A. C. (1961). Pressure–volume curves in live, intact dogs. *Am. J. Physiol.* **201**, 471–474.

Ross, J., Jr., Linhart, J. W. and Braunwald, E. (1965). Effect of changing heart rate in man by electrical stimulation of the right atrium. Studies at rest, during exercise, and with isoproterenol. *Circulation* **32**, 549–558.

Sagawa, K. and Guyton, A. C. (1961). Pressure-flow relationships in isolated canine cerebral circulation. *Am. J. Physiol.* **200**, 711–714.

Sagawa, K., Ross, J. M. and Guyton, A. C. (1961). Quantitation of cerebral ischemic pressor response in dogs. *Am. J. Physiol.* **200**, 1164–1168.

Sagawa, K., Taylor, A. E. and Guyton, A. C. (1961). Dynamic performance and stability of cerebral ischemic pressor response. *Am. J. Physiol* **201**, 1164–1172.

Sagawa, K., Carrier, O. and Guyton, A. C. (1962). Elicitation of theoretically predicted feedback oscillation in arterial pressure. *Am. J. Physiol.* **203**, 141–146.

Sagawa, K. (1967). Analysis of the ventricular pumping capacity as a function of input and output pressure loads. *In* "Physical Basis of Circulatory Transport" (E. B. Reeve and A. C. Guyton, eds.), pp. 141–149, W. B. Saunders, Philadelphia.

Sarnoff, S. J., Mitchell, J. H., Gilmore, J. P. and Remensnyder, J. P. (1960). Homeometric autoregulation in the heart. *Circulation Res.* **8**, 1077–1091.

Sato, T., Yamashiro, S. M. and Grodins, F. S. (1971). Measurement of peripheral vascular properties by a frequency response method. *Am. J. Physiol.* **220**, 1640–1650.

Scher, A. M. and Young, A. C. (1963). Servoanalysis of carotid sinus reflex effects on peripheral resistance. *Circulation Res.* **12**, 152–162.

Scher, A. M., Franz, G. N., Ito, C. S. and Young, A. C. (1967). Studies on the carotid sinus reflex. *In* "Physical Basis of Circulatory Transport: Regulation and Exchange" (E. B. Reeve and A. C. Guyton, eds.), pp. 113–210, W. B. Saunders, Philadelphia.

Scher, A. M., Young, A. C. and Kehl, T. H. (1968). The regulation of stroke volume in the resting, unanesthetized dog. *Comput. Biomed. Res.* **1**, 315–336.

Shoukas, A. A. and Sagawa, K. (1970). Total systemic vascular compliance measured as incremental volume-pressure ratio. *Circulation Res.* **28**, 277–289.

Smith, O. A., Jr., Nathan, M. A. and Clarke, N. P. (1968). Central nervous system pathways mediating blood pressure changes. *In* "Neural Control of Arterial Pressure" (J. E. Wood, ed.), Hypertension, Vol. 16, pp. 9–20, American Heart Association, New York.

Snyder, M. F. and Rideout, V. C. (1969). Computer simulation studies of the venous circulation. *IEEE Trans. Bio-Med. Engr.* **BME-16,** 325–334.

Stegeman, J. and Tibes, U. (1969). Der Einfluss von Amplitude, Frequenz und Mittelwert Sinus förmiger Reizdrucke an den Pressoreceptoren auf den arteriellen Mitteldruck des Hundes. *Pflügers Arch.* **305,** 219–228.

Taylor, M. G. (1966). Use of random excitation and spectral analysis in the study of frequency-dependent parameters of the cardiovascular system. *Circulation Res.* **18,** 585–595.

Weiss, G. K. and Crill, W. E. (1969). Carotid sinus nerve: Primary afferent depolarization evoked by hypothalamic stimulation. *Brain Res.* **16,** 269–272.

Wilcken, D. E., Charlier, A. A., Hoffman, J. I. E. and Guz, A. (1963). Effects of alterations in aortic impedance on the performance of the ventricles. *Circulation Res.* **14,** 283–293.

Chapter 6

Some Computer Models in Cardiovascular Research

JAN E. W. BENEKEN

Research Group on Cardiovascular Physics,
Institute of Medical Physics TNO, Da Costakade, Utrecht, The Netherlands

1. INTRODUCTION

A. DEFINITION

The word "model" has been used and misused and has been subject to many interpretations. A comprehensive definition has been given by Fitzhugh (1969): "A model is something simple made by a scientist to help him understand something complicated. A model can consist of mathematical equations, an imaginary molecular structure obeying laws of physics, or a machine

173

which is physically different from the original phenomenon but which simulates its behaviour."

The purpose of this chapter is to review applications of modelling techniques in different areas which are related to the cardiovascular system, and to present a careful look into the future. No attempt is made to give a complete literature review; however, a few examples will be given in each area. The discussion will be limited to models designed to support theoretical considerations and of models designed for clinical or experimental applications.

The section on heart and heart muscle deals with the behaviour of muscle models in comparison with actual muscle behaviour, and with some attempts to approximate the shape of both ventricles. In the section on haemodynamics, some models of the arterial system are discussed in relation to clinical applications. Model studies on the venous system are limited in number but show promising results. A separate section is devoted to models of cardiovascular control. The transport function of the circulation receives much attention. In many disciplines the time has come for model applications related to transport phenomena. This is the reason for presenting some basic material related to simulation of transport by the bloodstream. Parameter estimation with the aid of models may develop into an important method for the indirect determination of quantitative data from patients.

Computer applications concerning monitoring or signal processing, and model studies described without mentioning possible applications will not be discussed. Another equally important area had to be excluded from this contribution; this is preprogrammed simulators (sometimes using tape recordings) such as those for teaching routines in coronary care or anaesthesia.

B. GENERAL CONSIDERATIONS ON MODELS

Except for the one definition cited earlier, very few authors make an attempt to define their concept of models. On the other hand, many make subdivisions according to differences in approach or application. In order to emphasize the different points of view from which one can look at models, some of these considerations will be reviewed briefly.

Berman (1963) distinguishes four different purposes of models: to describe data, to describe responses of a system to a stimulus, to simulate, and to characterize a system. He also refers to the need for consistency and uniqueness in models and to the requirement that parameters can be determined with reasonable precision. Higinbotham et al. (1963) state that models can be useful both when a system is known but the answers are unknown, and when, from an unknown system, the answers are known, e.g. from experimental results. According to Priban (1968) "a model always begins as a mental image which we use to explain the observable phenomena". He sees the need for models arising from the fact that many aspects of biological systems are being studied individually and that interaction receives very little attention. In his opinion evaluation of the effectiveness of a treatment will also be an important area in which models need to be applied.

Rideout (1969) recognizes two different approaches: one is to start with a complicated model and subsequently simplify it when more information becomes available or when the influence of some parameters proves to be negligible in view of their range and the required precision. The other is to start with a simple model and add to it if further studies and checks make this necessary and possible. In most cases the second approach is the only possible one because of the complexity of biological systems.

Other distinctions can be made, e.g. between deterministic and statistical models. The first type is likely to yield more insight into physiological processes because it is based on cause and effect considerations.

The user's model and the research model are entirely different: a user's model will remain in use as long as the original requirements persist. For example, Vadot's (1963) computer for the calculation of valve defects or shunts is acceptable within a limited range of accuracy and as long as pulsatile phenomena are not considered to play an important role. The research model, on the other hand, may be considered an hypothesis in which, within the limits of the original purposes, most known facts are taken into account. This model will be updated each time new information becomes available.

In some publications, the cardiovascular system of an experimental animal is referred to as a model of the human cardiovascular system. In view of the general acceptance of the meaning of the word "model", it is possibly better to refer to certain aspects of the animal being an analog of some human aspects. Usually, a model is a simplifying and known representation of a system.

Finally, a single class of models is worth mentioning, viz. the didactic model. An excellent example of this class is the "vascular waterfall" concept used by Permutt (1965). Although not introduced as a didactic model, it contributed considerably to the understanding of flow through collapsible tubes.

It is interesting to observe that none of the above-mentioned distinctions are contradictory but rather supplementary. As a consequence of this, it will be clear that it is incorrect to speak of *the* model of a system. The number of models that can be set up for a system equals the number of different points of view or different aspects of the system. One of the prerequisites to devising a model of a system, therefore, is to define its purpose exactly; in other words, what questions must it help to answer? As an example, in models of the systemic arterial bed:

(a) For a description of the afterload on the left ventricle, the proper input impedance of the arterial tree is sufficient.

(b) To study haemodynamics and transmission characteristics, the bandwidth of lumped segments and the velocity profile may need to be considered and wall viscosity parameters may need to be included.

(c) Pulsatility may need to be included to study short-term cardiovascular control, but may be unnecessary if long-term control is to be studied.

(d) Similarly in the case of transport by the blood stream; when simulating slow processes, like the uptake and distribution of anaesthetics, the inclusion of pulsatility, resulting in a large number of series compartments, is superfluous, while in the study of dye transport it is usually essential.

(e) For the study of thermoregulation or heat flow, pulsatility is of minor importance.

(f) In the case of a teaching model it entirely depends upon what is to be demonstrated as to whether a distributed system transmission line or a single compliance (Windkessel) needs to be used.

A number of different ways exist to materialize models. In haemodynamic research most models will originate as mathematical models representable by means of an analog, digital or hybrid computer, or by means of an electrical or hydraulic analog.

The analog computer operates rapidly because it solves the equations simultaneously, so that real time (or faster) operation is possible. In general, the time scale can be chosen at will, thus allowing either speeding up or slowing down of the simulation with respect to the original system. The analog computer is moderately flexible and permits an easy man–machine interaction. Its accuracy is limited, but in most cases acceptable. It is important to realize that the accuracy must be such that reproducible results are obtained from the computer model, despite the fact that considerable uncertainty exists about the basic parameters. The disadvantage of the analog computer is the absence of memory facilities often needed for transport delays or optimization procedures using experimental data.

Simulation of larger systems on the digital computer is usually slow, because of its principle of series operation. The flexibility in making program changes depends very much on the program; changing programs is usually fast. The digital computer is basically the more accurate, but the accuracy of the digital simulation may be exchanged for speed of operation by such techniques as selecting numerical methods and sampling rates.

The hybrid computer is a nearly ideal research tool, in that it combines the speed and flexibility of an analog computer with the memory and logical capability of a digital computer and is particularly suited for parameter estimation procedures and large simulations. The concept of parameter estimation and optimal control by means of models is the basis for development of patient adapted models which may be used in the future to determine optimal medical treatment. Because of the availability of digital computers, as well as the relative simplicity and reliability with which they can perform routine operations, clinical applications will probably involve digital computers. During the development phase of these parameter estimation schemes, the hybrid computer will be indispensable because of its versatility; extensive studies of parameter sensitivities must be made, for example in order to design an optimal model with a minimum number of parameters to be determined.

The electrical analog (see, for example, Noordergraaf, 1969) is relatively inexpensive and is particularly suitable for models requiring a large number of segments. It has a limited capability for introducing parameter changes, usually in steps. The application of such analogs has as yet been restricted to the description of linear systems.

The hydraulic analog, using pumps and tubing, is very useful for didactic purposes. Some hydraulic components can easily be introduced (d.c. resistance); others are more difficult to implement (compliances, or resistances with correct frequency dependence). A major application is the testing of prosthetic valves and artificial hearts.

2. HEART AND HEART MUSCLE

A. HEART MUSCLE

Warner (1959) published a computer model of the cardiovascular system in which he represented the action of the heart by time-varying compliances. Since then, many others have used the same principle (e.g. Beneken, 1963; Dick and Rideout, 1965), which is very attractive because the time course and amplitude of the compliance can be changed easily. The need for a description which is more firmly based on actual cardiac muscle properties arises when control phenomena acting on the heart or changes in intrinsic cardiac properties have to be taken into account. Robinson (1963) was the first to characterize the properties of the heart pump starting from muscle properties. In 1965, he published a further analysis schematically separating the left ventricular volume into contractile and series elastic fractions. His model included homeometric autoregulation and the Frank-Starling mechanism.

A detailed description of cardiac muscle mechanics was developed by Grupping (1963) and by Beneken and Grupping (1965). The description in terms of a three-element model (Fig. 1) incorporates the force-velocity relation

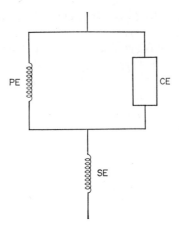

FIG. 1. Voigt three-element model of cardiac muscle, as used by Grupping (1963). PE = parallel elastic element, CE = contractile element, SE = series elastic element.

of the contractile element (CE). Grupping also introduced a dimensionless active state factor α, so that:

$$K_C = \alpha k K_{OC}, \tag{2.1}$$

α active state factor, dependent only on time

k velocity factor, dependent only on CE velocity, V_C (Hill relation)

K_{OC} fully activated CE force dependent only on CE length, L_C

$\alpha = 0$ non-active muscle

$\alpha = 1$ fully active muscle

$k = 0$ shortening velocity V_C is maximal

$k = 1$ shortening velocity is zero.

In non-active muscle α was assumed zero and for the fully activated muscle, the factor was, by definition, equal to one. In other words, Grupping assumed the contractile element at rest to be freely extensible. The transition of the activation factor from zero to unity occurred abruptly; the decay of the active state factor was gradual.

Beneken (1965) used the same force-velocity relation with some modifications in the length-force relations of the three elements, based on more reliable information from the literature. Some evidence was available indicating that the end-diastolic pressure-volume relation was subject to variation. The parallel elastic element, which by definition has constant properties, could not account for these. Therefore Beneken assumed that the non-activated contractile element was not freely extensible; this was expressed by giving the active state factor a small value instead of zero at rest. More recent evidence on this point was presented by Donders and Beneken (1971).

In 1967 Beneken and De Wit adapted the force-velocity relation of the contractile element to include a relation with the time after stimulation, as measured by Sonnenblick (1965). Assuming a fixed time course of the active state factor, a formula for the force-velocity relation was derived analytically with the active state factor as a time-varying parameter to fit Sonnenblick's measurement data. The upper half of Fig. 2 represents the new relation. Extrapolation of the hyperbolic curves into the lower half gave values for the lengthening velocities which were too low when incorporated in a complete ventricular model. Steeper lengthening velocity curves, as shown in the lower half, were required. No data on this were available to support or disprove

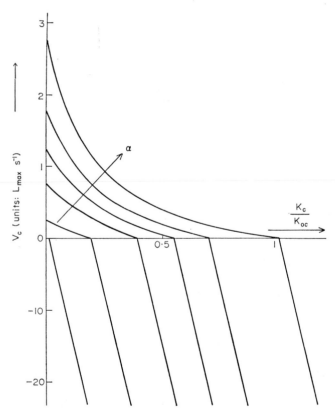

Fig. 2. Force-velocity relation of contractile element (CE). α = active state factor; V_C, K_C = velocity and force of CE, respectively; K_{OC} = force of CE when fully activated and when no shortening or lengthening occurs. K_{OC} is only a function of CE length; L_{max} = length at maximum developed force. Reproduced from Beneken and De Wit (1967) by permission of W. B. Saunders Co.

7*

these assumptions. This illustrates how model synthesis can indicate gaps in knowledge.

Donders and Beneken (1971) concluded from a comparison of model and actual muscle behaviour that a fan-shaped arrangement of lengthening-velocity curves, in which high values of the active state factor give a less steep slope, yields better results. This implies that it is more difficult to stretch the fully activated contractile element than the non-activated CE. Figure 3

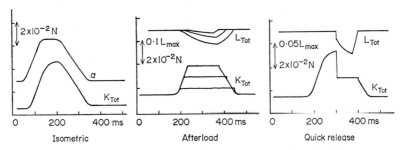

Isometric	Afterload	Quick release

FIG. 3. Three representative contraction patterns obtained with a computer model of cardiac muscle after Beneken and De Wit (1967). Length of muscle equals $0.92\ L_{max}$, where L_{max} represents the length at which maximum force is developed; cross-sectional area $1 \times 10^{-6}\ m^2$. Preload $0.4 \times 10^{-2}N$.

shows examples of the behaviour of the model of Beneken and De Wit (1967). Donders and Beneken (1971) discussed this model in great detail and its merits and limitations were shown. Descriptions of heart muscle behaviour are still phenomenological in that they are based on measurements interpreted in terms of two or more element models. They are very useful for checking the internal consistency of measured data. The muscle properties are highly non-linear, which makes synthesis by computer very meaningful. The following example will illustrate this.

Phase-plane tracings from real muscle were compared with those from the model (Fig. 4). Both show the same feature of the common pathway. By starting from different initial muscle lengths, the points on this common pathway are reached at different times after stimulation. This means that the relation between length and velocity, at a given constant total load, is for some period independent of time. Donders and Beneken (1971) showed that this common pathway can only exist if there is a plateau in the time course of the active state factor. Decay of this factor is the cause of the dissociation of the traces at the right-hand side. When this model was proposed these relationships were not known. The fact that the model produced results similar to those obtained with the muscle means that these muscle experiments did not, basically, generate new knowledge, i.e. the information was

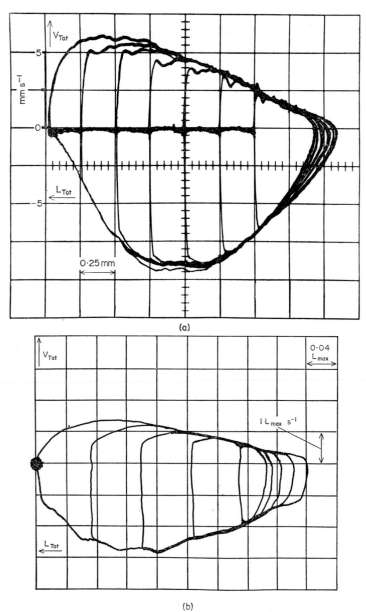

(a)

(b)

FIG. 4(a). Velocity-length phase-plane tracings from afterloaded contractions. Total load was held constant. Initial muscle length was reduced between contractions (Brutsaert and Sonnenblick, 1969).

(b). Similar phase-plane tracings taken from the muscle model by Beneken and De Wit (1967). Observe common pathway regardless of different initial lengths.

already present, though hidden in the original data on which the model was based. However, due to the complexity, this conclusion could not be reached without the model study. This is the sort of interaction between physiological and model experiments that can be very fruitful.

Another intrinsic property of heart muscle, the influence of the interval between beats on the amplitude of the contraction was implemented by Beneken and De Wit (1967). The following empirical formula describes the change in contraction height as a result of an interval change at $t = t_N$.

$$H(t) = a + b.f_N + c(f_N - f_{N-1})U(t - t_N)\left\{1 - 2\exp\left[-\frac{(t - t_N)}{\tau}\right]\right\}, \quad (2.2)$$

where $H(t)$ is a multiplication factor for the active state factor α, and equals unity for the normal heart rate

f_N is heart rate (inverse of interval) at $t = t_N$

$U(t - t_N)$ is a unit step function, which equals zero at $t < t_N$ and equals unity at $t > t_N$

a, b, c and τ are constants.

When this relation is included the muscle model exhibits similar responses to sudden rate changes (e.g. extrasystoles) as does heart muscle. Johnson and Kuohung (1968) developed the "trigamma" system on a basis of a number of compartments that must be passed by some transmitter substance. Their results also compare favourably with actual muscle behaviour during rate changes.

B. VENTRICULAR SHAPE

To model ventricular behaviour, the shape of the cavity and the thickness of the wall have to be considered, as well as the muscle behaviour. Both Grupping (1963) and Robinson (1965) used a cylindrical approximation, and Grupping also took wall thickness into account. Beneken (1965) approximated the left ventricular wall by a spherical shell and the right ventricular free wall as a thinner spherical shell wrapped around part of the outer surface of the thick-walled left ventricle. This made it possible to take into account the interaction between left and right ventricles. An estimation of the volume of the trabeculae carneae and the papillary muscles was made and added as dead space to the inner volume. The rough inner surface facilitates a more complete emptying. For example, if dead space is 30 per cent of the end-diastolic blood volume, this increases the ejection fraction of the ventricle by more than 40 per cent for the same muscle shortening.

The cylindrical and spherical approximations of the left ventricle also assume a homogeneous isotropic wall material. However, the wall of the ventricles is composed of muscle fibres which have a very specific directional distribution. Streeter *et al.* (1969) collected quantitative information about fibre orientation in the left ventricle during systole and diastole. Heart muscle can, in its operating range, shorten by 20 per cent with appreciable remaining developed force. It is generally accepted that the left ventricular ejection fraction in the normal heart is about 0·6. Sallin (1969) showed that a 20 per cent fibre shortening allows a maximum ejection fraction of 0·488 for a sphere with circularly arranged muscle fibres, but did not consider the contribution of the trabecular space. Even a helical arrangement of fibres around a sphere or a cylinder allows no larger ejection fractions, but helical fibres around an ellipsoid of revolution can allow an ejection fraction of 0·612 for 20 per cent fibre shortening (Sallin, 1969).

Mirsky (1970) made a thorough study of the effects of anisotropy and non-homogeneity on left ventricular wall stresses and took some of Streeter's findings into account. A few assumptions are that the medium is orthotropic and that three mutually orthogonal planes of elastic symmetry exist. Anisotropy, such that the meridional Young's modulus is 10 times smaller than the radial or circumferential moduli, resulted in 20 per cent greater stress in the midwall than in the isotropic case. Inhomogeneity was included by assuming that the Young's modulus at the midwall is 10 times larger than at the endo- and epicardial surfaces. This resulted in a 40 per cent increase in midwall stress. A particularly interesting finding was that in the non-homogeneous case compressive forces arise at the endocardial surface leading to crenation.

All these studies serve to increase the understanding of the mechanics of the left ventricle. The results may eventually make it possible to compute muscle fibre properties from pressure-volume relations of the intact heart.

3. Haemodynamics

This subject was recently reviewed by McDonald (1968) who looked at modelling efforts from a physiological point of view. Noordergraaf (1969) also covered the same area and we refer to this comprehensive study instead of rewording the same material. However, some clinical applications will be discussed briefly.

A. arterial haemodynamics

The mathematics of pulsatile flow based on Womersley's work (1957), extended to include the sleeve effect and the necessary electrical networks are expertly described by Noordergraaf (1969). Snyder *et al.* (1968) described a model of the arterial tree using an equal volume principle to determine segment length. In this way the aorta and larger arteries are represented in more detail than the smaller arteries. Since the bandwidth of a lumped segment is inversely proportional to its length, the representation of the central segments

is valid over a wider frequency range. The values of the longitudinal impedance components were based on the difference–differential approximation of
the Navier-Stokes equations (Rideout and Dick, 1967).

The incorporation of the viscous properties of the arterial wall in the
transverse impedance is discussed by Westerhof and Noordergraaf (1970). A
five-element network (Fig. 5) simulates the frequency dependence of Young's
modulus as well as stress relaxation, creep and hysteresis.

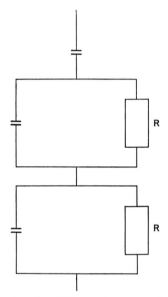

Fig. 5. Five-element network which as transverse impedance represents the
visco-elastic arterial wall properties. (After Westerhof and Noordergraaf, 1970.)

All these models of the arterial tree use a linear pressure–volume relation
for the arterial segments. Dick *et al.* (1968) performed intermodulation
measurements and concluded that non-linearities in the arterial wall are small.
In a hybrid computer study, using a perturbation scheme (Beneken and
Rideout, 1968), Rideout and Sims (1969) showed clearly that, with small
non-linearities distributed along a tube, the amplitude of the harmonics
generated in a travelling wave tends to increase with distance from the input.

These models of the arterial system mentioned above, contain a large
number of segments. The theory is rather complex and, therefore, models
can help to evaluate certain refinements of the theory. In other words, these
models are based on and start from the theory and produce information that
may agree with actual measurements and, thus, improve insight in the
properties of this system.

Another category of models starts from measurements on the arterial system, or parts of it, which are then interpreted in terms of model components. These models are necessarily simpler than those discussed above because, in general, not enough information is contained in the measurements to find all the constants of a complicated model. These simple models are usually set up for a very specific purpose, as is shown by the following examples. Watt and Goldwyn (1967) interpret the time course of diastolic aortic pressure waves in terms of a four-component network consisting of two elastic chambers connected by an inertance and terminated by a resistance representing the peripheral resistance (Fig. 6). The numerical values of these

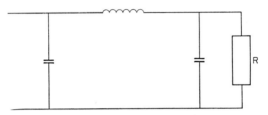

FIG. 6. Electrical representation of a four-component model of the arterial system as used by Watt and Goldwyn (1967).

components and the end-systolic pressure and flow (initial conditions) can be found from the diastolic pressure curve, but only one pressure is available and no information on the impedance level of the network can be extracted. It is, therefore, unlikely that a unique solution for the R, L, and C values will be found. Three sets of L and C values are given from measurements on three patients with different diseases. However, the R values have been made equal to unity and, unfortunately, the consequences of this normalization are not discussed. To indicate the potential danger of such methods let us suppose a patient changes his peripheral resistance alone, to one-half its previous value between two measurements. If the measurements are compared after normalization with respect to R they will indicate that the compliances (Fig. 6) had been reduced to one-half the original value and that the inertance value had been doubled. A peripheral vasodilatation is thus indistinguishable from a central vasoconstriction.

Despite these objections the method is straightforward and if one parameter is independently determined (e.g. peripheral resistance) it may prove clinically useful.

Defares and Van der Waal (1969) describe a method to determine systemic arterial compliance and peripheral resistance in man, based on non-invasive measurements of systolic and diastolic arterial pressure, and the systolic interval. The underlying model concept is the simple Windkessel-peripheral resistance CR-circuit. However, aortic pressures seldom show an exponential decay and the clinical usefulness of their scheme still has to be evaluated. A combination of the two methods might overcome some of the individual disadvantages.

A third practical application of a simplified model is described by Rothe and Nash (1968). Pressure and flow in the renal artery of dogs are measured simultaneously. A signal equivalent to the renal pressure is used as the input signal of a four-component model of the renal artery. The difference between the flow signal from the model and the actual flow signal is minimized by manual adjustment of the main renal artery resistance (R) and inertance (L) followed by automatic adjustment of renal compliance (C), of conductance (G) between artery and glomeruli and of glomerular pressure (P_g). Drug-induced changes in the latter three quantities (C, G and P_g) are automatically followed by the model; assuming the former two components (R and L) stay unchanged. The paper pays attention to the uniqueness of the solution and to parameter sensitivity and indicates limitations and suggestions for improvements. This study is an excellent example of the use of a simple but meaningful model.

Wesseling *et al.* (1972) have tried to determine the parameters of human arm arteries. The arteries between the axilla and the wrist were represented by four lumped-parameter segments (Fig. 7). The components were related to vessel length l, cross-sectional area S and radius/wall-thickness ratio h according to:

$$R = \frac{8\pi\eta l}{S^2} \tag{3.1}$$

$$L = \frac{\rho l}{S} \tag{3.2}$$

$$C = \frac{3Sl(h+1)^2}{E(2h+1)}, \tag{3.3}$$

with η and ρ representing the blood viscosity and density, respectively, and E the Young's modulus of the wall material. In Fig. 7, R_L represents the

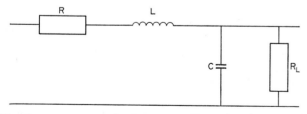

Fig. 7. The human arm arteries between axilla and wrist are represented by four of these segments in series (Wesseling *et al.*, 1972).

resistance to the flow of blood leaving the vessel segment through side branches. Assuming h to be known and the length of each segment to be measurable from the outside one has the quantities S, E and R_L to be determined for each segment. Signals were obtained from an external pulse pick-up element in the axilla and at the wrist. The axillary signal was used as an input pressure to the four segments and the output pressure of the model compared with the signal obtained from the wrist. The difference is minimized by adjusting the model parameters from which the vessel properties can be derived. Results are discussed in Section 6 of this chapter.

B. VENOUS SYSTEM

In a recent special issue on venous studies (IEEE-BME-16, no. 4, 1969) half the papers dealt with model studies. Such studies have developed rather slowly for the veins. The reason for this is the complexity caused by low transmural pressures leading to collapse of some veins during certain phases of the cardiac cycle and difficulties in making reliable measurements of flow and transmural pressure. Many recent studies of veins deal with flow through collapsible tubes, as exemplified by the term "vascular waterfall" (Permutt, 1965). Other studies are due to Holt (1969), Conrad (1969), Katz et al. (1969), Moreno et al. (1969), and many others. Under certain conditions, the flow through a collapsing tube depends solely on the input pressure and the pressure outside the tube, while the pressure at the downstream end has no influence. Similarly in the case of a waterfall, the height of the water below the fall does not in general influence the flow. A rigorous mathematical treatment of the subject is given by Kresch and Noordergraaf (1969). The implications of venous collapse on overall circulatory behaviour were discussed by Guyton as early as 1955, in terms of venous return curves.

All the known major effects that affect the venous circulation are quantitatively taken into account by Snyder and Rideout (1969). Besides resistance to flow, inertance, compliance and the influence of collapse, the following phenomena are included in their hybrid computer model: gravitational forces, venous valves, changes in transmural pressure due to respiration and muscle action, and changes in venous tone mediated by the sympathetic nervous system. This model, incorporating various control loops, also contains the pulmonary and the systemic arterial circulation as well as the atria and ventricles. This very extensive model shows many similarities with the actual circulation which makes it a powerful tool for further total circulation studies when done in close relation to animal studies.

An entirely new approach to the venous system is the digital computer model by Dickinson (1969). The system is subdivided into a number of identical compartments, each has an inflow from its distant neighbour and an inflow from an assumed high impedance flow source. Outflow occurs only into the proximal compartment. Thus the inferior and superior venae cavae and the right heart are described but the model is incomplete and some of the assumptions are not realistic. It is interesting that this model gives a reasonable prediction of the point in the system at which the pressure changes the least when the body is tilted. No attention is paid to the possible effects of incorporating actual dimensional data. Continuation of the study in that direction might yield interesting results.

4. MODELS OF OVERALL CARDIOVASCULAR CONTROL

Model studies of the overall cardiovascular system involving a closed loop with constancy of total blood volume originate from Guyton (1955), who used the fact that venous return and cardiac output must be equal when the circulatory system is in a steady state. Venous return is impeded by increasing the right atrial pressure and cardiac output is raised by the same pressure increase. The principle is visualized by plotting both the venous return curve and the cardiac output curve as functions of mean right atrial pressure in one graph (Fig. 8). The course of these curves is dependent on a great many

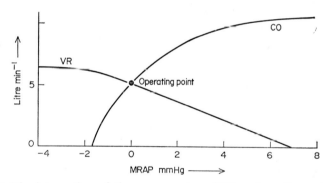

FIG. 8. The intersection of the venous return (VR) and cardiac output (CO) curves determines the operating point (Guyton, 1955).

parameters such as peripheral resistance, venous resistance, blood volume, and heart function. Most of these relations are known and their influence on cardiac output and other circulatory variables can be evaluated (Guyton, 1963). Grodins (1959) published a compartmental study of the cardiovascular system based on twenty-three independent simultaneous equations, the solution of which gave mean values for the variables. Cardiac activity was represented by a linear relation between end-diastolic ventricular volume and stroke work. The results from this model compare favourably with those of physiological experiments. Warner (1959) used six compartments to represent the circulatory system. A total of 18 equations were needed for the solution which also included the pulsatile character of the variables. Ventricular contraction and relaxation were represented by compliance changes. In 1963, Defares *et al.* published an extensive mathematical description of the entire uncontrolled system. The time course of ventricular compliance change is phenomenological and based on a number of publications concerning the effect of pre- and afterload on cardiac output and the time course of some variables.

Most of the studies, mentioned above, were begun to allow the future incorporation of control mechanisms; this was also the case for the closed system study by Beneken (1965). In this, attention was paid to the quantitative effect of certain parameter changes and to the fact that in a closed system cardiac output is less dependent on peripheral resistance change than in the case of an open system with a constant mean left atrial pressure. This phenomenon is called "apparent control" because it is effective without the operation of any reflex mechanisms.

Amongst the various control mechanisms the baroreceptor reflex has received much attention; a comprehensive compilation of studies on this reflex appeared in Kezdi (1967). The subject remains under study following different procedures and serving various objectives (Öberg and Sjöstrand, 1969; Hyndman, 1970 and see Chapter 5).

In 1967, Beneken and De Wit published an analog computer model of the cardiovascular system, consisting of nineteen compartments, which incorporated a representation of the baroreceptor effects on heart rate and peripheral resistance and some aspects of blood volume control (Fig. 9). Drastic blood volume changes resulted in behaviour comparable with that of animals in haemorrhagic shock. The model also indicated the possible existence of a threshold for coronary perfusion pressure, below which continuous impairment of heart function will take place. This hypothesis was later supported by measurement results from animal experiments (Beneken *et al.* 1969).

The long-term regulation model devised by Guyton and Coleman (1967) is original and unique (Fig. 10). It incorporates not only immediate baroreceptor action but also its long-term adaptation (Block 23, 24 and 25). Furthermore, long-term autoregulation is included by increase or decrease of the vasculature in response to cardiac output changes (Block 9) and due to normal destruction of old vasculature (Blocks 10, 11 and 12). Blocks 1 to 8 represent the basic system in terms of venous return and cardiac output. The properties of this model are evaluated against results from animal experiments, particularly on the effects of reduced renal and cardiac function. The control of cardiac output during exercise was studied (Topham and Warner, 1967) with an analog computer model. Differences in response of the actual

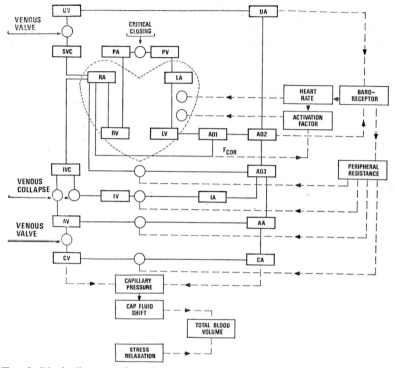

Fig. 9. Block diagram of cardiovascular system model. AO 1, 2 and 3 represent aortic segments; UA and UV: arteries and veins of head and arms; IA and IV: arteries and veins of intra-abdominal organs; AA and AV: remaining intra-abdominal arteries and veins; CA and CV: arteries and veins of the legs; IVC and SVC: inferior and superior vena cava. (From Beneken and De Wit, 1967.)

system and the model were reduced by adjusting the model parameters. The approach is very interesting, but more corresponding variables should be mutually compared in order to produce a unique solution. Pickering *et al.* (1969) describe a cardiovascular control model for the confirmation of diagnosis of cardiopulmonary disease.

In Section 3 the hybrid computer model of Snyder and Rideout (1969) was discussed. As well as a detailed representation of the venous system, heart rate control, peripheral resistance and venomotor control are incorporated. Furthermore, the effects of gravity, breathing and muscular contraction on transmural pressures and driving pressures are taken into account. Figure 11 shows results from a simulation of a case of aortic stenosis, while the Valsalva manoeuvre and a tilt from horizontal to vertical and back is imitated. The comparison of such results with clinical data might yield additional information for a better diagnosis.

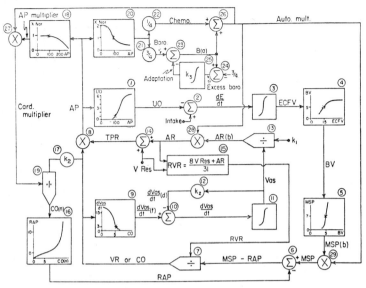

Fig. 10. A complex system analysis of long-term cardiovascular control. The functions of some of the blocks is discussed in the text. (From Guyton and Coleman, 1967.)

The control of the circulatory system serves the purpose of adaptation to the varying needs of the entire body. Variation in need may arise internally, e.g. illnesses causing fever, anatomical changes like cardiac valve defects, infections, etc. or may arise externally. Examples of the latter are tilting, heat load, altitude change, exercise. Without any changes in the internal and external influences, the cardiovascular system would operate at a fixed operating point (or possibly in a small operating range due to interaction with respiration) and no single study on the relations between circulatory variables could be made.

In more technical terms, the operating point of the cardiovascular system is entirely determined by the complete set of parameter values. The term parameter is used in its broadest sense, i.e. not only resistances and compliances but also total blood volume, intra-thoracic pressure, and the time-varying elastances used to represent cardiac action, are considered as parameters. In other words, all those quantities needed to specify numerically the haemodynamic aspects of the system are called parameters. For a given set of parameter values, the (time-varying) variables such as pressures, flows, volumes, and concentrations, will have certain values, in the stationary state. A change in a variable, e.g. cardiac output, cannot be accomplished directly, but must be made indirectly by changing one or more parameters. This is the

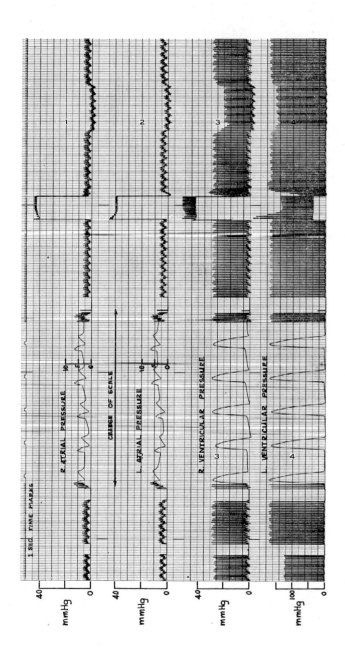

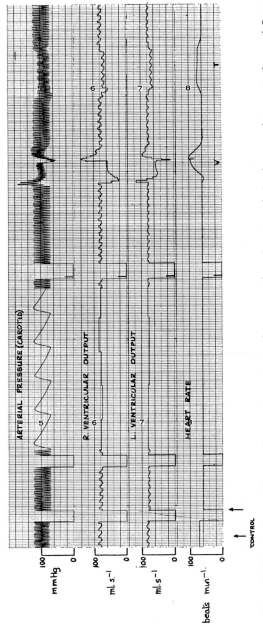

Fig. 11. Simulation of the cardiovascular system with an aortic valve stenosis having a resistance to forward flow of 133 dyne sec cm^{-1} which is 10 times larger than assumed to be normal. The second arrow indicates the introduction of the heart defect, V indicates a Valsalva manoeuvre and T indicates a tilt from horizontal to vertical and back. (Unpublished work by Dr. M. Snyder.)

way cardiovascular control is achieved. No direct alteration of variables takes place; it occurs indirectly by control loops acting on parameters. Many feedback loops are present to improve stable operation and to respond appropriately to changing conditions. An interesting observation on various circulatory control models is that no set-points are needed to guarantee stable operation under a variety of conditions. Although at the moment no conclusive evidence can be presented to negate the set-point concept in relation to the cardiovascular system, it seems unlikely that set-points will be found. Investigators have found it difficult to specify the form of set-point references such as those for pressure, flow or even pH. However, we can conceive of a biochemical reaction, the reaction constants of which are highly dependent on pH or temperature (cf. Section 5). The set-point approach requires the determination of a difference between set-point and controlled variable, whereas the cardiovascular system is envisaged here as being in a dynamic equilibrium state, with changes in parameters resulting from changes in variables without the need for information regarding previous, normal, reference, (or otherwise named) values of the quantities concerned.

Systematic studies of these and other aspects of the cardiovascular system will produce an improvement in understanding which is the basis for better diagnosis and therapy.

5. Transport by the Bloodstream

Transport studies with models were used in 1963 (Papper and Kitz) to describe the uptake and distribution of anaesthetics. They did not take into account any effect of the anaesthetic agent on the circulatory parameters, though the need for this was recognized by Landahl (1963). Beneken and Rideout (1968) described a systematic approach to transport by the bloodstream using a multiple model.

A. theory

In a lumped parameter approximation of an elastic tube, the following three equations relate pressure p, volume q, and flow f (Fig. 12):

$$q_{2tot} = q_{2tot}(0) + \int (f_2 - f_3) \, dt \qquad (5.1)$$

$$p_2 = \frac{1}{C_2} (q_{2tot} - q_{2u}) = \frac{q_2}{C_2} \qquad (5.2)$$

$$p_1 - p_2 = R_2 f_2 + L_2 \frac{df_2}{dt}, \qquad (5.3)$$

q_{2u} is the unstressed volume of the 2nd compartment and q_2 is the excess-volume above q_{2u}. C, R, and L represent the compliance, the resistance to flow and the inertance (see Section 3), respectively.

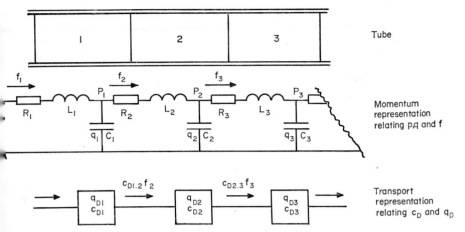

FIG. 12. Multiple model representation of a tube subdivided into three compartments. Electrical representation of the relations between pressure p, volume q, and flow f in each of the tube compartments. R, L and C are resistance to flow, inertance and compliance. To each compartment values are assigned for the concentrations of a substance, c_D, and the total amount of the substance, q_D.

Assuming instantaneous and complete mixing of a substance D (e.g. dye) in the blood, the compartmental approach can be used to study transport in the following way. Denoting q_D and c_D as the volume and concentration of the substance D in the blood, the following two simple relations hold:

$$q_{D2} = q_{D2}(0) + \int (c_{D1,2} f_2 - c_{D2,3} f_3)\, dt, \qquad (5.4)$$

with

$$c_{D1,2} = c_{D1} \quad \text{if} \quad f_2 > 0$$
$$= c_{D2} \quad \text{if} \quad f_2 < 0,$$
$$c_{D2,3} = c_{D2} \quad \text{if} \quad f_3 > 0$$
$$= c_{D3} \quad \text{if} \quad f_3 < 0,$$

$$c_{Dn} = \frac{q_{Dn}}{q_{ntot}}. \qquad (5.5)$$

Equation (5.4) is the continuity equation for D in compartment 2 (Fig. 12). For positive values of the flow f_2 and f_3, the volume of dye per unit time transported into compartment 2 is $c_{D1} f_2$ while $c_{D2} f_3$ is the dye volume per unit time leaving compartment 2. Equation (5.5) defines the concentration assuming complete mixing. The computer implementation of these equations and the need for only two additional equations (5.4 and 5.5) for each substance studied, were described by Beneken and Rideout (1968). However the transport of dye may be modelled by using a combination of complete mixing chambers and "plug" flow chambers as suggested by Henig (1961), and as commonly used in chemical engineering models (Himmelblau and Bischoff, 1968). This concept was the basis for a hybrid computer simulation of dye transport in the entire circulatory loop by Rideout and Schaefer (1970), in which a digital "memory wheel" was used in order to include effects of flow reversal and of vessel collapse in the plug flow parts of the model.

Simulations based on equations (5.1) to (5.5), using a number of compartments in series, produced concentration curves quite similar to actual curves although the shape depends on the number of compartments used (De Waal, 1969). The larger the number of subdivisions the smaller the spread in the simulated tube (Fig. 13). De Waal also showed the reason for this difference, for the special case in which the flow f is constant, i.e. $f = f_1 = f_2 = f_3$. In this case (5.4) with addition of the Laplace operator s, becomes

$$q_{D2} = \frac{1}{s} f(c_{D1} - c_{D2}),\qquad (5.6)$$

and from (5.5)

$$q_{D2} = c_{D2} \cdot q_{2\text{tot}}.\qquad (5.7)$$

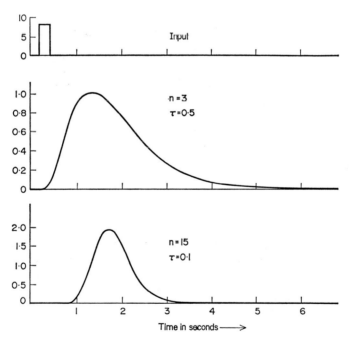

FIG. 13. Simulation of dye transport following single bolus injection. Representation of the same tube, $q_{\text{tot}}/f = 1·5$ sec, with 3 and 15 segments. (From De Waal, 1969.)

From (5.6) and (5.7) we have

$$\frac{c_{D2}}{c_{D1}} = \frac{1}{1+s\,\dfrac{q_{tot}}{f}} = \frac{1}{1+s\tau}, \tag{5.8}$$

when

$$\frac{q_{tot}}{f} = \tau. \tag{5.9}$$

This means that a compartment with total blood volume q_{tot} and with flow f through it has a concentration transfer ratio c_{D2}/c_{D1} equal to that of a first order low-pass filter with a time constant $\tau = q_{tot}/f$. If this compartment is subdivided into n identical compartments in series, each one of those will have a volume q_{tot}/n, while the flow through each will remain f. The transfer ratio of the small compartments from (5.8) and (5.9) will be

$$\frac{c_n}{c_{n-1}} = \frac{1}{1+s\,\dfrac{q_{tot}}{nf}} = \frac{1}{1+\dfrac{s\tau}{n}}. \tag{5.10}$$

The transfer ratio of the n identical compartments becomes:

$$\frac{c_n}{c_1} = \left(\frac{1}{1+\dfrac{s\tau}{n}}\right)^n = e^{-s\tau} \qquad \text{if } n\to\infty. \tag{5.11}$$

Thus c_n/c_1 represents a pure time delay with no filtering distortion when n is very large.

This effect can also be seen by comparing the $n = 3$ and the $n = 15$ case in Fig. 13; the curve for $n = 15$ is much sharper and thus resembles the input pulse more closely.

It appears that the two different descriptions (single or multi-compartment) produce two entirely different transfer ratios. In some cases, it may be possible to find a value for n, such that the actual and the model transfer ratio agree sufficiently well. A combination of a pure time delay with a limited number of first order segments obeying equation (5.10) may yield satisfactory results (Rideout and Schaefer, 1970). However, to date no reliable criterion has been developed to optimize the segment size for transport simulation.

Some of these limitations of transport simulation were eliminated by Tilanus (1971). Consider in a segment of a tube the volume q_{Dx} of a substance D between x and $x+dx$ (Fig. 14).

This volume is determined by the inflow and outflow of the substance, which is proportional to the main fluid flow f, and by diffusion of the material

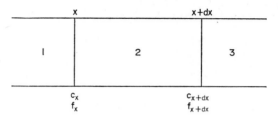

Fig. 14. Subdivision of tube segments for derivation of the transport differential equation (5.14).

at x and at $x+dx$, which is proportional to the concentration gradient $\partial c/\partial x$, the diffusion coefficient D and the cross-sectional area A.

$$q_{Dx} = q_{Dx}(0) + \int \left(c_x f_x - c_{x+dx} f_{x+dx} - D \frac{\partial c_x}{\partial x} A + D \frac{\partial c_{x+dx}}{\partial x} A \right) dt, \quad (5.12)$$

since

$$c_{x+dx} = c_x + \frac{\partial c_x}{\partial x} dx,$$

and

$$\frac{\partial c_{x+dx}}{\partial x} = \frac{\partial c_x}{\partial x} + \frac{\partial^2 c_x}{\partial x^2} dx,$$

and

$$f_{x+dx} = f_x + \frac{\partial f_x}{\partial x} dx,$$

and

$$c_x = \frac{q_{Dx}}{A \, dx},$$

we find after arranging (5.12)

$$\frac{\partial c_x}{\partial t} = D \frac{\partial^2 c_x}{\partial x^2} - \frac{f_x}{A} \frac{\partial c_x}{\partial x} - \frac{c_x}{A} \frac{\partial f_x}{\partial x}. \quad (5.13)$$

When the flow f is constant, the last term on the right-hand side reduces to zero, which leaves the one-dimensional diffusion equation (Norwich and Zelin, 1970)

$$\frac{\partial c}{\partial t} = D \frac{\partial^2 c}{\partial x^2} - v \frac{\partial c}{\partial x}, \quad (5.14)$$

with v representing the fluid velocity.

Since the dispersion that takes place in flowing blood depends not only on the character of the flow, e.g. laminar or turbulent, but also on the path length, D is a quantity that has to be experimentally determined. Norwich and Zelin obtained values of order 90 cm sec^{-2}. If a volume m of indicator is injected in a very short time when $t = 0$, the solution of (5.14) becomes:

$$c(x, t) = \frac{m}{2A(\pi Dt)^{\frac{1}{2}}} e^{-(x-vt)^2/4Dt}. \tag{5.15}$$

This is a normal distribution function symmetrical with respect to x when t is constant, and which is asymmetrical with respect to time at a given x. This second situation resembles the actual technique of measuring at a fixed position which produces the well-known skewed dilution curve.

The same approach as that used above for a distributed system can be applied to a lumped parameter system such as that shown schematically in Fig. 15.

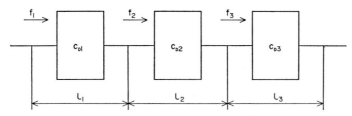

FIG. 15. Lumped parameter representation of tube segments for derivation of the transport equation (5.18). (See also Fig. 12.)

Diffusion between compartments, assumed to be well mixed, is proportional to the concentration difference, cross-sectional area A, diffusion constant D and inversely proportional to the length l, over which diffusion must take place. The difference-differential form of equation (5.12) for compartment 2 in Fig. 15 is:

$$q_{D2} = q_{D2}(0) + \int \left\{ f_2 c_{D1} - f_3 c_{D2} + \frac{A_{12}D}{\frac{1}{2}(l_1+l_2)}(c_{D1}-c_{D2}) \right.$$
$$\left. - \frac{A_{23}D}{\frac{1}{2}(l_2+l_3)}(c_{D2}-c_{D3}) \right\} dt \tag{5.16}$$

since $c_{D2} = q_{D2}/(A_2 l_2)$.

This can be written as:

$$\frac{dc_{D2}}{dt} = \frac{f_2 c_{D1} - f_3 c_{D2}}{A_2 l_2} + \frac{1}{A_2 l_2} \left\{ \frac{A_{12}D}{\frac{1}{2}(l_1+l_2)}(c_{D1}-c_{D2}) \right.$$
$$\left. - \frac{A_{23}D}{\frac{1}{2}(l_2+l_3)}(c_{D2}-c_{D3}) \right\}. \tag{5.17}$$

This equation is the lumped-parameter diffusion equation to be applied in the presence of main flow f. This need not be stationary but can be pulsatile with flow reversal, in which case a set of conditions must be observed similar to those accompanying equation (5.4). The major assumption, however, is

still complete mixing within the compartments. The meaning of equation (5.17) readily becomes apparent when a special case is considered, for example with constant cross-sectional area: $A_{12} = A_2 = A_{23} = A$; constant flow: $f_2 = f_3 = f$; and segments of equal length: $l_1 = l_2 = l_3 = l$.
In this case equation (5.17) simplifies and becomes:

$$\frac{dc_{D2}}{dt} = \frac{f}{Al}(c_{D1} - c_{D2}) + \frac{D}{l^2}(c_{D1} - 2c_{D2} + c_{D3}).$$ (5.18)

The correspondence with equation (5.14) is easy to understand. The first term on the right-hand side of equation (5.18) corresponds to the first derivative term and the second term corresponds to the second derivative term of c with respect to x in equation (5.14).

The relative importance of the two right-hand terms in equation (5.18) can be estimated by considering the introduction of dye in compartment 1 only, leaving $c_{D2} - c_{D3} - 0$. The contribution from the flow term to the rate of rise of c_{D2} is 27 c_{D1} and from the diffusion term 10 c_{D1} for the case where: $f = 80$ cm^3 sec^{-1}; $l = 1$ cm; $A = 3$ cm^2; $D = 10$ cm^2 sec^{-1}. The value for D is in accordance with Tilanus (1971) and shows that the diffusion term has significant effect.

In this example, the length l was chosen arbitrarily for no criterion is available from the literature on which to base segment length for transport studies, except the two criteria developed by Tilanus. The first one deals with errors introduced by dividing a normal distribution curve into a number of steps of constant concentration, and the second criterion deals with the bandwidth of the compartments.

Diffusion between parts of a distributed system depends on the concentration gradient $\partial c/\partial x$, as in equation (5.14). In a lumped-parameter system, the diffusion is governed by the concentration difference, as in equation (5.17). In order to evaluate the influence of segment length l on the accuracy of the transport simulation we must compare the concentration gradient with the difference quotient (Tilanus, 1971).

Rewriting equation (5.15) and introducing $\sigma = (2Dt)^{\frac{1}{2}}$, $x_o = x - vt$ and $h = \frac{1}{2}l$ which implies a fixed time and site of observation x_o,

$$c(x) = \frac{m}{A\sigma}\frac{1}{(2\pi)^{\frac{1}{2}}} e^{-\frac{1}{2}(x/\sigma)^2}.$$ (5.19)

The difference quotient at x_o is:

$$\frac{\Delta c}{\Delta x} = \frac{\Delta c}{2h} = \frac{m}{A\sigma}\frac{1}{(2\pi)^{\frac{1}{2}}} \frac{e^{-\frac{1}{2}[(x_o+h)/\sigma]^2} - e^{-\frac{1}{2}[(x_o-h)/\sigma]^2}}{2h}$$

$$\approx -\frac{m}{A\sigma}\frac{1}{(2\pi)^{\frac{1}{2}}} e^{-\frac{1}{2}(x_o/\sigma)^2}\left\{1 - \frac{h^2}{2\sigma^2} + \frac{h^2 x_o^2}{6\sigma^4}\right\}.$$ (5.20)

From equation (5.19) we derive

$$\frac{dc}{dx} = -\frac{m}{A\sigma}\frac{1}{(2\pi)^{\frac{1}{2}}}\frac{x_o}{\sigma^2}\, e^{-\frac{1}{2}(x_o/\sigma)^2} \tag{5.21}$$

The difference between difference- and differential-quotient must be small compared with the differential quotient:

$$\left| -\frac{h^2}{2\sigma^2} + \frac{h^2 x_o^2}{6\sigma^4} \right| \frac{dc}{dx} \ll \frac{dc}{dx},$$

or

$$\left| -\frac{h^2}{2\sigma^2} + \frac{h^2 x_o^2}{6\sigma^4} \right| \ll 1,$$

or

$$h^2 \ll \frac{6\sigma^4}{\left| x_o^2 - 3\sigma^2 \right|}. \tag{5.22}$$

In Fig. 16, the normal density function and the relation of equation (5.22) are depicted.

Segment length considerations, when x_o is further than 2σ from the peak concentration, are less important. Within these $+2\sigma$ and -2σ limits (95 per

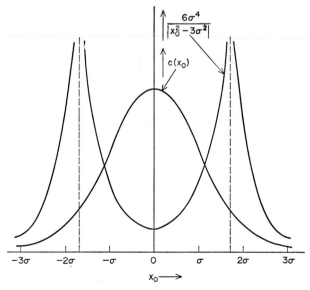

FIG. 16. Graphical representation of a normal distribution curve according to (5.19) and (5.22). The minimum value of the right-hand side of (5.22) between $+2\sigma$ and -2σ is $2\sigma^2$ at $x_o = 0$.

cent of the area under the density function curve) the smallest value for the right-hand side of equation (5.22) is $2\sigma^2$, and is found at $x_0 = 0$. In other words:

$$h^2 \ll 2\sigma^2.$$

Since it was assumed that the segment length $l = 2h$ and $\sigma = (2Dt)^{\frac{1}{2}}$ we find the first limitation of the segment length

$$l^2 \ll 16Dt. \tag{5.23}$$

The consequences of this will be dealt with after discussion of the second criterion based on bandwidth considerations (Tilanus, 1971).

As mentioned above, since equation (5.15) is the solution of the diffusion equation (5.14), it can be considered as a normal distribution function. However, the variance σ^2 increases linearly with time, $\sigma^2 = 2Dt$ causing the skewness of $c(x,t)$ with respect to t.

In order to estimate the frequency content of the concentration curve, we neglect the time-dependent variance and assume $x = 0$. If K_1 is a constant we write

$$c(t) = K_1 e^{-\frac{1}{2}(t/\theta)^2}, \tag{5.24}$$

with

$$\theta = (2Dt)^{\frac{1}{2}}/v. \tag{5.25}$$

The frequency content of a signal, from equation (5.24), is:

$$c(\omega) = K_2 e^{-\frac{1}{2}(\theta\omega)^2}, \tag{5.26}$$

which also resembles a normal distribution function with a variance equal to $1/\theta^2$.

No direct information is available on the bandwidth needed for transferring the signal $c(t)$. Therefore, a constant a is incorporated, the value of which must be determined. This constant represents the number of standard deviations of $c(\omega)$ that must be covered,

$$\omega_{\max} = \frac{a}{\theta} = \frac{av}{(2Dt)^{\frac{1}{2}}}. \tag{5.27}$$

From equation (5.18) we learn that the characteristic frequency when diffusion takes place, is

$$\omega_{cD} = f/Al + 2D/l^2,$$

which is larger than ω_{co} obtained when $D = 0$.

We now make $\omega_{\max}$ in equation (5.27) equal to ω_{co}.

The time constant for $D = 0$, using equation (5.9) for the nth compartment, is

$$\tau_n = \frac{q_{\text{tot}}}{f} = \frac{l_n A}{vA} = \frac{l_n}{v} \tag{5.28}$$

since a flat velocity profile was assumed.
The maximum length now follows from equation (5.27)

$$l_{n\,\text{max}}^2 = 2Dt/a^2 \tag{5.29}$$

where t is time after injection.

It appears that the requirement for proper spatial resolution of equation (5.23) is much less stringent than the requirement for acceptable frequency transfer characteristics of the segment, since a is certainly larger than 1. We will continue with the bandwidth criterion and determine the permissible segment length. We know that

$$\frac{1}{v} \sum_{i=1}^{n} l_i = t, \tag{5.30}$$

and that

$$t = t_n + \sum_{i=1}^{n-1} t_i, \tag{5.31}$$

where

$$t_i = l_i/v, \tag{5.32}$$

this being the average time a particle takes to pass through segment i.
From the last four equations we find

$$l_{n\,\text{max}}^2 - \frac{2D}{a^2 v} l_{n\,\text{max}} - \frac{2D}{a^2 v} \sum_{i=1}^{n-1} l_i = 0. \tag{5.33}$$

The meaning of equation (5.29) and equation (5.33) is that the segment lengths for transport simulation can increase either with time after injection or with distance downsteam from the injection site. The reason is obvious. Dye concentration curves further downstream show greater dispersion and therefore, have reduced frequency content. To transfer this signal, a narrower bandwidth is adequate which means that longer segments can be tolerated.

To evaluate this theory and the criteria developed for the determination of segment lengths, at least three tests must be performed. First of all the applicability of equation (5.14) to actual indicator dilution curves must be tested. The result of such a test is shown in Fig. 17(a), where comparison is made between an actual curve and a numerical solution of equation (5.14) using a digital computer. Good agreement is obtained.

C.F.D.—I

The second test is the demonstration that with subdivisions beyond a certain limit, no further improvement is found in the model representation. Close to the injection site the segment lengths tend to become extremely short as seen from equation (5.29). In order to estimate the smallest number of segments needed a piece of tubing extending from a point 10 cm from the injection site to one 10 cm further downstream was simulated. The input signal was derived from a digital computer which solved equation (5.14) for the first 10 cm. The output signal is shown in Fig. 17(b), for representations of the second 10 cm length by 8, 14 or 25 segments. There are only minor differences between the 14- and the 25-segment representation. This indicates that for $a = 2\sqrt{3}$ the bandwidth of the individual segment is acceptable.

The third test is the comparison between analog simulation and the digital solution of equation (5.14) shown in Fig. 18. The curve from Fig. 17(b) for $a = 2\sqrt{3}$ compares well with the digital solution for a tube 20 cm long.

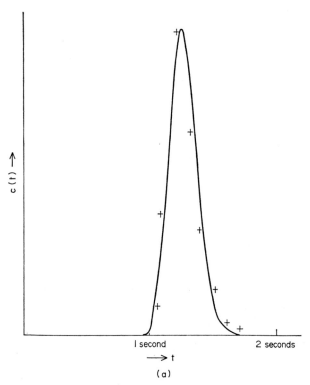

(a)

FIG. 17a. Indicator dilution curve measured in a tube (full line), 50 cm in length, with flow at a mean velocity of 45 cm sec^{-1}. Digital computer solution of (5.14) using the actual length and velocity data and taking $D = 10$ cm^2 sec^{-1} (crosses).

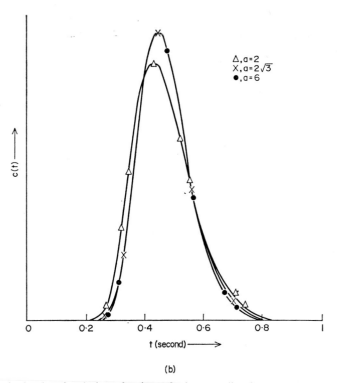

(b)

FIG. 17b. Analog simulation of a piece of tube extending from a point 10 cm down-stream from the injection site to one 10 cm further downstream. The input signal was derived from a digital computer. Curves show output signals from an analog computer model consisting of 8, 14 and 25 segments. The corresponding values for a are 2, $2\sqrt{3}$ and 6, respectively. No further improvement is obtained by going from 14 to 25 segments for the same tube length. (From Tilanus, 1971.)

These results indicate that the theory and the criteria for selecting segment lengths yield a useful method for simulating transport by the blood stream. The number of segments needed is very high. The extent to which simplifying assumptions can be made to reduce the number of segments depends entirely on the problem and no general rule can be given.

B. INDICATOR DILUTION

Bassingthwaighte *et al.* (1966) have described the dilution curve, obtained after a brief injection of indicator at some upstream position using a lagged normal density function b, which is a solution of:

$$b(t) = \frac{1}{\sigma(2\pi)^{\frac{1}{2}}} e^{-\frac{1}{2}[(t-t_c)/\sigma]^2} - \tau \frac{db(t)}{dt}. \tag{5.34}$$

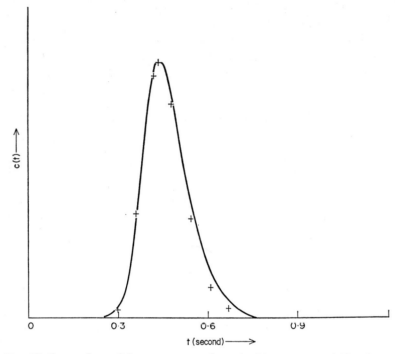

FIG. 18. Comparison of the output curve from the 14-segment model in FIG. 17(b) (full line) with a digital computer solution (crosses) for 20 cm length of tube. (From Tilanus, 1971.)

The concentration-time curves then become:

$$c(t) = m\, b(t)/f. \tag{5.35}$$

Observe the difference between the meaning of the spread σ in equation (5.34) and the meaning of σ in Section 5A. The dispersion of the curve, according to equation (5.35), is determined by σ and τ which makes direct comparison with the results in Section 5A very difficult. The measurements by Bassingthwaighte *et al.* (1966) showed a linear regression relation between both σ and τ, and the mean transit time was equal to $\tau + t_c$. For a description of the curve by equation (5.34) and equation (5.35) σ, τ and t_c are the essential parameters; they can be found by curve fitting procedures.

However, since the lagged normal density curve does not represent any physical system (Bassingthwaighte *et al.*, 1966) it does not readily lend itself to computer simulation in dynamic models. In this context dynamic models are those in which changes in variables over wide ranges result in corresponding changes of all other variables, according to equations describing the physical system. Thus, in the simulation proposed in Section 5A a change in flow rate will automatically result in a corresponding change in the indicator dilution curve. Equations (5.4) and (5.5), with $f_2 = f_3$ and with $q_{n \text{ tot}} =$ constant, are the basis for a steady state model, whereas combination with equations (5.1) to (5.3) makes the model dynamic.

If blood and indicator flow through a vascular bed, the dispersion of indicator is partly the result of particles traversing different pathways. The distribution of indicator-particle transit time is found by measuring the concentration at the venous side of a vascular bed after rapid arterial injection. The distribution of transit times is the vascular system's unit impulse response or its time domain transfer function. The steady-state transfer function was determined by Coulam et al. (1967) from the quotient of output and input concentration-time functions after they had been transformed into the frequency-domain (by Fourier transform). In order to eliminate interference due to recirculation the upstream indicator dilution curve was terminated. This was done in a smooth fashion using an integrated Gaussian distribution function thus introducing little high-frequency content. The corresponding down-stream termination was found using an iterative procedure; the first approximation was used to determine the transfer function, which in its turn led to a better estimation of the termination function.

The validity of the procedure was tested with signals derived from an analog computer simulation with a known transfer function. The method was also applied to actual vascular beds, where the convolution of the transfer function with the upstream concentration-time function yielded a time function that agreed well with the down-stream concentration function, this being another test of the validity of the method.

Friedman and Downing (1968) investigated with an analog computer the influence of central shunts on the measurement of flow through peripheral vascular beds. The mathematical description is based essentially on equations similar to equations (5.4) and (5.5), i.e. with no other dispersing factors. Experiments with animals in which a shunt was created across the left heart supported the simulation results in that essentially no difference was found between the systemic flow estimated from femoral artery and from pulmonary artery dilution curves.

For a computer representation of indicator dilution in the entire circulation, the theory discussed in Section 5A and the transfer function approach by Coulam et al. (1967) should be combined. It is very unlikely that theory will ever be able to predict the transfer across a vascular bed, but on the other hand a theory including diffusion predicts transport in vessels reasonably accurately, thus facilitating the simulation of shunts and their influence on indicator dilution. For use in dynamic models that correctly represent the effect of parameter changes on overall behaviour, the relation of the vascular bed transfer function to flow through the bed must still be investigated.

C. TRANSPORT OF ANAESTHETICS

Mathematical and analog models were used long ago to study the uptake and distribution of anaesthetics (Papper and Kitz, 1963). A detailed description of a mathematical model is given by Eger (1963a), the results of which are compared with published data concerning the uptake of nitrous oxide, cyclopropane, Halothane and ether as a function of time. Good agreement was obtained. The effect of changes in circulatory or respiratory quantities on alveolar concentration and the uptake in various body compartments was also systematically studied by Eger (1963b). Much attention was paid to the concentration effect, which refers to the fact that alveolar concentration does not change in proportion with the amount of anaesthetic taken up by the blood. This effect is included in Eger's mathematical model, whereas incorporation in electrical analogs is very difficult. The concentration effect is small for low concentrations of anaesthetic agents.

Electrical analogs were described by Severinghaus (1963) and Mapleson (1963). The former study distinguishes not only lung gas and lung tissue compartments, but also separate compartments for arterial blood, brain, organs, skin, fat and poorly perfused tissues. Mapleson includes, besides lung gas and lung tissue compartments, only the viscera, lean and fat tissue. Both models have good didactic and reasonable predictive applications. However, besides Eger's objection concerning the omission of the concentration effect, all these models have limitations in that they do not incorporate the effect of anaesthetic concentration itself on the function of the cardiovascular and respiratory system. These effects alter both the cardiac output and blood volume distribution, which in their turn influence the uptake and distribution of the anaesthetic (Landahl, 1963). A study of the effects of shock and excitement on the rate of cerebral equilibration, using Eger's mathematical model, was published by Munson et al. (1968). The proportional change in blood flow to different tissues as assumed in the model is mentioned by these authors as one of the limitations of this study. Waud and Waud (1970) used a computer model to predict the time course of the cerebral anaesthetic concentration when administered intermittently. A delay of 45 sec was found to which must be added another 6 sec to allow for the lung-to-brain circulation time. However, these circulation times and the influence of the anaesthetic on the system itself were not incorporated.

A complete description, incorporating for each segment, both the haemodynamic relations, equations (5.1), (5.2) and (5.3), and the transport equations (5.3) and (5.4), together with a sufficient number of segments would overcome most of the disadvantages of the models mentioned above. However, each model should be set up with attention to the specific needs and the special circumstances which it should simulate. This allows for some simplification which will be discussed later.

The amount of anaesthetic in compartment n, α_n, can be expressed as:

$$\alpha_n = \rho_{nb}\lambda_b q_{n\,tot} + \rho_{nt}\lambda_{nt}q_{nt}, \tag{5.36}$$

where ρ_{nb} and ρ_{nt} are the partial pressures of the anaesthetic in the nth compartment in blood and tissue, respectively,

λ_b and λ_{nt} the solubility constant of the anaesthetic in blood and in the tissue of the nth compartment, respectively,

and $q_{n\,tot}$ and q_{nt} the blood and tissue volume, respectively.

This extension of equation (5.5) is needed because anaesthetics also dissolve in the tissues, while an indicator is assumed to remain in the blood stream. It is assumed that the partial pressures in blood and tissue equilibrate rapidly, and they are made equal, ρ_n.

Equation (5.36) then becomes:

$$\rho_n = \frac{\alpha_n}{\lambda_b q_{n\,tot} + \lambda_{nt}q_{nt}}. \tag{5.37}$$

Diffusion of anaesthetic from one compartment to another is assumed to be negligible, leaving the blood stream as the only means of changing the amount of anaesthetic within a compartment.

$$\alpha_n = \alpha_n(0) + \int(\rho_{ni}\lambda_b f_{ni} - \rho_{no}\lambda_b f_{no})\,dt, \tag{5.38}$$

where $\alpha_n(0)$ is the initial amount of anaesthetic (at $t = 0$),

ρ_{ni} and ρ_{no} the partial pressures in the in- and outflowing blood, respectively,

and f_{ni} and f_{no} the inflow and outflow of blood, respectively.

The time needed for the equilibration of anaesthetics is in the order of hours, but time needed to reach a steady state in the circulatory system after a parameter change is usually two orders of magnitude less, and the main frequency of pulsatile flow is one further order of magnitude lower. This is the reason for using nonpulsatile flow and constant blood volume, i.e.

$$f_{ni} = f_{no} = f_n.$$

Since we assume no concentration gradient within any compartment, we have: $\rho_{no} = \rho_n$, and we may therefore write:

$$\rho_n = \rho_n(0) + \frac{\lambda_b f_n}{\lambda_n q_{n\,tot} + \lambda_{nt}q_{nt}}\int(\rho_{ni} - \rho_n)\,dt, \tag{5.39}$$

where

$$\rho_n(0) = \frac{\alpha_n(0)}{\lambda_b q_{n\,tot} + \lambda_{nt}q_{nt}}. \tag{5.40}$$

For each compartment such a non linear equation is needed, with additional equations to relate f_n to the total cardiac output and to incorporate the effect of the anaesthetic on various parameters.

Studies based on this were published by Zwart et al. (1972) and by Smith et al. (1972a,b). Besides compartments representing the lungs, the left heart and arterial blood, the right heart and the venous blood, they also considered nine further compartments representing the systemic vascular bed and the interacting tissue structures (Fig. 19).

The equation for the partial pressure in the right heart and venous blood (subscript v) is slightly different from equation (5.39):

$$\rho_v = \rho_v(0) + \frac{\lambda_b}{\lambda_b q_{v\,tot} + \lambda_v q_{vt}} \int \left[\sum_{m=1}^{9} f_m \rho_{m0} - \rho_v \sum_{m=1}^{9} f_m \right] dt. \qquad (5.41)$$

In the lung, which includes the gas-blood interface, the following gives the partial pressure:

$$\rho_1 = \rho_1(0) + \frac{1}{q_a + \lambda_b q_{l\,tot} + \lambda_{lt} q_{lt}} \int [\dot{q}_a(\rho_{insp} - \rho_1) + \lambda_b f(\rho_v - \rho_1)] \, dt, \qquad (5.42)$$

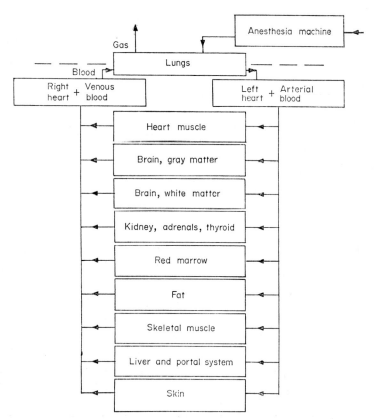

Fig. 19. Subdivision of the human body into compartments for uptake and distribution studies of Halothane. (After Zwart et al., 1972.)

where q_a is mean lung gas volume (residual volume plus one half tidal volume),

$\dot{q}_a$ alveolar ventilation rate,

P_{insp} partial pressure of anaesthetic in inspired gas mixture

and f is cardiac output.

The computer representation of Fig. 19 was used by Zwart *et al.* (1972) to study the difference between the uptake and distribution of Halothane predicted with a steady-state model (no interaction of Halothane concentration on parameters) and with a dynamic model (Fig. 20). For the dynamic model (Fig. 20) it was assumed that the cardiac output falls in proportion

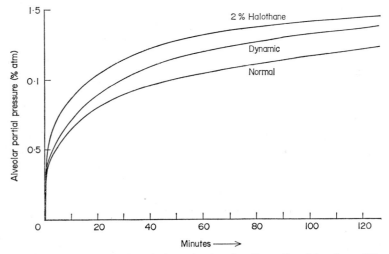

FIG. 20. Concentration of Halothane in the alveoli predicted by three different models.
Normal: Circulation where there is no effect of Halothane. Two per cent Halothane: circulatory parameters adjusted as if this concentration were present from the onset. Dynamic model: continuous effect of the increasing partial pressure of Halothane on the circulatory parameters. (Unpublished work by N. T. Smith and A. Zwat.)

to the partial pressure of Halothane in the heart muscle, and that the conductances (reciprocal of flow resistances) of the various vascular beds varied in proportion to the arterial Halothane partial pressure, as shown by the data reviewed by Smith and Smith (1971). The first publication of a dynamic model of this sort (Ashman *et al.*, 1970) included only the reduction of cardiac output. The difference between the corresponding partial pressures in their static and dynamic model are only slight. There is still some uncertainty on the exact location and structure where the anaesthetic acts. The dynamic

8*

model was used by Smith *et al.* (1972a) to test various hypotheses. The variation in the peripheral resistances in response to Halothane administration is either a local effect or mediated by the central nervous system. In the first case, the resistance variation might be related to the arterial partial pressures, whereas in the second case a relation with brain partial pressures is more likely. For the same reasons cardiac output variations can be related either to the partial pressure in the brain or cardiac muscle. Smith *et al.* (1971a) conclude from their model studies that when alveolar concentration alone is known it is practically impossible to distinguish between these hypotheses, and that other variables must be measured.

It can be concluded that the use of models in anaesthesiology is extremely valuable for research and that in this field teaching models can be very effective because good agreement between them and the real system can be obtained readily. The combination of models of uptake and distribution with existing teaching manikins like Sim One (Denson and Abrahamson, 1969) can be expected to be extremely valuable.

D. THE RADIOCARDIOGRAM AND THE RENOGRAM

The rapid or continuous injection of radio-isotopes with external recording of radio-activity as a function of time at one or more locations on the body is often performed to estimate cardiac and/or pulmonary blood volume and to investigate renal function. The method of analysis used is essentially the same as for indicator dilution technique, i.e. multi-compartmental analysis.

Kuwahara *et al.* (1967) approximated the entire circulation by four compartments: right heart, lungs, left heart, and body; and two transport delays, one for the pulmonary and one for the systemic circulation. A good agreement between the ^{131}I-serum albumin radiocardiogram and a simulated radiocardiogram was shown, but no information was presented on the accuracy, reproducibility or uniqueness of the solution.

A more technical presentation is the electronic radiocardiogram analog simulator by Roux *et al.* (1969). Much attention was paid to the indirect determination of left-to-right, or right-to-left, shunts. Recirculation was eliminated by comparing only the first part of the curve with the simulation result. The entire circulation is simulated by 11 mixing chambers obeying equations (5.4) and (5.5). Very good agreement was obtained between simulation and experimentally obtained results, for example with respect to the ejection fractions of the two ventricles in cases with shunts.

A generalized multi-compartment transport model was described by Gregg (1963). As an example, a two- or three-compartment kidney analog was presented, showing that for certain purposes (the concentration of tracer in renal blood) no improvement resulted from using the more complicated model; a good illustration of the importance of keeping such models as simple as possible. It was also demonstrated that in some cases problems concerning the uniqueness of the solutions can be solved by setting boundary values for a number of parameters. The introduction of these limitations excludes some alternative solutions.

A thorough study of renal function led to a model predicting renal blood flow from the disappearance of Diodrast (an iodine-containing material) from the plasma (Wilson *et al.*, 1970). Their equations express material balance between uptake and discharge with no transport delays except that between the renal artery and vein. This study illustrates a sound use of models, for analysis of the relations between different variables led to the design of experiments to estimate the validity of the model. A digital parameter estimation scheme was used to determine k_2 and k_9 (Fig. 21) from plasma and red blood cell Diodrast concentrations. Independent methods were used to determine k_2 and k_9, and to check the values found indirectly from the model. Good agreement was found suggesting that such a model might serve as a basis for clinical applications.

Another promising approach is discussed by Gianunzio and Rideout (1970)

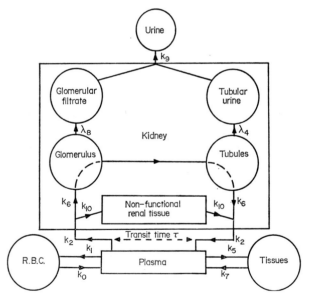

Fig. 21. Diagram of renal model to describe the disappearance of an indicator after impulse injection. k_0, k_1: flows of Diodrast-containing fluid between interior of red cell and plasma: k_5, k_7: flows of Diodrast-containing fluid between plasma and tissue cells; k_6: plasma flow to and from glomerular portion to peritubular portion of kidney; k_{10}: plasma flow to rest of kidney; $k_2 + k_6 + k_{10}$: total renal plasma flow; λ_4 and λ_8: tubular and glomerular extraction, respectively. (From Wilson *et al.*, 1970).

and Gianunzio (1971). In this model, 12 different compartments are defined to represent renal arteries and veins, the tubules, Henle's loop, interstitial fluid compartments, etc. Both active and passive sodium transport is taken into account, as well as the specific architecture of the nephron. Evaluation of the model depends on the comparison of clinical renograms with those from the model.

E. TEMPERATURE REGULATION

Another aspect of transport by the blood stream, which does not include the transport of foreign material, such as indicator, anaesthetic or radio-isotopes, is heat transport. In 1966, Stolwijk and Hardy published a theo-retical study of temperature regulation in man in which they distinguished seven body compartments: head-skin, head-core, trunk-skin, trunk-muscle, trunk-core, extremity-skin and extremity-core. Heat exchange between various compartments took place through conduction or convection by the blood, the temperature of which was assumed to be the same as the central temperature. Heat losses by radiation and evaporation were included. One basic assumption regarding thermal control is the existence of a set point reference for the head-core, mean skin, and muscle temperature. For the seven body compartments and the central blood compartment, eight heat-balance equations are presented, the solution being found by an analog computer. The results compare favourably with measurements on humans under time-varying heat loads, and it was stressed that these model studies should be carried out in close relation to the physiological experiments.

A study of local thermal control mechanisms could benefit from the work of Mitchell and Myers (1968) who describe the heat exchange phenomena in terms of the counter current principle for limbs where arteries and veins are in close proximity.

Another study of total body temperature regulation was published by Atkins and Wyndham (1969). Their "physical" model approximating the human body consists of four concentric cylinders representing the core, the muscles, the deep skin and fatty tissues, and the outer skin. Blood flow ensures convection of heat between the cylinders. Arterial blood has its own temperature which can be different from the core temperature, and heat loss is by radiation, convection and evaporation. Temperature receptors are located in the outer skin and in the arterial blood representing the receptors near the skin surface and within the spinal cord and hypothalamus. The control system acts upon blood flow, heat production and sweat rate. The complete set of equations was programmed on an analog computer, which evaluated the relative importance of arterial blood temperature and skin temperature in the control of sweat rate and blood flow. Comparison of experimental with computer results revealed a strong effect on these two mechanisms of arterial blood temperature. There was no discussion on long-term metabolic control.

An interesting difference exists between this approach and that of Stolwijk and Hardy (1966). For, although both simulations show good agreement with experiments, the Stolwijk and Hardy approach requires three temperature set points and the Atkins and Wyndham model operates without any set points whatsoever. In Section 4, some attention was paid to such differences. It seems that temperature regulation in the human body might also be described as a system in a dynamic equilibrium state.

6. PARAMETER ESTIMATION

Until recently models have mostly been used as hypotheses; that is the relevant known information was incorporated and assumptions were made about some unknown aspects. These assumptions were subsequently evaluated experimentally after the model was shown to behave realistically. Another promising model application is found in relation to parameter-estimation methods. In an estimation scheme the models generally receive input signals from the real system (forcing time functions) while other signals obtained from the system are compared with corresponding model signals. The difference between them is then minimized by adjusting the model parameters. Figure 22 represents this schematically.

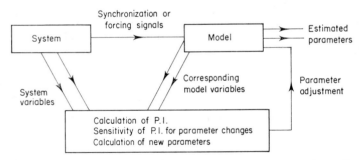

FIG. 22. Schematic representation of a parameter-estimation procedure. The model is synchronized with or forced by an input signal derived from the system. Corresponding variables from the system and the model are used to find the performance index. (P.I.). New parameter values are introduced until the P.I. is optimal. The estimated parameters are then available from the model.

Rothe and Nash (1968) applied the principle to study the properties of the renal arteries. Renal arterial pressure was used as an input signal, and renal arterial flow and the corresponding model flow were used to calculate the performance index (see also Section 3). An initial indication of the applicability of a certain procedure comes from a "model-to-model" estimation. One or more time-functions of the model are recorded and then a number of parameter values are changed. Subsequently, the original time-functions are used to force the modified model or as functions to calculate the performance index. The time taken and the number of iterations needed to return to the original parameter settings is a measure of the efficiency of the estimation scheme.

Van Herk (1969) used a digital model with three compartments for the cardiovascular system; one segment represented the heart. The time course of one pressure cycle was specified at 21 discrete time intervals and the initial conditions of the two remaining pressures, and of the peripheral resistance, were also set. The other parameters, including the time course of ventricular elastance, were known. Representation of the two heart valves complicated the calculations considerably. Extension to a seven-compartment model failed because of computational difficulties related to the choice of the least-squares estimation method.

Sims (1970) used the parameter-estimation method together with animal data in a ten-compartment model with three peripheral resistances to represent the arterial tree and a time-varying compliance to represent the action of the heart. Three pressures and two flows were used to optimize the ten compliances and the three peripheral resistances. The other resistances, and all the inertances, were calculated and held constant. The optimization procedure used a least-square error criterion while the step-size determination was a combination of the steepest descent method and the differential correction (Gauss) method, an algorithm designed by D. W. Marquardt (1963).

A model-to-model test, performed after disturbing the 13 parameters, needed only eight iterations to return most parameters to within 3 per cent of their original values. The approach appeared to be less sensitive for parameter deviations of components downstream from the most distal measuring site. Subsequently the optimization of the 13 parameters was performed with signals from dogs, there being three pressures and two flows measured simultaneously. Reasonably acceptable matches of the time courses of the variables in the model and animal were obtained. Improved prediction of delay times might have been obtained if the inertances and viscous wall properties had also been estimated during the same run. Simulation of cardiac action could be improved, and the aortic flow signal could be used as a forcing function, which would also improve the match between model and animal and improve the estimated parameters even more (Sims, 1970). Although all problems were not solved, Sims' study clearly indicates the power of estimation techniques to determine parameters indirectly.

The method for measuring renal blood flow described by Wilson et al. (1970)

is another example of parameter estimation. This work is discussed in Section 5D (Fig. 21).

Katz *et al.* (1970) used a seven-compartment model of the inferior vena cava; six had constant compliances and one (the infra-hepatic) compartment had a compliance which was a function of transmural pressure. This model was driven by right atrial pressure and hepatic flow, with the intra-abdominal and intra-thoracic pressures from animal experiments as boundary conditions. Blood pressures at the caval bifurcation, just below the liver, and in the intra-thoracic vena cava were used to generate the performance index; this was the time integral of the absolute values of the differences between the corresponding animal and model variables. The purpose of this was the determination of thirteen parameters (seven compliances, six resistances) for the vena cava model. So far results from one experiment have been reported, the procedure is rather insensitive to parameter deviations in the region where the performance index is near its optimum, for optimization trials, using identical data, resulted in a 10 per cent parameter variation.

Wesseling *et al.* (1972) described a non-invasive method to measure the properties of the arm arteries using a four-compartment model. Pulse wave contours were measured externally in the axilla and at the wrist. The axillary signal, though uncalibrated, forms the input signal and the output signal is compared with the wrist pulse. The integral of the squared error over four heart cycles was the performance index. The haemodynamic quantities (resistance, compliance, inertance, and resistance to flow in side branch shunts) were expressed in terms of vessel cross-sectional area, Young's modulus of the vessel wall and conductance of the side branches. The four compartments, therefore, involve 12 parameters. Since the signals are uncalibrated, another parameter, the amplitude ratio of axillary and wrist signals is optimized. Parameter adjustment is carried out manually, and the values determined are within the physiological range and reasonably reproducible (see also Section 3A).

The above studies indicate that parameter estimation techniques are powerful tools. Both in physiology and in clinical medicine it is often impossible to obtain certain quantitative information from the intact system, either because measurements will seriously interfere with the system or because certain regions are inaccessible. If sufficient qualitative insight into the system is available a model can be designed and the quantitative data obtained by parameter estimation.

In setting up a model for parameter estimation attention must be paid to the uniqueness of the ultimate solution. It is obvious that if two or more numerically different models match the real system equally well, no quantitative conclusion concerning the real system can be drawn. Occasionally, some solutions can be discarded if they lie beyond limits determined from *a priori* information. Theoretically, only n independent data points are needed to determine n parameters. The number of independent samples that can be taken from a signal is proportional to the frequency content of that signal, this means that, in a given case, the time course of a single variable alone could be sufficient to estimate many parameters. However, biological systems can probably never be exactly simulated by models so that the error criteria will never become zero. The inevitable presence of noise has the same effect. It is desirable therefore that more information be used than the theoretical lower limit. A thorough study of the choice of performance indices or of error criteria is needed.

Parameter estimation procedures, whether performed manually or by advanced computer methods, are generally rather complex. It must, however, be kept in mind that when a number of time-dependent variables are available, other methods such as network synthesis routines may be used fruitfully. When, as in clinical applications, the number of quantities to be measured must be kept a minimum, thorough evaluation may prove parameter estimation to be the most valuable tool.

7. Conclusion

In the preceding sections a large variety of models have been discussed all of which relate to studies of the cardiovascular system. It is a little disappointing to observe that many good model studies have thus far been applied in few situations. In some cases the models are too complex to be of practical use, while others are too simple to yield useful results. The most successful approach is possibly to start with a rather extensive model. The reason is that quantitative evaluation of the relative importance of certain factors is needed before simplifying assumptions are made. This evaluation can ideally be made with the model itself resulting in well-founded simplifications.

It is important to have an exactly defined problem including an answer to the question: "What if the problem is solved?" It will be obvious that to deal with questions like these, there must be very close co-operation between the biologist, whose primary interest is in the answer, and the computer scientist who handles the mathematics and simulation. They should understand each other's subject well enough to prevent both the over simplification of assumptions and misinterpretation of results. This is a matter of mutual responsibility and requires patience from both sides.

The majority of the models published so far serve mainly to improve understanding. In the near future, it is believed that models will be used with more direct relation to patient diagnosis and care. The models will be matched to individual patients in order to obtain better insight into the disorder and to serve as prognostic aids in relation to the proposed treatment. The major contribution of model studies to diagnosis is likely to be a more exact statement of the quantities that need to be measured and the improvement of data acquisition by parameter estimation procedures. Patient care need not depend on information that is directly and easily obtainable, and it is now possible to specify what other information is worth using.

ACKNOWLEDGEMENTS

The helpful and stimulating suggestions made during the preparation of this manuscript by Jan J. H. Donders, Jan Kuiper, Vincent C. Rideout, N. Ty Smith, and Karel H. Wesseling are gratefully acknowledged.

REFERENCES

Ashman, M. N., Blesser, W. B. and Epstein, R. M. (1970). A non-linear model for the uptake and distribution of Halothane in man. *Anesthesiology* **33**, 419–429.

Atkins, A. R. and Wyndman, C. H. (1969). A study of temperature regulation in the human body with the aid of an analogue computer. *Pflügers Arch.* **307**, 104–119.

Bassingthwaighte, J. B., Ackerman, F. H. and Wood, E. H. (1966). Application of the lagged normal density curve as a model for arterial dilution curves. *Circulation Res.* **18**, 398–415.

Beneken, J. E. W. (1963). Investigation on the regulatory system of the blood circulation. *In* "Circulatory Analog Computers" (A. Noordergraaf, G. N. Jager and N. Westerhof, eds), N. Holland Publishing Co., Amsterdam.

Beneken, J. E. W. (1965). A mathematical approach to cardiovascular function. The uncontrolled human system. Int. rep. 2.4.5/6. Institute of Medical Physics TNO, Utrecht.

Beneken, J. E. W. and De Wit, B. (1967). A physical approach to hemodynamic aspects of the human cardiovascular system. *In* "Physical Bases of Circulatory Transport" (E. B. Reeve, A. C. Guyton, eds), W. B. Saunders, Philadelphia.

Beneken, J. E. W. and Grupping, J. C. M. (1965). Electronic analog computer model of the human circulatory system. *In* "Medical Electronics" (F. H. Bostem, ed.) pp. 770–785, Desoer, Brussels.

Beneken, J. E. W., Guyton, A. C. and Sagawa, K. (1969). Coronary perfusion pressure and left ventricular function. *Pflügers Arch.* **305**, 76–95.

Beneken, J. E. W. and Rideout, V. C. (1968). The use of multiple models in cardiovascular system studies: Transport and Perturbation. *IEEE Trans. Bio. Med. Eng.* **15**, 281–289.

Berman, M. (1963). The formulation and testing of models. *Ann. N.Y. Acad. Sci.* **108**, 182–194.

Brutsaert, D. L. and Sonnenblick, E. H. (1969). Force-velocity-length-time relations of the contractile elements in heart muscle of the cat. *Circulation Res.* **24**, 137–149.

Conrad, W. A. (1969). Pressure flow relationships in collapsible tubes. *IEEE Trans. Bio. Med. Eng.* **16**, 284–295.

Coulam, C. M., Warner, H. R., Marshall, H. W. and Bassingthwaighte, J. B. (1967). A steady state transfer function analysis of portions of the circulatory system using indicator dilution technique. *Comput. Biomed. Res.* **1**, 124–138.

Defares, J. G., Osborn, J. J. and Hara, H. H. (1963). Theoretical synthesis of the cardiovascular system. Study I: The controlled system. *Acta Physiol. Pharm. Neerl.* **12**, 189–265.

Defares, J. G. and Van der Waal, H. J. (1969). A method for the determination of systemic arterial compliance in man. *Acta Physiol. Pharm. Neerl.* **15**, 329–343.

Denson, J. S. and Abrahamson, S. (1969). A computer controlled patient simulator. *J. Amer. Med. Ass.* **208**, 504–508.

De Waal, B. M. J. (1969). An analog model of transport in the blood circulation. Int. rep. Institute of Medical Physics TNO, Utrecht.

Dick, D. E., Kendrick, J. E., Matson, G. L. and Rideout, V. C. (1968). Measurements of non-linearity in the arterial system of the dog using a new method. *Circulation Res.* **22**, 101–111.

Dick, D. E. and Rideout, V. C. (1965). Analog simulation of left heart and arterial dynamics. *Proc. 18th ACEMB*, Philadelphia, p. 78.

Dickinson, C. J. (1969). A digital computer model of the effects of gravitational stress upon the heart and venous system. *Med. Biol. Eng.* **7**, 267–275.

Donders, J. J. H. and Beneken, J. E. W. (1971). Computer model of cardiac muscle mechanics. *Cardiovascular Res.* Suppl. 1, 34–50.

Eger, E. I. (1963a). A mathematical model of uptake and distribution. *In* "Uptake and Distribution of Anaesthetic Agents" (E. M. Papper and R. J. Kitz, eds.), McGraw-Hill, New York.

Eger, E. I. (1963b). Applications of a mathematical model of gas uptake. *In* "Uptake and Distribution of Anaesthetic Agents" (E. M. Papper and R. J. Kitz, eds.), McGraw-Hill, New York.

Fitzhugh, R. (1969). Mathematical models of excitation and propagation in nerve. *In* "Biological Engineering" (H. P. Schwan, ed.), pp. 1–85, McGraw-Hill, New York.

Friedman, P. J. and Downing, S. E. (1968). Estimation of systemic blood flow by the indicator dilution technic in the presence of central shunts. *Am. J. Cardiol.* **22**, 672–677.

Gianunzio, J. (1971). A model of renal function. Ph.D. Thesis: University of Wisconsin.

Gianunzio, J. and Rideout, V. C. (1970). A multiple model of sodium transport in the cardiovascular-renal system. *Proc. 23rd ACEMB*, Washington.

Gregg, E. C. (1963). An analog computer for the generalized multi-compartment model of transport in biological systems. *Ann. N.Y. Acad. Sci.* **108**, 128–146.

Grodins, F. S. (1959). Integrative cardiovascular physiology: A mathematical synthesis of cardiac and blood vessel hemodynamics. *Quart. Rev. Biol.* **34**, 93–123.

Grupping, J. C. M. (1963). Regulatory systems of the blood circulation. An analog model of the human heart. Int. rep. 2.4.5/5. Institute of Medical Physics TNO, Utrecht.

Guyton, A. C. (1955). Determination of cardiac output by equating venous return curves with cardiac response curves. *Physiol. Rev.* **35**, 123–129.

Guyton, A. C. (1963). "Circulatory Physiology: Cardiac Output and its Regulation" W. B. Saunders, Philadelphia.

Guyton, A. C. and Coleman, Th. G. (1967). Long-term regulation of the circulation: Interrelationships with body fluid volumes. *In* "Physical Bases of Circulatory Transport" (E. B. Reeve and A. C. Guyton, eds), pp. 170–201, W. B. Saunders, Philadelphia.

Higinbotham, W. A., Sugarman, R. M., Potter, D. W. and Robertson, J. S. (1963). A direct analog computer for multi compartment systems. *Ann. N.Y. Acad. Sci.* **108**, 117–121.

Henig, T. (1961). An analog computer simulation of the blood circulation. *Proc. 3rd Int. Ass. Analog Computation*, Presses Academiques Européenes, Brussels.

Holt, J. P. (1969). Flow through collapsible tubes and through *in situ* veins. *IEEE BME* **16**, 274–283.

Himmelblau, D. M. and Bischoff, K. B. (1968). "Process Analysis and Simulation; Deterministic Systems", John Wiley, New York.

Hyndman, B. W. (1970). A digital simulation of the human cardiovascular system and its use in the study of sinus anhythmia. Ph.D. Thesis: Imperial College, London.

Johnson, E. A. and Kuohung, P. W. (1968). The tri-gamma system. A model of the intrinsic mechanism of control of cardiac contractility. *Math. Bioscience* **3**, 65–89.

Katz, A. I., Chen, Y. and Moreno, A. H. (1969). Flow through a collapsible tube. *Biophys. J.* **9**, 1261–1279.

Katz, A. I., Fromm, N. C. and Moreno, A. H. (1970). Parameter optimization for a model of the cardiovascular system. *Proc. Summer Computer Simulation Conf.*, pp. 889–898, Association Computer Machinery, New York.

Kezdi, D. (1967). "Baroreceptors and Hypertension", Pergamon Press, Oxford.

Kresch, E. and Noordergraaf, A. (1969). A mathematical model for the pressure-flow relationship in a segment of vein. *IEEE Trans. Bio. Med. Eng.* **16**, 296–307.

Kuwahara, M., Iwai, S., Takayasu, M., Nohara, Y. and Hirakawa, A. (1967). Radio cardiogram analysis by analog computer simulation. *Digest 7th Int. Conf. on Med. and Biol. Eng.*, Stockholm.

Landahl, H. D. (1963). On mathematical models of distribution. *In* "Uptake and Distribution of Anaesthetic Agents" (E. M. Papper and R. J. Kitz, eds), McGraw-Hill, New York.

McDonald, D. A. (1968). Hemodynamics. *Annu. Rev. Physiol.* **30**, 525–556.

Mapleson, W. W. (1963). Quantitative prediction of anesthetic concentration. *In* "Uptake and Distribution of Anaesthetic Agents" (E. M. Papper and R. J. Kitz, eds.), McGraw-Hill, New York.

Marquardt, D. W. (1963). An algorithm for least-squares estimation of nonlinear parameters. *J. Soc. ind. appl. Math.* **11**, 431–441.

Mirsky, I. (1970). Effects of anisotropy and non-homogeneity on left ventricular stresses in the intact heart. *Bull. Math. Biophys.* **32**, 197–213.

Mitchell, J. W. and Myers, G. E. (1968). An analytical model of the counter current heat exchange phenomena. *Biophys. J.* **8**, 897–911.

Moreno, A. H., Katz, A. I. and Gold, L. D. (1969). An integrated approach to the study of the venous system with steps toward a detailed model of the dynamics of venous return to the right heart. *IEEE Trans. Bio. Med. Eng.* **16**, 308–324.

Munson, E. S., Eger, E. I. and Bowers, D. L. (1968). The effects of changes in cardiac output and distribution on the rate of cerebral equilibrium. *Anesthesiology* **29**, 533–537.

Noordergraaf, A. (1969). Hemodynamics. *In* "Biological Engineering" (H. P. Schwan, ed.), pp. 391–545, McGraw-Hill, New York.

Norwich, K. H. and Zelin, S. (1970). The dispersion of indicator in the cardio-pulmonary system. *Bull. Math. Biophys.* **32**, 25–43.

Öberg, P. A. and Sjöstrand, U. (1969). Studies on blood pressure regulation II. On line simulation as a method of studying the regulatory properties of the carotid sinus reflex. *Acta Physiol. Scand.* **75**, 287–300.

222 JAN E. W. BENEKEN

Papper, E. M. and Kitz, R. J. (1963). "Uptake and Distribution of Anesthetic Agents", McGraw-Hill, New York.

Permutt, S. (1965). Vascular waterfall. *Proc. 18th ACEMB*, 11–7, Philadelphia.

Pickering, W. D., Nikiforuk, P. N. and Merriman, J. E. (1969). Analogue computer model of the human cardiovascular control system. *Med. Biol. Eng.* **7**, 401–410.

Priban, J. (1968). Forecasting failure of health. *Spectrum* **48**, 9–12.

Rideout, V. C. (1969). Computer simulation of physiological processes. *Proc. A.S.M.E. Comput. Conf.* A.S.M.E., New York.

Rideout, V. C. and Dick, D. E. (1967). Difference differential equations for fluid flow in distensible tubes. *IEEE Trans. Bio. Med. Eng.* **14**, 171–177.

Rideout, V. C. and Katra, J. A. (1969). Computer simulation of the pulmonary cardiovascular system. *Simulation* **12**, No. 5.

Rideout, V. C. and Schaefer, R. L. (1970). Hybrid computer simulation of the transport of chemicals in the circulation. Presented at AICA-IFIP Conference, Munich.

Rideout, V. C. and Sims, J. B. (1969). Computer study of the effects of small non-linearities in the arterial system. *Math. Bioscience* **4**, 411–426.

Robinson, D. A. (1963). Ventricular dynamics and the cardiac representation problem. In "Circulatory Analog Computers" (A. Noordergraaf, G. N. Jager and N. Westerhof, eds), pp. 56–73, N. Holland Publishing Co., Amsterdam.

Robinson, D. A. (1965). Quantitative analysis of the control of cardiac output in the isolated left ventricle. *Circulation Res.* **17**, 207–221.

Rothe, C. F. and Nash, F. D. (1968). Renal arterial compliance and conductance measurement using on-line self adaptive analog computation of model parameters. *Med. Biol. Eng.* **6**, 53–69.

Roux, G., Lansiart, A., de Vernejoul, P. and Kellershohn, C. (1969). Simulation analogique electronique de radio cardiogrammes. *Med. Biol. Eng.* **7**, 57–70.

Sagawa, K. (1969). Overall circulatory regulation. *Annu. Rev. Physiol.* **31**, 295–330.

Sallin, E. A. (1969). Fibre orientation and ejection fraction in the human left ventricle. *Biophys. J.* **9**, 954–964.

Severinghaus, J. W. (1963). Role of lung factors. In "Uptake and Distribution of Anaesthetic Agents" (E. M. Papper and R. J. Kitz, eds), McGraw-Hill, New York.

Sims, J. B. (1970). A hybrid-computer-aided study of parameter estimation in the systemic circulatory system. Ph.D. Thesis: University of Wisconsin.

Smith, N. T., Zwart, A. and Beneken, J. E. W. (1972). An analog computer multiple model of the uptake and distribution of Halothane, Innovation in Medicine. *Proc. 11th Annual Biomedical Symposium*, San Diego.

Smith, N. T., Zwart, A. and Beneken, J. E. W. (1972). Interaction between circulatory effects and uptake and distribution of Halothane. *Anesthesiology*, in press.

Smith, N. T. and Smith, P. (1971). Circulatory effects of modern inhalation anesthetic agents. In "Handboek der exp. Pharmokologie", Band XXX, Section 4.3, (M. B. Clenoweth, ed.), Springer-Verlag, Berlin.

Snyder, M. F. and Rideout, V. C. (1969). Computer simulation studies of the venous circulation. *IEEE Tans. Bio. Med. Eng.* **16**, 325–334.

Snyder, M. F., Rideout, V. C. and Hillestad, R. J. (1968). Computer modelling of the human systemic arterial tree. *J. Biomechanics* **1**, 341–353.

Sonnenblick, E. H. (1965). Determinants of active state in heart muscle: Force, velocity, instantaneous muscle length, time. *Fed. Proc.* **24**, 1396–1409.

Stolwijk, J. A. J. and Hardy, J. D. (1966). Temperature regulation in man: A theoretical study. *Pflügers Arch.* **291**, 129–162.

Streeter, D. D., Spotnitz, H. M., Patel, D. J., Ross J. and Sonnenblick, E. H. (1969). Fibre orientation in the canine left ventricle during diastole and systole. *Circulation Res.* **24**, 339–347.

Tilanus, E. W. (1971). Analysis and simulation of transport phenomena in the blood stream. M.Sc. Thesis: Technical University, Eindhoven.

Topham, W. S. and Warner, H. R. (1967). The control of cardiac output during exercise. *In* "Physical Bases of Circulatory Transport" (E. B. Reeve and A. C. Guyton, eds), pp. 77–90, W. B. Saunders, Philadelphia.

Vadot, L. (1963). Application d'une analogie électrique à l'étude des corrections des malformations cardiaques combinées. *In* "Medical Electronics" (F. Bostem, ed.), pp. 809–815, Desoers, Brussels.

Van Herk, M. (1970). Parameter estimation applied to the human circulatory system. M.Sc. Thesis: Technical University, Eindhoven.

Warner, H. R. (1959). The use of analog computer for analysis of control mechanisms in the circulation. *Proc.I.R.E.* **47**, 1913–1916.

Watt, T. B. and Goldwyn, R. M. (1967). Arterial pressure contour analysis for the clinical estimation of human vascular properties. *Proc. 7th ICMBE*, Stockholm, p. 54.

Waud, B. E. and Waud, P. R. (1970). Calculated kinetics of distribution of nitrous oxide and methoxyflurane during intermittent administration in obstetrics. *Anesthesiology* **32**, 306–316.

Wesseling, K. H., De Waal, B. M. J., De Wit, B and Beneken, J. E. W. (1972). Arm arterial parameters from externally measured pulsewave contours. Submitted for publication.

Westerhof, N. and Noordergraaf, A. (1970). Arterial visco elasticity: A generalized model. *J. Biomechanics* **3**, 357–379.

Wilson, D. M., Apter, J. T. and Schwartz, F. D. (1970). A model for measuring renal blood flow from plasma disappearance of iodopyracet. *J. appl. Physiol* **28**, 79–88.

Womersley, J. R. (1957). An elastic tube theory of pulse transmission and oscillating flow in mammalian arteries. WADC Tech. Report TR 56–54.

Zwart, A. Smith, N. T. and Beneken, J. E. W. (1972). Multiple model approach to uptake and distribution of Halothane. *Comp. Biomed. Res.*, in press.

Chapter 7

The Meaning and Measurement of Myocardial Contractility

J. R. BLINKS

Department of Pharmacology, Mayo Medical School,
Rochester, Minnesota, U.S.A.

and

B. R. JEWELL

Department of Physiology, University College,
London, England

1. NATURE OF THE PROBLEM

During the past decade there has been a relatively rapid introduction into the cardiovascular literature of a body of concepts and terminology formerly restricted almost wholly to work on the mechanics of skeletal muscle. With this, considerable attention has been given to the problem of quantifying "myocardial contractility", a term that had previously been widely used with little consideration of its precise meaning. Unquestionably, the application of the principles of muscle mechanics to the study of the function of the heart has furthered the understanding of cardiovascular dynamics. However, it is equally true that misunderstanding and misapplication of these principles have been widespread in the cardiovascular literature. Some of the most widely quoted work in the field is based on highly questionable assumptions or inappropriate experiments, and it is very difficult for the newcomer to avoid being drawn into the trap of building on foundations that are likely to crumble.

It is the purpose of this chapter to review the major principles of muscle mechanics relevant to the study of myocardial function, and to provide a basis for the critical evaluation of methods for the description and measurement of the contractile performance of heart muscle. In this, emphasis will be placed on principles rather than applications, and since quantitative results are most readily obtained from studies on preparations of isolated heart muscle, the greater share of attention will be devoted to them.

Before we go into the principles of muscle mechanics required to frame a specific definition of what does and what does not constitute a change in contractility, let us consider some of the problems that have necessitated the introduction of those concepts into studies of heart muscle. Most of us feel quite confident on an intuitive level that we know what is meant by "myocardial contractility" and what would constitute a change in contractility. However, awkward questions sometimes arise when specific situations are considered. For example, should a change in the performance of the heart resulting from a change in end-diastolic fibre length be considered a change in myocardial contractility? Most people would probably answer that it should not, but would be hard-pressed to provide a rigorous defence for that position. Those who answer that it should be are invited to ponder the question of the influence of the change in fibre length that occurs as a ventricle ejects blood during the course of a single beat. Is myocardial contractility to be considered as something that is normally changing during the course of each contraction? To take the stand that it is changing presents obvious problems, but so does taking the alternative position, as will be seen later in this discussion (Section 3A 3). Clearly, it would be useful to have a specific and generally accepted definition of what constitutes a change in myocardial contractility. A change must be recognized in order to be measured meaningfully.

Changes in myocardial contractility are often expressed in terms of variations in some experimentally measured quantity that is used as an index of contractility. The index chosen for one experimental situation may not be applicable to another, and the quest for a generally useful index of contractility is a topic that we shall deal with later. One criterion that an index of contractility ought to satisfy is that it not be subject to modification by factors outside the myocardium. An example of an index that does not meet this requirement is ventricular stroke work (i.e. the product of the stroke volume and the mean pressure against which this is ejected), which has been used frequently as the chief or even the sole measure of myocardial contractility in haemodynamic studies. The feature of stroke work that probably accounts for its appeal is that it combines in a single measure the two most distinctive features of muscular contraction—tension development and shortening. The fact that these two tend to change in opposite directions when the load on a muscle is altered lends a further superficial plausibility to the use of stroke work as an index of contractility. However, the fact that there is an inverse relation between tension development and shortening does not mean that ventricular stroke work will remain constant as the resistance to ejection is varied. The ventricle does no external work when it ejects blood with no opposing pressure, and it does none when the pressure is so high that ejection is prevented altogether. If the pressure is varied from one of these extremes to the other, stroke work will rise from zero to a maximum and then fall to zero again. The fact that stroke work is highly subject to modification by the pressure opposing ejection means that in an experimental situation where both pressure and stroke work change, the change in stroke work cannot be depended upon to bear a fixed relation to the magnitude or even to the direction of any change in contractility. This should certainly make one have serious reservations about the use of ventricular stroke work as an index of contractility, yet that measure has been employed so widely that few authors seem to have felt the need to justify its use.

Recently a good deal of attention has been given to the notion that the maximum velocity of shortening of the unloaded muscle (v_{max}) could serve as a generally applicable index of contractility. There are serious problems with this as well, but a discussion of these requires that we first consider in detail certain basic concepts of muscle mechanics.

2. BASIC CONCEPTS OF MUSCLE MECHANICS

The sliding filament hypothesis is now accepted as the mechanism of contraction of striated muscle (i.e. skeletal and cardiac muscle), largely as a result of the efforts of A. F. Huxley, H. E. Huxley, and their collaborators. Muscles of this type are made up of interdigitating arrays of thick filaments (myosin) and thin filaments (actin, tropomyosin, and troponin), which are arranged in a way that gives skeletal and cardiac muscle a characteristic striated appearance. Stimulation of the muscle causes cross bridges to appear between the overlapping parts of the two arrays of filaments (Fig. 1(a)). These produce a sliding motion of one set of filaments relative to the other, which

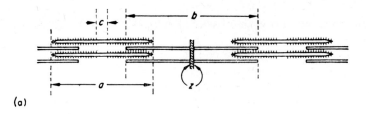

(a)

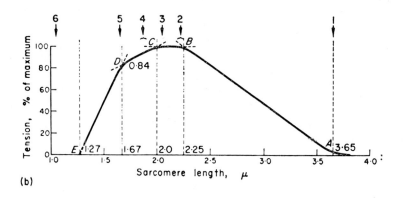

(b)

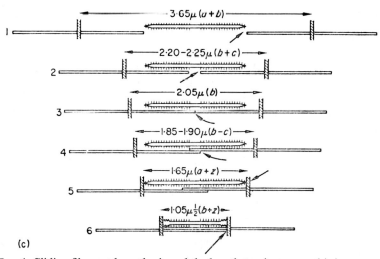

(c)

Fig. 1. Sliding filament hypothesis and the length-tension curve. (a) Arrangement of filaments in striated muscle. The following are the standard filament lengths in frog muscle fibres: a = thick filament (myosin), 1·60 μ; b = thin filament (actin + tropomyosin + troponin) extending through the z line, 2·05 μ; c = projection-free zone in the middle of thick filaments, 0·25–0·20 μ. (b) Length-tension curve from part of a single frog skeletal muscle fibre (schematic summary of results). The arrows along the top show the various critical stages of overlap that are portrayed in (c). (c) Critical stages in the increase of overlap between thick and thin filaments as the sarcomere length decreases. (From Wilkie, 1968, and based on the work of Gordon *et al.*, 1966.)

will result in active shortening of the muscle, tension development, or both, depending on the mechanical loading conditions. Fuller accounts of the sliding filament hypothesis and its implications will be found in numerous general texts (e.g. Wilkie, 1968; Bendall, 1969; H. E. Huxley, 1965, 1969).

A. RESTING AND ACTIVE MUSCLE

A muscle fibre is brought very rapidly from a state of rest to a state of activity by the passage of an action potential over its surface membrane. The rapid change in membrane potential during the rising phase of the action potential is thought to trigger off a release of calcium into the sarcoplasm, mostly from intracellular stores (probably the sarcoplasmic reticulum), where it is held at high concentration. The rise in sarcoplasmic Ca^{++} concentration results in the appearance of cross bridges between the overlapping parts of the actin and myosin filaments, and the muscle is capable of active shortening and tension development: it is then said to be in the active state. (The mechanism of calcium activation is discussed in detail in two excellent articles by Ebashi and co-workers (1968, 1969).) In cardiac muscle, at least in some species, the initial rise in sarcoplasmic Ca^{++} concentration triggered off by the rising phase of the action potential is augmented and prolonged by the entry of calcium from the extracellular fluid during the plateau phase of the action potential.

The muscle fibre is restored to its resting state by the action of metabolically-powered pumping mechanisms that lower the sarcoplasmic Ca^{++} concentration to a subthreshold level by returning the calcium to the intracellular stores or by extruding it from the cell. The gradual fall of Ca^{++} concentration leads to a waning of the active state, as judged by the ability of the muscle to bear tension and to shorten; in a later section we shall consider ways in which the state of activity or degree of activation of the muscle can be measured at various times after stimulation.

B. LENGTH-TENSION RELATION

If sliding of the filaments is prevented by an external mechanical restraint, the formation of cross bridges will result in a rise of tension in the muscle to a level that will be determined by the number of cross bridges per sarcomere. The latter depends on the amount of overlap between the interdigitating arrays of filaments (Fig. 1(c)), and the tension developed by a single frog muscle fibre has been shown to depend in a precise way on the geometry of the sarcomere (Fig. 1(b) and (c)). Thus the study of the length-tension relation in cardiac muscle may be expected to give useful information about the relative numbers of cross bridges formed at various muscle lengths. Although the decline in force at short sarcomere lengths has been attributed to mechanical interference with the sliding motion of the filaments (see Fig. 1(c)), another contributing factor has recently come to light (Taylor and Rüdel, 1970); this is that there is partial failure of the excitation-contraction coupling mechanism (described in the previous section) at short muscle lengths. To what extent this may also account for the form of the ascending limb of the length-tension curve in cardiac muscle is not at present known. This is an important point, because cardiac muscle normally works on the ascending limb of this curve.

C. FORCE-VELOCITY RELATION

When the loading conditions permit sliding of the filaments, the muscle shortens at a velocity that is inversely related to the force opposing motion. Alternatively, it may be stated that the muscle generates a force or tension that is inversely related to the speed at which it is shortening. The underlying mechanism for this might be conceived of as follows. The tension in a muscle depends on the fraction of the pool of potential cross bridges that is attached at a given time. When an active muscle is allowed to shorten, cross bridges must be detached and reformed as the thick and thin filaments slide past one another. The process of breaking and remaking a cross bridge must take a finite time, so the faster the muscle is shortening the smaller will be the fraction of cross bridges attached at any given time, and the lower will be the tension in the muscle. A force-velocity curve shows this inverse relation, often approximately hyperbolic, between the force opposing shortening (tension in the muscle) and the velocity of shortening. The intercept on the force axis (which we will designate F_i) is the maximum tension that can be developed by the muscle under the prevailing conditions; it will be determined by the number of cross bridges formed when no sliding takes place. The intercept (v_i) on the velocity axis is the speed of shortening when there is no force opposing motion. This will be the maximum velocity of shortening of the muscle under those conditions. It reflects the maximum rate of turnover of cross bridges, and according to some current theories should be independent of the number of cross bridges participating (as long as internal forces opposing shortening do not arise). Thus the force-velocity relation of a muscle gives potentially useful information about things happening at the cross bridges, though as we shall see later the actual characterization of this relation in terms of force-velocity curves is a complicated business because of interaction with the length-tension relation, and the fact that both relations are time-dependent.

D. ANALOG MODELS OF MUSCLE

Although it is useful to think in terms of what is happening at crossbridges when one is considering the length-tension and force-velocity relations, it is not possible to make measurements at anything near that level in cardiac muscle. Studies must be made on the whole heart or on isolated preparations (e.g. papillary muscles) that are much more complex than a single sarcomere or even a single cell. Until now work in this field has been dominated by the classical approach to muscle mechanics that was evolved by A. V. Hill and others at University College London for the study of the mechanical properties of whole frog muscles. This approach depends heavily on a particular conceptual model of muscle, which has a contractile component and one or more passive elastic components (Fig. 2). Over the past 15 years, this approach

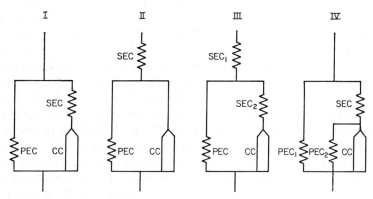

FIG. 2. Mechanical analog models of muscle. SEC = series elastic component PEC = parallel elastic component, and CC = contractile component.

has been shown to have many shortcomings when applied to skeletal muscle. Three essential premises of the classical approach that are now considered to be incorrect are:

(i) that the force-velocity relation of the contractile component is an "instantaneous" relation, i.e. a force-velocity curve obtained by measuring the steady velocity of shortening of the muscle against different constant loads in a series of isotonic contractions can be used to predict the velocity of shortening of the contractile component in a situation where the force opposing shortening is changing rapidly;

(ii) that the contractile component is freely extensible at rest, contributing nothing to the resting length-tension relation of the muscle; and

(iii) that the series elastic component is a purely passive element with properties that are unaffected by the state of activity of the muscle.

The steadily-increasing body of evidence that none of these premises is strictly correct in the case of skeletal muscle has been reviewed by Simmons and Jewell (1972). Muscles appear not to switch simply and instantly from one point to another on the force-velocity curve; careful studies of the behaviour of single muscle fibres during isotonic releases have shown that there is a delay and a complex velocity transient before a steady velocity of shortening is achieved against a constant load (Civan and Podolsky, 1966; Armstrong *et al.*, 1966). A detailed study of the properties of resting muscle at short lengths (Hill, 1968) has revealed a form of resistance to stretch that could not be accounted for by the classical two- or three-component model in its simple form. Finally, it is becoming increasingly clear that the properties of the series elastic component cannot be regarded as being constant, even from moment to moment within a given muscle. Huxley and Simmons (1971) have obtained evidence that a significant fraction of the "series" compliance in frog muscle fibres resides in the crossbridges between thick and thin filaments: as more crossbridges are established in parallel with one another the measured stiffness of the series elastic component increases. Other sources of series compliance must exist (e.g. non-overlapping parts of myofilaments Z discs, ends of fibres, lack of parallel arrangement of myofibrils, tendon) and it is probable that these contribute much more to the total series compliance in cardiac than in skeletal muscle. This might lead one to predict that the series compliance in preparations of cardiac muscle would obey premise (iii) much more closely than appears to be the case for skeletal muscle. On the other hand, it could be argued that the "non-crossbridge" sources of series compliance may also be affected by the state of activity of the muscle unless there is complete temporal and spatial homogeneity in the activation of myofibrils throughout the muscle. Indeed, Noble and Else (1972) and Pollack *et al.* (1972) have recently shown that in the cat papillary muscle the stiffness of the series elastic component depends critically on the time after stimulation that the measurement is made.

In the skeletal muscle field, the classical approach to muscle mechanics has been almost completely superseded by a new approach that aims to account for the physical behaviour of muscle in terms of the properties of structures (e.g. sliding filaments and crossbridges) known to be present in the living muscle. This new approach is justified in the case of skeletal muscle, where highly sophisticated techniques now allow mechanical measurements to be made at the sarcomere level. However, there seems to be little hope that comparable measurements could ever be made on cardiac muscle because of the lack of suitable preparations. Those of us working in the latter field therefore face an awkward dilemma: should we continue to use the classical approach in spite of its known limitations, or should we switch to the contemporary approach that is being used in the skeletal muscle field in spite of the technical limitations alluded to above? (There is one other possibility and that is to turn a blind eye to both of these approaches and to treat measurements of tension and length changes in preparations of cardiac muscle as a useful operational description of the properties of the muscle.) The classical approach currently dominates the study of cardiac muscle mechanics, and is likely to continue to do so for some time. Provided that its limitations are not lost sight of, we believe that approach still provides a useful conceptual framework for understanding many aspects of muscle function. Accordingly, we have oriented this chapter around it, while at the same time trying to call attention to its limitations. Readers who are interested in finding out more about the new approach that is being used in the skeletal muscle field may find it helpful to study the article by Simmons and Jewell (1972) on this subject.

The essential basis of the classical approach is that an isolated muscle behaves as if it were made up of a contractile component, which is freely extensible at rest and responsible for the active length-tension and force-velocity relations discussed previously, plus at least two passive elastic components, one in series with the contractile component and the other in parallel with it. The two possible arrangements of these three components, known as Model I (also referred to as the Maxwell model) and Model II (also referred to as the Voigt model) are illustrated in Fig. 2. More complex models incorporating a fourth component have also been proposed: these are shown as Models III and IV. In principle, at least, it is possible to obtain enough information from release experiments on resting and active muscle to decide which of the four models illustrated is most appropriate for a given preparation (Brady, 1968). (It should be noted that different models may give the best fit for results from a series of preparations of the same type.) Once this choice has been made, raw length-tension and force-velocity data obtained from the whole muscle can be analysed to give information about the properties of the contractile component. This aspect of cardiac muscle mechanics has been dealt with by Hefner and Bowen (1967) and more recently in a detailed article by Pollack (1970). Those who are not prepared to adopt quite such a rigorous approach to the choice of a suitable model may make use of the simplest model that will give a reasonably accurate simulation of the properties of all preparations—we have already argued that Model I fills this role (Jewell and Blinks, 1968).

3. Measurements of the Mechanical Properties of Cardiac Muscle

In the previous section, our main aim was to emphasize the importance of the length-tension relation and the force-velocity relation in understanding the basic mechanisms of contraction. We deliberately ignored the complications that result from the interaction of these two relations, and from the fact that both relations change continuously as the activity of the muscle waxes and wanes after stimulation. In this section, we must come to grips with the problems that arise in a situation where one is dealing with the interaction of the three prime variables force, length, and time, and the derived variable velocity. A reasonably complete description of muscle performance seems to require the use of all four variables, and since all of these may be changing simultaneously during a contraction, the description is necessarily complex. Approaches to the study of muscle function generally boil down to studies of the relation between two of the four variables with varying degrees of attention given to the control of the other two. There are

TABLE 1.

Relations used in the study of muscle mechanics

General relation	Particular relation	Designation
F vs t	F vs t F_1 vs t	Isometric contraction curve Active state curve for tension-bearing ability
l vs t	l vs t	Isotonic contraction curve
v vs t	v vs t v_1 vs t	First derivative of isotonic contraction curve Active state curve for shortening ability
F vs l	Peak F vs l l_{min} vs F F_{max} vs l'	Active tension vs length (isometric) Contracted length vs tension (isotonic) Length dependence of tension-bearing ability
v vs l	v vs l v_{max} vs l'	"Phase plane diagram" for shortening Length dependence of shortening ability
F vs v	F vs v	Force-velocity curve from afterloaded isotonic contractions Force-velocity curve from isotonic release contractions Force-velocity curve from isometric contractions

Legend for symbols used in the table and in the text relating to it

t = time after stimulation

F, l, v = force, length and velocity, of the muscle

F', l', v' = force, length and velocity, of the contractile component

F_1 = tension-bearing ability of the contractile component at given l' and t

F_{max} = maximum value of F_1 at a given l'

v_1 = velocity of shortening of the contractile component against zero load at given l' and t

v_{max} = maximum value of v_1 at a given l'

l_{max} = muscle length at which the greatest tension is developed in isometric contractions

l_{min} = shortest muscle length achieved in a freeloaded or afterloaded contraction.

six possible combinations among the four variables and these delineate six general categories into which most experimental approaches fall. Table 1 lists these categories, together with brief designations of type of experimental measurements that fall in each. The various experimental approaches involved will be discussed in some detail in the sections that follow. Symbols are defined in the legend to Table 1.

A. FORCE-TIME RELATION

(1) *Isometric contraction curve* (F vs t)

It is a simple matter to obtain isometric contraction curves by connecting the muscle to a force transducer and recording the output of the latter on fast-moving paper. Under these conditions it is impossible to obtain perfectly isometric contractions of the muscle because there must always be some

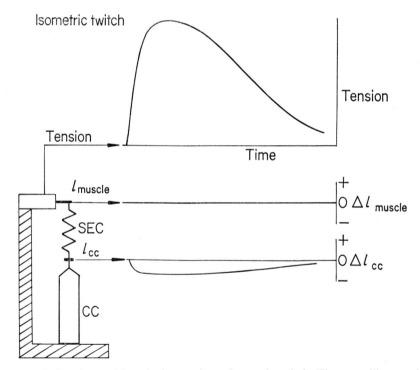

FIG. 3. Tension and length changes in an isometric twitch. These are illustrated for a two-component model in which SEC = series elastic component and CC = contractile component. The lines indicate (from above downwards) the tension in the muscle, the change in length of the muscle, and the change in length of the contractile component during an isometric contraction.

compliance in the force transducer, and, more particularly, in the connections between it and the muscle. Even when the greatest care is taken to keep this stray compliance to a minimum, the isometric contraction is still a complex event because the contractile component undergoes a cycle of length changes as a result of its interaction with the series elastic component in the muscle (Fig. 3). This is therefore a situation in which all four variables are changing simultaneously, but that does not mean (as we shall explain in Section 3A 3) that the isometric contraction cannot be a useful means of looking for changes in myocardial contractility.

Summary of state of variables

F vs t under examination.
F' vs t can be estimated by calculation on the basis of an assumed model.
l' and v' will be changing in a way that varies with the model.

(2) *Active state curve for tension-bearing ability* (F_i vs t)

Because the length of the contractile component changes continuously during an isometric contraction, the tension recorded in such contractions would not be expected to be equal to the tension-bearing ability of the contractile component at each instant. It is known that the contractile component produces less force when it is shortening than it does at constant length, and that it resists being stretched with a greater force than it produces at constant length. It has therefore been argued that the rise and fall of tension in an isometric contraction would be a good deal faster if the contractile component did not undergo length changes due to its interaction with the series elastic component. A curve showing the time course with which the tension in the contractile component of the frog sartorius muscle would change if it could be held at constant length during a contraction is shown in Fig. 4, which includes an isometric twitch for comparison. The tension indicated by this curve at any given instant after stimulation (designated F_i in this chapter) has been referred to as the "intensity of the active state", which A. V. Hill (1949) defined as the tension that the contractile component can just bear at the given instant without shortening or lengthening. This is a straightforward definition of the tension-bearing ability of the contractile component, but some confusion has been caused in the cardiac muscle literature by the use of the expression "intensity of the active state" to refer also to the shortening ability of the contractile component at a given instant after stimulation. In this chapter we have not used the term "intensity of the active state" in this general sense; instead we have described the state of activity (degree of activation) of the muscle at any given instant in terms of either tension-bearing ability (F_i) or shortening ability (v_i), in order to give a clear indication of the

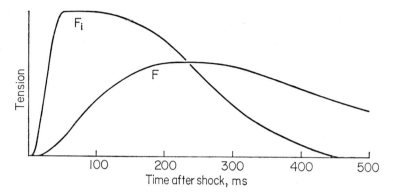

FIG. 4. F is the tension change in a typical isometric twitch of a frog skeletal muscle at 0°C, and F_i is the supposed time course of the "intensity of the active state" of the muscle, which is defined as the tension that the contractile component could bear without shortening or lengthening. (Adapted from Hill, 1970.)

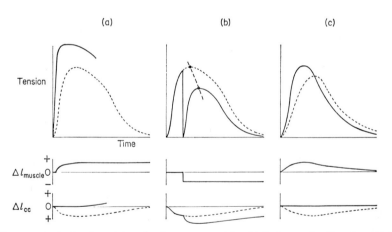

FIG. 5. Methods of studying the time course with which the tension-bearing ability of the contractile component changes after stimulation, as developed by (a) Hill (1949), (b) Ritchie (1954), and (c) Brady (1968). Schematic representations of results obtained from frog skeletal muscle (a) and (b), and cat papillary muscle (c). Each panel shows (from above downward) tension, change of length of the muscle, and change of length of the contractile component. The dotted lines show what would happen in an isometric twitch, and the solid lines indicate what happens when the muscle length is changed as required by the different techniques.

mechanical property under consideration. Shortening ability (v_i) is defined in Table 1 as the velocity of shortening of the contractile component against zero load at given contractile component length and at a given time after stimulation. (We recognize that the term "shortening ability" is not an unambiguous description of v_i, but we have been unable to think of a better one.)

Three techniques have been used to examine the tension-bearing ability of the contractile component at various times after stimulation (Fig. 5); the first gives information about the onset of the active state, the second about its decline, and the third about its complete time course.

(a) *Quick stretch technique* (Hill, 1949, 1970). This has been used mainly to examine the onset of the ability to bear tension in skeletal muscle, and less successfully for this purpose in cardiac muscle (Abbott and Mommaerts, 1959; Brady, 1965). The object of the method is to stretch the muscle during the early part of a contraction in order to offset the internal shortening of the contractile component that would otherwise take place. The technique as applied to skeletal muscle is illustrated schematically in Fig. 5(a).

Summary of state of variables

F_i vs t under examination.

$v' = 0$ because l' is presumed to be fixed during the early part of the contraction.

(b) *Quick release technique* (Ritchie, 1954). This method has been used in both skeletal and cardiac (Brady, 1966) muscle to examine the disappearance of the ability to bear tension. The technique is illustrated schematically in Fig. 5(b); it makes use of the fact that at a tension peak (e.g. the peak of an isometric twitch) the rate of change of tension is zero; therefore the contractile component is neither shortening nor lengthening, and the tension in the muscle at that instant provides a measure of the "intensity of the active state" (F_i). The quick release technique is used to produce tension peaks at various times after stimulation. The muscle is first stretched to the top of its length-tension curve (Fig. 1(b), point 2), so that small changes in contractile component length will alter the ability to develop tension as little as possible. After it has been stimulated and allowed to develop tension, the muscle is released a short distance and then allowed to redevelop tension at the new length. The peak of each curve of tension redevelopment gives the value of F_i at that instant, and a large part of the decay of the active state can be followed by releasing the muscle at various times after stimulation. Note that this technique cannot give information about the intensity of the active state at times earlier than the normal peak of the isometric contraction curve.

Summary of state of variables

F_i vs t under examination.

$v' = 0$ but l' is slightly different for different measurements.

(c) *Length clamping technique* (Brady, 1968). This technique is the most sophisticated of the three in that the aim is to determine the tension-bearing ability at each instant during a single contraction by adjusting the length of the muscle continuously so that the contractile component is held at constant length. The method involves use of an active lever system under the control of an on-line computer or an equivalent device that calculates the required length adjustment from moment to moment during the contraction (Fig. 5(c)). This requires prior determination of the stress-strain relation of the SEC in that particular muscle, and the whole procedure depends critically on the adoption of the correct analog model of the muscle, and the assumption (now recognized to be incorrect) that the properties of the SEC remain constant throughout the contraction.

Summary of state of variables

F_i vs t under examination.

$v' = 0$ because l' is fixed throughout the contraction.

(3) *Relative merits of methods for studying force-time relation*

The methods just described are those that have been developed to examine how the tension-bearing ability of the contractile component varies with time after stimulation. Their usefulness is severely limited by the fact that the time course of activity is affected by length changes that take place in the contractile component while it is active; shortening at any time during the contraction leads to an earlier disappearance of the active state. The only technique that avoids length changes in the contractile component is Brady's method, but this is much too elaborate for routine use. The curves he has obtained showing how tension-bearing ability varies with time have differed only slightly from simple isometric contractions (they differ much less than the curves shown for skeletal muscle in Fig. 4) and it can be argued that isometric contractions recorded under conditions in which the amount of series compliance outside the muscle has been kept to a minimum provide a useful, easily obtained, and reasonably reliable indication of the way in which the tension-bearing ability of the contractile component varies with time. In fact a good deal of useful information can be inferred from high-speed records of isometric contractions, provided one assumes (see note below) that the properties of the passive elastic components are unchanged by inotropic interventions. For example:

(i) Peak tension. A large increase in peak tension can safely be taken as reflecting an increase in the maximum tension-bearing ability (F_{max}), though small changes are difficult to interpret in these terms.

(ii) Rise of tension. If the tension rises faster in the early part of an isometric contraction, the contractile component must be shortening faster. This indicates that shortening ability (v_i) builds up more rapidly after excitation, but it does not necessarily follow that maximum v_i (v_{max}) is increased as well.

(iii) Time-to-peak and total duration of contraction. Small changes are again difficult to interpret, but large changes indicate corresponding alterations in the time to maximum activity and the duration of activity.

Note that although it has been found that most inotropic interventions do not detectably alter the properties of the passive elastic components, it is not safe to assume this always to be so, for the extensibility of the series elastic component is known to be reduced by hypertonic solutions (Wildenthal *et al.*, 1969) and by cooling (Yeatman *et al.*, 1969). Furthermore, to the extent that the series compliance resides in the crossbridges, one might expect it to be altered by interventions that alter the number of attached bridges.

B. LENGTH-TIME RELATION

(1) *Freeloaded isotonic contraction curve (l vs t)*

A muscle is said to be freeloaded when it bears the same force during activity as it does at rest. If the contractile component is freely extensible at rest, the load is borne in the resting muscle by passive elastic components, but it is progressively transferred to the contractile component as the active muscle shortens. Freeloaded isotonic contractions are complicated for this reason, and also because the initial length from which contractions begin depends on the load on the muscle (Fig. 6(a)). They have not been widely used in studies of the mechanical properties of cardiac or skeletal muscle.

(2) *Afterloaded isotonic contraction curve (l vs t)*

A muscle is said to be afterloaded when the load it shortens against is greater than the load it bears at rest. The resting length of the muscle is established by the presence of a preload, and the afterload is not lifted until the muscle has developed a corresponding amount of tension, as is illustrated in Figs 6(b) and 7. The time required to develop this tension will depend on the afterload, heavier afterloads being lifted at later times after stimulation. Figure 7 shows an interesting feature that might have been predicted from what we have said in Section 3A(1)—that the decay of tension during relaxation

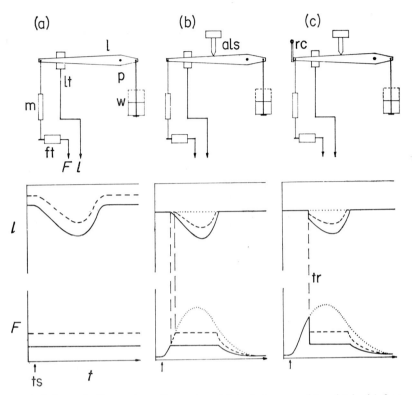

FIG. 6. Schematic illustration of experimental technique used to obtain (a) free-loaded, (b) afterloaded, and (c) timed-release isotonic contraction curves. Each panel shows (from above downward) the experimental setup, records of muscle length, and records of tension in the muscle. In each case, records of contractions against two different loads are shown by solid and dashed lines. Dotted lines indicate tension developed in isometric contractions. Abbreviations: m = muscle, lt = length transducer, ft = force transducer, l = lever, p = pivot axis, w = weights used to load lever, als = afterload stop, rc = release catch, ts = time of stimulation, tr = time of release. F, l and t are force, length and time.

occurs earlier if the muscle has shortened than it does if shortening has been prevented, the effect being more or less proportional to the amount of shortening. This important influence of shortening of the active muscle on the time course of activity will be discussed further in Section 3F. During the initial isometric phase of an afterloaded contraction, internal length changes take place (i.e. shortening of the contractile component with extension of the series elastic component), and in all models except model I there will be some transfer of the preload to the contractile component. The isotonic contraction

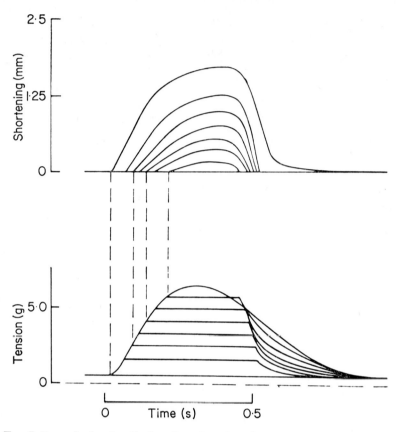

Fig. 7. Records showing the length and tension changes that take place in a cat papillary muscle in afterloaded isotonic contractions against a series of different loads (21 °C, frequency 30 min^{-1}). Initial length, 9 mm (preload 0·4 g); increasing afterload (0·8 g in increments). Note that in this figure, unlike the previous one, decreases in length are recorded as upward deflections. (From Sonnenblick, 1962.)

curve that is recorded when external shortening takes place shows the length-time relation of the muscle when it is shortening against a constant load. The length-time relation of the contractile component will differ from this and the load on the contractile component will change in ways that will depend on the model assumed for the muscle. Afterloaded contractions have been widely used to examine the force-velocity relation of cardiac muscle, but with insufficient attention to the problems of interpreting the results in terms of what is happening to the contractile component. These problems have been examined in detail by Noble *et al.* (1969) and Pollack (1970).

(3) *Timed-release isotonic contraction curve* (*l* vs *t*)

As we have seen in the preceding section, one of the problems with simple afterloaded contractions is that the time after stimulation at which external shortening begins depends on the afterload (Figs. 6(b) and 7). This problem can be avoided by delaying the onset of external shortening until a preset time after stimulation, when the muscle is suddenly allowed to shorten against an afterload (Fig. 6(c)—the isotonic release technique, Jewell and Wilkie, 1960). Isotonic shortening can be examined against a range of loads up to a value set by the tension in the muscle at the time of release. Although this technique gets around the problem of the varying time of onset of shortening in afterloaded contractions against different loads, the other problems discussed previously cannot be avoided; i.e. internal length changes and redistribution of tension between the passive elastic components and the contractile component will still occur, and to an extent that will depend on the model assumed for the muscle. Caution is therefore required in the interpretation of release contraction curves, just as in that of other types of isotonic contraction curves. Further information about the isotonic release technique will be given in Section 3F.

Summary of state of variables for the methods in this section

l vs *t*   under examination.

l' vs *t*   can be estimated by calculation on the basis of an assumed model.

F' and *v'* will be changing in a way that varies with the model.

C. VELOCITY-TIME RELATION

(1) *First derivative of the isotonic contraction curve* (*v* vs *t*)

Clearly all the problems that arise in the interpretation of isotonic contraction curves will also arise when the first derivatives of those curves are being analysed. Nevertheless, velocity-time plots do offer a convenient method of making accurate velocity measurements, especially peak velocities, provided that problems inherent in electronic methods of differentiation are not overlooked (see Philbrick Manual, 1966). They also prevent the experimenter from being fooled into thinking that shortening velocities during isotonic contractions are more constant with respect to time than is actually the case (see Fig. 8).

Summary of state of variables

v vs *t*   under examination.

v' vs *t*   can be estimated by calculation on the basis of an assumed model.

F' and *l'* will be changing in a way that varies with the model.

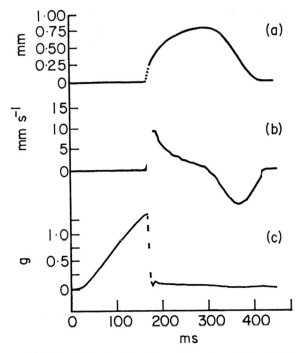

FIG. 8. Records of length, first derivative of length, and tension in an isotonic release contraction of rabbit papillary muscle (29·5°C, frequency 30 min^{-1}). Velocity of shortening declines rapidly with time. (Redrawn from Edman and Nilsson, 1968.)

(2) *Active state curve for shortening ability* (v_i vs t)

The isotonic release technique provides a method of examining the ability of the contractile component to shorten at various times after stimulation. Various aspects of the ability to shorten can be measured, but the one that has proved most useful is the velocity of shortening against the smallest load that it is practicable to use—this will approximate v_i. The muscle length and velocity of shortening both change rapidly during a release contraction (Fig. 8), and when releases are made at different times after stimulation, a question arises about the muscle length at which each velocity of shortening be measured if it is to refer to a fixed contractile component length. The answer will depend on the model assumed for the muscle, as will the accuracy of the assumption that $F' \approx 0$.

This method has been used extensively to follow the time course of activity in cardiac muscle (e.g. Fig. 9), but it should be pointed out that it suffers from the same drawback as two of the methods for determining the time

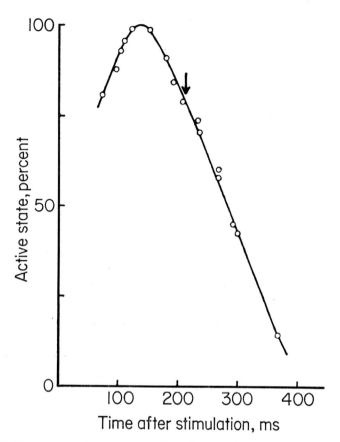

FIG. 9. Time course of active state of cardiac muscle, as revealed by ability to shorten during isotonic release contractions (v_i vs t). All the measurements of v_i were made at the contractile component length existing at the peak of an isometric twitch, and v_i is plotted as a percentage of v_{max}. The arrow shows the time at which peak tension was reached in an isometric twitch. Rabbit papillary muscle, 72 contractions per minute, 29 °C. (From Edman and Nilsson, 1968.)

course with which tension-bearing ability changes after stimulation: the time course obtained for the decay of shortening ability depends on the amount of shortening that has taken place up to the time at which the measurement of v_i is made.

Summary of state of variables

v_i vs t under examination.

$F' \approx 0$ and l' is fixed if the data are analysed on the basis of an assumed model.

D. FORCE-LENGTH RELATION

(1) Active tension vs length (peak F vs l)

Length-tension relations of cardiac muscle are usually examined by setting the length of the resting muscle to a series of different values, and measuring the peak tension developed in isometric contractions at each of those muscle lengths. The problem of controlling the velocity of shortening of the contractile component is solved by measuring the tension at the peak of the contraction when this velocity is zero. If the time to peak tension were independent of muscle length, time could also be eliminated as a variable, but unfortunately this is usually not the case—stretch increases the time to peak tension, sometimes substantially (e.g. Blinks, 1970). This procedure gives the length-tension curves for resting and active muscle. The relation of active tension to the length of the contractile component (peak F' vs l') can be obtained from these curves by correcting for the contribution of the parallel elastic component and by allowing for internal shortening of the contractile component during the development of tension. The procedure for making these corrections will depend on the model assumed for the muscle.

Summary of state of variables

Peak F vs l under examination.

Peak F' vs l' can be estimated by calculation on the basis of an assumed model.

$v' = 0$ but t will vary somewhat with muscle length.

(2) Contracted length vs tension (l_{min} vs F)

Another way to approach the study of the length-tension relation of the active muscle is to measure the minimum length reached in freeloaded or afterloaded isotonic contractions against a series of different loads. The velocity of the contractile component is fixed because it will be zero when the muscle length reaches its minimum, but peak shortening may occur at different times after stimulation (see Fig. 7), so time cannot be eliminated as a variable except by chance. Although it has been reported that length-tension curves obtained by this and the previous method are the same (Sonnenblick, 1965a) or almost the same (Brutsaert and Sonnenblick, 1969), other work indicates a clear difference between them (Taylor, 1970). Such a difference is to be expected if shortening is limited by the brevity of the active state.

Summary of state of variables

l_{min} vs F under examination.

l_{min} vs F' can be estimated by calculation on the basis of an assumed model.

$v' = 0$ and t may be different for different measurements.

(3) *Length-dependence of tension-bearing ability* (F_{max} vs l')

This curve would show how F_{max}, as might be determined by Brady's length-clamping technique, depends on contractile component length. As far as we are aware, the muscle literature does not yet include any such curves.

Summary of state of variables

F_{max} vs l' under examination.

$v' = 0$ but t probably different for different measurements.

E. VELOCITY-LENGTH RELATION

(1) *"Phase-plane diagrams" for shortening* (v vs l)

Some use has been made in recent papers (Sonnenblick, 1965b; Brutsaert and Sonnenblick, 1969) of so-called phase-plane diagrams in which the velocity of shortening is displayed as a continuous function of the muscle length during isotonic shortening (Fig. 10). It has been found that over a substantial portion of the shortening phase, the velocity of shortening against a given load is a function simply of the muscle length and not of time after stimulation. Although an alternate explanation (the chance cancellation of the effects of changes in length and time) seems more plausible to us, this finding could be interpreted as indicating the existence of a plateau of activity during the isotonic contraction. If true, this would be surprising, because other evidence (e.g. Fig. 9) indicates that the degree of activation changes continuously during a contraction. However, it must be remembered that results such as Fig. 9 show how v_i varies with time at a fixed contractile component length. Because the degree of activation at a given instant after stimulation depends on both the contractile component length at that instant (Section 3D) and the amount of shortening that has taken place up to that instant (Section 3A 3), we do not know enough to predict the time course of activity that would be expected in isotonic contractions. It remains to be seen whether phase-plane diagrams obtained under a wide variety of conditions will substantiate the suggestion that there might be a plateau of activity during isotonic contractions. Although velocity-length curves do not appear to us to be particularly valuable (in the way that a force-velocity curve is) in revealing a basic property of the muscle because time is an undetermined variable, they do provide a convenient way of measuring the velocity of shortening at a particular muscle length. The analysis of phase-plane diagrams to give information about the velocity-length relation of the contractile component again requires the assumption of a model of the muscle.

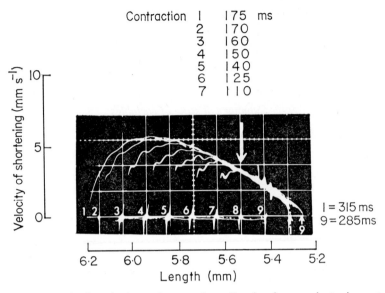

FIG. 10. Velocity-length phase-plane tracings. Starting from an isotonic contraction with no afterload, initial muscle length (6·2 mm) was decreased prior to each succeeding contraction. Total load was maintained constant at 0·35 g throughout the experiment. The results were fully reversible when the initial length was re-established. Times after stimulation, at which a common velocity-length relation (arrow) was achieved by contractions 1 through 7, are listed above the arrow. Note that over a wide range and independent of time, all curves follow a common pathway regardless of the initial length from which the shortening began. Also note the terminal velocity-length dissociation later during the contraction. Time to peak tension of a stable isometric beat of the same muscle at 0·35 g preload was 320 msec. The delay from stimulus to onset of tension development averaged 25 msec. Temperature, 29 °C. (Figure and caption reproduced from Brutsaert and Sonnenblick, 1969.)

Summary of state of variables

v vs l under examination.

v' vs l' can be estimated by calculation on the basis of an assumed model.

F' will vary with muscle length in a way that will depend on the model.

t is an undetermined variable.

(2) *Length-dependence of the ability to shorten* (v_{max} vs l')

This curve would show how the maximum velocity of shortening of the contractile component varies with the length of that component. The muscle literature includes no curves that actually show this relation, though estimates of v_{max} made by extrapolating force-velocity curves from afterloaded isotonic contractions (see Section 3F 1) have sometimes been plotted as functions of muscle length (e.g. Sonnenblick, 1965b).

Summary of state of variables

v_{max} vs l' under examination.

$F' = 0$ but t would probably be different for different measurements.

F. FORCE-VELOCITY RELATION

Any description of the force-velocity relation of cardiac muscle, if it is to be complete, must take account of the following facts:

(i) the force-velocity relation varies with the muscle length,

(ii) the force-velocity relation varies with the degree of activation of the muscle,

(iii) the degree of activation varies with time after stimulation,

(iv) the degree of activation at a given time after stimulation is influenced by the sequence of length and tension changes that the muscle has undergone up to that instant.

The influence of muscle length on the force-velocity relation can be depicted in a three-dimensional graph having the co-ordinates force, velocity, and length. The force-velocity-length relation of the muscle at a given degree of activation will then be a surface in the space defined by the three axes. To take account of point (iii), one must imagine this surface as changing with time after stimulation, the surface first growing out of the length axis as the active state develops and then collapsing towards it again as the active state decays. While this is a useful way of visualizing how the force-velocity relation depends on muscle length and on the degree of activation of the muscle, it will be impossible to arrive at a precise definition of these surfaces experimentally because of point (iv). The dependence of the degree of activation on the sequence of length and tension changes undergone by the muscle means that the surfaces will be deformed by any attempt to define them experimentally, and the nature of the deformation will depend on the particular method used to collect the data.

The experimenter who wishes to study the force-velocity relation of cardiac muscle is therefore placed in an impossible position, for he cannot hope to arrive at a complete description of this relation. The question that then arises is what type of force-velocity curves should be determined if one wants to examine the effects of an inotropic intervention on myocardial contractility. The three approaches that have been used are as follows:

(1) *Force-velocity curves from afterloaded isotonic contractions* (F vs v)

Afterloaded isotonic contractions against a series of different loads (see Figs. 6(b) and 7) have been used extensively as a means of obtaining force-velocity curves for cardiac muscle. The velocities measured have usually been the peak velocities, rather than initial velocities of shortening. The main problem with this approach is that the velocity measurements are made at different times after stimulation, and perhaps at different contractile component lengths. We have already argued that this approach is therefore not suitable for any serious investigation of the force-velocity relation (Blinks and Koch-Weser, 1963; Jewell and Blinks, 1968). However, Brutsaert and Sonnenblick (1969) have reported recently that the force-velocity curve that can be obtained by measuring the peak velocities of shortening of the muscle in afterloaded isotonic contractions against various loads has two special unexpected features: first, it represents the behaviour of the contractile component at a more or less constant length; second, the curve is substantially independent of time after stimulation. The first feature was noted when allowance was made for internal shortening of the contractile component at the expense of the series elastic component during the isometric phases of the afterloaded contractions; the contractile component length at which peak shortening velocity was reached was found to be only slightly dependent on the load. The second special feature ascribed to these curves (the independence of time) depends on two things: (i) the demonstration (Fig. 10) that in afterloaded contractions the velocity of shortening is a function simply of the muscle length and not of time over a substantial portion of the contraction phase; and (ii) the assumption that this would be the case at the times at which peak shortening velocities are reached in afterloaded contractions against all loads. These two features certainly simplify the interpretation of curves that otherwise would be of questionable significance. The problem is, however, that neither feature would have been predicted on the basis of known properties of muscle, and neither is the result of deliberate experimental control. These special features seem to be the result of chance interactions among uncontrolled variables, and it remains to be seen to what extent this piece of good luck can be relied upon. As has been noted already, the apparent dependence of the velocity of shortening simply on muscle length during a substantial portion of the isotonic contraction is a puzzling feature of this work in view of all the other published evidence indicating that the degree of activation of cardiac muscle must be changing throughout a contraction. Until this conflict is resolved and the special features mentioned above are shown to apply over a wider range of conditions, we feel that it would be best to keep an open mind on the validity of this approach to the problem of examining the force-velocity relation of cardiac muscle.

Summary of state of variables

F vs v under examination.

F' vs v' can be estimated by calculation on the basis of an assumed model.

l' may be more or less fixed for all measurements (by chance).

t is an unspecified variable.

(2) *Force-velocity curves from isotonic release contractions* (F vs v)

In principle, isotonic release contractions (see Fig. 6(c)) provide the best way of examining force-velocity relations in cardiac muscle, because the experimenter can control both the time after stimulation and the contractile component length at which all the velocity measurements are made. In fact, it is not possible to control both of these parameters entirely, and a choice must be made between making the measurements at a fixed time after stimulation (and accepting slight variations of contractile component length), and making the measurements at a fixed contractile component length (with slight variations in the time after stimulation). Edman and Nilsson (1968, 1969) have advanced convincing arguments in favour of the latter approach, the key point being that the properties of the contractile component vary more steeply with length than they do with time after stimulation under the conditions existing in release studies. In spite of their obvious theoretical advantages, release contractions are not ideal: first, each measurement of velocity has to be made while the velocity is changing rapidly; second, there is the problem that shortening of the muscle causes a curtailment of the active state, which may aggravate the first problem. There is some evidence (K. A. P. Edman, personal communication) that the very rapid shortening, the inertial oscillations, or both, following a quick release may have a greater deactivating influence than the shortening that occurs in simple afterloaded isotonic contractions. Edman and his co-workers (1968, 1969) have been able to get around this difficulty by damping the movement of their lever system, and it seems likely that this procedure may greatly enhance the usefulness of the isotonic release technique in the study of force-velocity relations in cardiac muscle. Better control of contractile component length would be possible if an active lever system could be used in the manner described by Brady (1968) to clamp the length of the contractile component during the isometric phase preceding each release; it would then be possible to measure the velocity of shortening of the contractile component against different loads at an almost fixed contractile component length and at a fixed time after stimulation.

Summary of state of variables

F vs v under examination.

F' vs v' can be estimated by calculation on the basis of an assumed model

l' or t can be fixed, but the other will be slightly different for different measurements.

(3) Force-velocity curves from isometric contractions (F vs v)

It is possible to obtain a force-velocity curve by analysing the tension rise in an isometric contraction, provided that (i) an analog model established by other methods is available for the muscle under investigation, and (ii) the characteristics of its elastic components are known (Macpherson, 1953). This approach has been tried by Sonnenblick (1964) on cardiac muscle, but there are serious problems in evaluating the results. The range of times over which the force-velocity data are accumulated extends from the first detectable increase in tension to the peak of the isometric contraction, and during this period the degree of activation is generally considered to build up from nothing to its maximum level and then to begin to fall again. If this is so, then the force-velocity curve suffers from the same uncertainties as the one that is plotted from measurements of the initial velocity of shortening in afterloaded isotonic contractions against various loads. This problem is compounded by the fact that during the period over which the measurements are made the stiffness of the series elastic component is probably changing (see Section 2D). For this reason, force-velocity curves obtained from isometric contractions are probably considerably less reliable than those determined by more straightforward techniques.

Summary of state of variables

F' vs v' is estimated by calculation from an isometric contraction curve on the basis of a previously determined model.

l' and t are uncontrolled variables.

G. GENERAL COMMENTS

In this account of the measurement of the mechanical properties of cardiac muscle we have not attempted to discuss the multitude of other factors that need to be taken into consideration as far as more general experimental conditions are concerned. For further information on these, the reader is referred to our earlier reviews (Blinks and Koch-Weser, 1963; Jewell and Blinks, 1968). Notice should also be taken of the recent paper by Parmley et al. (1969), which draws attention to special problems that may be encountered in experiments where the mechanical loading conditions are varied. Any experimental protocol for a study of cardiac muscle mechanics should be drawn up in a way that takes care of matters of this sort.

4. THE SEARCH FOR A SIMPLE INDEX OF CONTRACTILITY

It is probably not meaningful to attempt to provide a rigorous definition for the term "myocardial contractility" as such. One can only describe the contractile state of the heart, and as we have seen a complete description requires the use of at least four variables (force, velocity, length, and time) all of which may be changing simultaneously during the course of a contraction. On the basis of such a description, then, it is possible to frame an explicit definition of a change in contractility. In such a definition it is probably useful to draw a distinction between changes in performance resulting from alterations in one or more of the four specified physical variables (e.g. initial length or afterload) and those attributable to other factors (e.g. drugs or frequency of contraction). Changes of the latter type would then be regarded as changes in contractility, while those of the former type would not. This is in practice often equivalent to defining a change in contractility as a change in the performance of the heart that does not result from a change in initial length or afterload; the reason is that of the other two variables (time and velocity), one (time) cannot be controlled, and the other (velocity) is seldom under direct control. Of course it should not be regarded as sufficient to decide that a change in the performance of the heart represents a change in contractility; the nature of the change still must be described, and the best description is a complete one in terms of the changes in the relations among all the variables concerned.

Of the many possible relations among these variables, we feel the most informative are probably shown by curves of the following types:

(i) the curve relating active tension to contractile component length (F' vs l'),

(ii) families of instantaneous force-velocity curves (F' vs v' at fixed or nearly fixed l' and t),

(iii) curves indicating the time course of the active state in terms of tension-generating capacity (F_i vs t) or the ability to shorten (v_i vs t).

Taken together, these three types of curves give a reasonably complete description of the performance of the muscle, and it seems likely that most changes in contractility will be detected by them. They also provide a logical framework for an interpretation of the change, because according to current concepts each curve has a very direct relevance to an important aspect of the contractile process.

Obviously, it is not often possible or practical to go to the length of determining all these curves to follow changes in myocardial performance, and an evident need exists for simple indices of contractility. But what index should one use? Because of the complexity of the interactions among the relevant variables, it seems unlikely that any simple index of contractility can be expected to be universally applicable. If the index is really simple, its information content is unlikely to be adequate. Simple indices can be regarded as windows that give us glimpses, or silhouettes, of a complex four-dimensional relation. Different indices gives views of the relation from different vantage-points, and it is only to be expected that the window giving the most revealing silhouette may vary with the nature of the change being looked at. Also it seems safe to assume that multiple views will allow us to piece together a better picture of what is going on than any single one is likely to. In recent years considerable effort has been directed toward the development of simple indices that would reflect changes in contractility and not be influenced by changes in fibre length or afterload. We are not convinced that it will be possible to find such an index, and have serious doubts about two that have been proposed in recent years.

(a) $(dP/dt)/IIT$

In 1963, Siegel and Sonnenblick proposed that the ratio of maximum rate of development of isometric tension to the area under the rising phase of the tension-time curve $(dP/dt)/IIT$ might serve as a generally useful index of myocardial contractility. They reported this index to be independent of fibre length, but sensitive to all the inotropic interventions they tested either in the isolated cat papillary muscle or in the dog ventricle from which outflow was momentarily occluded with a balloon. The ratio $(dP/dt)/IIT$ has the dimensions of s^{-2} and is highly sensitive to changes in the time to peak tension. The reason that Siegel and Sonnenblick (1963) found the ratio to be uninfluenced by fibre length was presumably related to the fact that under the particular conditions of their experiments, time to peak tension was not influenced by fibre length. Under most circumstances, muscle length has a substantial influence on the time course of contraction (e.g. Blinks, 1970), and we have found the ratio $(dP/dt)/IIT$ to be influenced as much as several fold by changes in muscle length. If this is the case generally, the utility of this particular index would seem to be rather low.

(b) v_{max}

More recently v_{max} has received a great deal of attention as an index of contractility, also because of its supposed independence of muscle length. v_{max} is generally taken to mean the maximum velocity of shortening of the contractile component when the external force opposing shortening is zero. Strictly speaking, this is not an adequate definition, because the maximum velocity achievable will depend somewhat on when during the contraction cycle shortening is allowed to begin. A more rigorous definition would specify

v_{max} as the maximum value achieved by v_i (the instantaneous velocity of contractile component shortening against zero load) during the contraction. We have already indicated that this can be tentatively regarded as a reflection of the maximum rate of turnover of cross bridges, and as such it is a valuable index of a basic property of the muscle. The measurement of v_{max} presents some problems, however, because it is impracticable to work with zero external force opposing shortening. v_{max} must therefore be estimated by extrapolation from force-velocity data that extend down to the smallest load with which it is practicable to work. All of the uncertainties associated with the determination of the force-velocity curve (see Section 3F) are compounded when the curve is extrapolated beyond the range of experimental observations. An additional important question that must be considered is what analog model should be used for the extrapolation. Noble et al. (1969) and Pollack (1970) have shown that this question is crucial, and it is clear from their analyses that the most appropriate analog model must be known for a given preparation before any accurate estimation can be made of v_{max}.

The great advantage claimed for v_{max} as an index of myocardial contractility has been its supposed independence of muscle length. We have already expressed scepticism about data and arguments that have been offered in support of this claim (Jewell and Blinks, 1968), and evidence is now accumulating that in the cat papillary muscle v_{max} varies steeply with muscle length over most of the ascending limb of the length-tension curve (R. Forman and L. E. Ford, personal communication). While it is possible that v_{max} remains constant over a narrow range of muscle lengths close to the optimal one (l_{max}), its utility as an index of myocardial contractility that is independent of length in the intact heart will be diminished if the muscle fibres normally operate at lengths shorter than that. The quantitative evidence on this point is not yet good enough for us to arrive at any reliable conclusion.

5. CONTRACTILITY IN THE INTACT HEART

Readers of this chapter who hope to find an explicit "how to do it" account of methods for the estimation of contractility in the intact heart will be disappointed. This is not because the authors regard the subject as unimportant, for it is clearly highly relevant to certain aspects of experimental haemodynamics, and also of great practical importance in clinical medicine. Rather, the reason lies in the generally unsatisfactory state of the art, and the authors' belief that ad hoc treatments of the problem based on a thorough understanding of the principles of muscle mechanics are far less likely to come to grief than the automatic or indiscriminate application of techniques devised or advocated by others. This follows directly from our opinions stated earlier that no single index of contractility is likely to be universally applicable, and that the selection of an index (or indices) must depend upon the nature of the change to be demonstrated as well as the constraints imposed by the system under investigation. Thus, we prefer to avoid advocating any specific techniques for the assessment of contractility in the whole heart, and to limit our treatment of the problem to pointing out certain of the difficulties to be encountered in work of this sort.

It is hardly surprising that attempts to apply concepts of muscle mechanics to the study of the intact heart have followed closely behind similar work on isolated heart muscle. In particular, there is a rapidly accumulating body of literature on the estimation of force-velocity relations in the intact ventricle. We have serious misgivings about the value of the information that has been or is likely to be gained from such estimates, chiefly because of the large number of simplifying assumptions that must be made in order to extract force-velocity data from pressure-volume measurements made on the intact heart. Consider the following questions:

(i) In order to estimate the end-diastolic volume from measurements of end-diastolic pressure in the beating heart is it appropriate to use the pressure-volume relation determined by static measurements on a dead or KCl-depolarized ventricle?

(ii) How precise a measure of the ventricular volume at a given instant during systole can be made by subtracting the integrated output flow-rate from the estimated end-diastolic volume?

(iii) Is it reasonable to estimate the instantaneous radius from the instantaneous ventricular volume by assuming that the cavity of the left ventricle is a sphere (or other simple figure of rotation)?

(iv) Is it reasonable to estimate ventricular wall thickness by assuming that the ventricular mass is distributed uniformly around this cavity of idealized shape?

(v) Is it appropriate to calculate the mean wall stress when it is known that large variations in tangential stress occur across the wall of a thick-walled container?

(vi) If there is some purpose in calculating mean wall stress, which modification of the Laplace equation should be used, and what radius should be used in making the calculation?

(vii) What evidence is there that the characteristics of the series elastic components of isolated papillary muscles from the right ventricle of the cat have any similarity to those of the intact left ventricle of the dog or man?

(viii) What meaning can be attached to a force-velocity curve that has been derived from a single isochoric ("isovolumic") beat, when it is known that the level of activity in the muscle probably varied throughout the period during which the force-velocity data were being accumulated?

(ix) How much is this problem compounded by asynchrony of activation of various parts of the muscle mass, which exists in the normal ventricle, and is accentuated in certain disease states?

(x) Do force-velocity data obtained from the intact ventricle allow any useful inferences to be made about what is happening in the muscle fibres when it is known that their orientation is totally different in the various layers that make up the ventricular wall and the velocities of shortening in different muscle bundles must vary?

Some of these questions have been discussed in some of the papers concerned with such measurements, but in general we have not found the answers reassuring. In the absence of a more rigorous approach to these uncertainties, we feel that there is little point in going to the trouble of extracting force-velocity data from measurements on the intact heart except to satisfy oneself that the behaviour of the whole ventricle is reasonably consistent with what is known about that of isolated heart muscle. In this connection it may be appropriate to consider why it ever might be important to know about the force-velocity relation of a muscle. Three possible reasons come to mind.

(i) The first, and in our minds the most important, is that the precise shape of the curve, and the details of the way in which it may be influenced by various interventions, are bound to figure centrally in the development of theories of muscular contraction. For this purpose so much depends on quantitative measurement and freedom from interference by extraneous factors that studies on the intact heart can be dismissed as having no reasonable promise whatever. It is highly questionable whether even studies on isolated heart muscle can be refined to the point of giving reliable information of this sort.

(ii) It provides a basis for understanding, and to some extent for predicting, the behaviour of the muscle under a variety of circumstances other than those in which the relation was determined. However, because of the uncertainties involved in determining force-velocity relations in the intact heart, it seems to us that a general knowledge of the properties of heart muscle might be as useful in this regard as would specific information about any given ventricle.

(iii) It has been proposed that force-velocity curves be used as an index of contractility in the intact heart, and such curves have been extrapolated to the maximum velocity of unloaded shortening (v_{max}) in the search for an index of contractility that is independent of preload. We have very mixed feelings in this matter. On the one hand, we believe it is highly desirable that the development of indices of contractility for the intact heart be based on the principles of muscle mechanics rather than on blind empiricism. On the other hand, we doubt very seriously that the sort of "force-velocity curve" that can be constructed from information obtained on the whole ventricle has a greater content of reliable information than many simpler indices. Our prejudice with respect to the use of v_{max} will be obvious, because we feel the extrapolation of the most reliable force-velocity curve is hazardous at best, and also because there is good reason to doubt that v_{max} is in fact independent of preload in heart muscle. It seems to us that more direct methods are likely to give indices of contractility that are just as reliable without pretending to be something that they are not.

6. SUMMARY

It is not possible to give a rigorous definition of "myocardial contractility" as such. One can only describe the contractile state of the heart, and this is best done in terms of the relations among three prime variables—force, length, and time—and a derived variable—velocity. A clear distinction must be made between changes in performance stemming from changes in those variables themselves (such as changes in initial length or in afterload) on the one hand, and changes in performance that are manifestations of changes in the relations among the variables in question (as might be induced by inotropic substances, nerve stimulation, or changes in the frequency or rhythm of contraction) on the other. Changes of the latter type constitute changes of contractility, whereas those of the former type do not.

A thorough description of a change in contractility is not easy, and usually will require the use of several of the six possible relationships between pairs of the variables force, velocity, length, and time. The two-dimensional relations that are most revealing in one circumstance may not be so in another, and it is evident that the use of several such relations will usually be more informative than that of any one alone. A simple, universally applicable index of contractility would obviously be of great value, but none of the attempts to devise one has yet met with notable success. We seriously question whether the goal of developing such an index is an attainable one.

The application of the principles of muscle mechanics to the intact heart has been useful in so far as it has confirmed that the performance of the whole heart is generally consistent with what is known about the contractile behaviour of isolated heart muscle. However, so many simplifying assumptions are required in experiments of this sort that we feel it unlikely that they can ever be expected to be capable of providing penetrating insight into fundamental mechanisms of contraction.

REFERENCES

Abbott, B. C. and Mommaerts, W. F. H. M. (1959). A study of inotropic mechanisms in the papillary muscle preparation. *J. gen. Physiol.* **42**, 533–551.

Armstrong, C. M., Huxley, A. F. and Julian, F. J. (1966). Oscillatory responses in frog skeletal muscle fibres. *J. Physiol.* **186**, 26–27.

Bendall, J. R. (1969). "Muscles, Molecules and Movement". Heinemann Educational Books, London.

Blinks, J. R. and Koch-Weser, J. (1963). Physical factors in the analysis of the actions of drugs on myocardial contractility. *Pharmacol. Rev.* **15**, 531–599.

Blinks, J. R. (1970). Factors influencing the prolongation of active state by stretch in isolated mammalian heart muscle. *Fed. Proc.* **29**, 611 Abs.

Brady, A. J. (1965). Time and displacement dependence of cardiac contractility: problems in defining the active state and the force-velocity relation. *Fed. Proc.* **24**, 1410–1420.

Brady, A. J. (1966). Onset of contractility in cardiac muscle. *J. Physiol.* **184**, 560–580.

Brady, A. J. (1968). Active state in cardiac muscle. *Physiol. Rev.* **48**, 570–600.

Brutsaert, D. L. and Sonnenblick, E. H. (1969). Force-velocity-length-time relations of the contractile elements in heart muscle of the cat. *Circulation Res.* **24**, 137–149.

Civan, M. M. and Podolsky, R. J. (1966). Contraction kinetics of striated muscle fibres following quick changes in load. *J. Physiol.* **184**, 511–534.

Ebashi, S. and Endo, M. (1968). Calcium ion and muscle contraction. *Prog. Biophys. Mol. Biol.* **18**, 123–183.

Ebashi, S., Endo, M. and Ohtsuki, I. (1969). Control of muscle contraction. *Quart. Rev. Biophys.* **4**, 351–384.

Edman, K. A. P. and Nilsson, E. (1968). The mechanical parameters of myocardial contraction studied at a constant length of the contractile element. *Acta Physiol. Scand.* **72**, 205–219.

Edman, K. A. P. and Nilsson, E. (1969). The dynamics of the inotropic change produced by altering pacing of rabbit papillary muscle. *Acta. Physiol. Scand.* **76**, 236–247.

Gordon, A. M., Huxley, A. F. and Julian, F. J. (1966). The variation in isometric tension with sarcomere length in vertebrate muscle fibres. *J. Physiol.* **184**, 170–192.

Hefner, L. L. and Bowen, T. E. (1967). Elastic components of cat papillary muscle. *Amer. J. Physiol.* **212**, 1221–1227.

Hill, A. V. (1949). The abrupt transition from rest to activity in muscle. *Proc. Roy. Soc. B.* **136**, 399–420.

Hill, A. V. (1970). "First and Last Experiments in Muscle Mechanics". University Press, Cambridge.

Hill, D. K. (1968). Tension due to interaction between the sliding filaments in resting striated muscle. The effect of stimulation. *J. Physiol.* **199**, 637–684.

Huxley, A. F. and Simmons, R. M. (1971). Mechanical properties of the cross-bridges of frog striated muscle. *J. Physiol.* **218**, 59–60.

Huxley, H. E. (1965). The contraction of muscle. *Scientific American* **213**, No. 6, 18–27.

Huxley, H. E. (1969). The mechanism of muscular contraction. *Science, N.Y.* **164**, 1356–1366.

Jewell, B. R. and Blinks, J. R. (1968). Drugs and the mechanical properties of heart muscle. *Annu. Rev. Pharmacol.* **8**, 113–130.

Jewell, B. R. and Wilkie, D. R. (1960). The mechanical properties of relaxing muscle. *J. Physiol.* **152**, 30–47.

Macpherson, L. (1953). A method of determining the force-velocity relation of muscle from two isometric contractions. *J. Physiol.* **122**, 172–177.

Noble, M. I. M., Bowen, T. E. and Hefner, L. L. (1969). Force-velocity relationship of cat cardiac muscle, studied by isotonic and quick-release techniques. *Circulation Res.* **24**, 821–833.

Noble, M. I. M. and Else, W. (1972). Limitations to the applicability of the A. V. Hill model of muscle to cat myocardium. *Circulation Res.* In press.

Parmley, W. W., Brutsaert, D. L. and Sonnenblick, E. H. (1969). Effects of altered loading on contractile events in isolated cat papillary muscle. *Circulation Res.* **24**, 521–532.

Philbrick Researches Inc. (1966). "Applications Manual for Computing Amplifiers". Nimrod Press, Boston.

Pollack, G. H. (1970). Maximum velocity as an index of contractility in cardiac muscle. *Circulation Res.* **26**, 111–127.

Pollack, G. H., Huntsman, L. L. and Verdugo, P. (1972). Cardiac muscle models: an overextension of series elasticity? *Circulation Res.* In press.

Ritchie, J. M. (1954). The effect of nitrate on the active state of muscle. *J. Physiol.* **126**, 155–168.

Siegel, J. H. and Sonnenblick, E. H. (1963). Isometric time-tension relationships as an index of myocardial contractility. *Circulation Res.* **12**, 597–610.

Simmons, R. M. and Jewell, B. R. (1972). Mechanics and models of muscular contraction. *In* "Recent Advances in Physiology" (R. J. Linden ed.), Churchill, London (to be published).

Sonnenblick, E. H. (1962). Force-velocity relations in mammalian heart muscle. *Amer. J. Physiol.* **202**, 931–929.

Sonnenblick, E. H. (1964). Series elastic and contractile elements in heart muscle: changes in muscle length. *Amer. J. Physiol.* **207**, 1330–1338.

Sonnenblick, E. H. (1965a). Instantaneous force-velocity-length determinants in the contraction of heart muscle. *Circulation Res.* **16**, 441–451.

Sonnenblick, E. H. (1965b). Determinants of active state in heart muscle: force, velocity, instantaneous muscle length, time. *Fed. Proc.* **24**, 1396–1409.

Taylor, R. R. (1970). Active length-tension relations compared in isometric, after-loaded and isotonic contractions of cat papillary muscle. *Circulation Res.* **26**, 279–288.

Taylor, S. R. and Rüdel, R. (1970). Striated muscle fibers: inactivation of contraction induced by shortening. *Science, N.Y.* **167**, 882–884.

Wildenthal, K., Skelton, C. L. and Coleman, H. N. III (1969). Cardiac muscle mechanics in hyperosmotic solutions. *Amer. J. Physiol.* **217**, 302–306.

Wilkie, D. R. (1968). "Muscle". Edward Arnold, London.

Yeatman, L. A. Jr., Parmley, W. W. and Sonnenblick, E. H. (1969). Effects of temperature on series elasticity and contractile element motion in heart muscle. *Amer. J. Physiol.* **217**, 1030–1034.

Chapter 8

The Fluid Mechanics of Heart Valves

B. J. BELLHOUSE

Fellow of Magdalen College, Oxford:
Department of Engineering Science, Oxford, England

1. INTRODUCTION

The heart acts as a double pump, with two pumping chambers (ventricles) and two collecting chambers (atria). The left ventricle pumps oxygenated blood round the body and back to the right atrium. The right atrium discharges to the right ventricle which pumps the de-oxygenated blood to the lungs and back to the left atrium, which in turn empties into the left ventricle. Each ventricle has an inlet and an outlet valve. The moving parts of these valves are thin (0·1 mm), flexible membranes called cusps. The outflow valves (in the aorta on the left side and the pulmonary artery on the right) are similar in appearance. Each cusp is approximately semi-circular and attached to the wall of the aorta (or pulmonary artery) around the curved edge. The valve has three cusps, and corresponding to each cusp there is a bulge in the wall of the aorta called a sinus.

The inlet valves lie between the atria and the ventricles and have to seal an orifice when the ventricles are contracting (systole). The inlet valve to the left ventricle is called the mitral valve, and has two major cusps attached around the perimeter of the mitral orifice. The inlet valve to the right ventricle has three cusps and is called the tricuspid valve.

2. THE AORTIC VALVE

Measurement of velocity in the dog and man (Bellhouse et al., 1967 and Schultz et al., 1968) show that blood flow in the aorta is laminar, and that in the normal valve reversed flow is less than 5 per cent of stroke volume. If the valve is stenosed, a turbulent jet is detected.

The absence of turbulence in the normal situation, despite a peak Reynolds number (based on diameter) of 10 000 indicates that the valve must present no obstruction to forward flow for most of systole. On the other hand, the small amount of reversed flow suggests that the valve is almost closed before the end of systole.

It is important that the cusps should close simultaneously if severe impact loads are to be avoided, and it is equally important that the coronary ostia (which lie within the sinuses of the aortic valve) are not obstructed by the cusps. McMillan et al. (1952) studied the action of aortic and pulmonary valves in a pulse duplicator. They reported that in their experiment the cusps did not open beyond a triangular shape and concluded that closure was obtained by reversed flow alone. Their observations were supported by ciné film but not by velocity measurement. Davila (1961) suggested that elastic recoil of the sinuses contributed to valve closure. Leonardo da Vinci (1513) predicted the formation of vortices between each cusp and its sinus, and appreciated that these would help to close the valve, but thought the vortices were shed and featured in the conversion of the kinetic energy of the fluid into heat, for he was unaware of the circulation of the blood.

Another cause of systolic valve closure is due to the unsteady flow. When flow is accelerating pressure in the aorta is highest at the ventricular end, but when the flow is decelerating the pressure gradient is reversed. If this pressure gradient could be used to establish a pressure difference across the valve cusps, then late-systolic closure of the valve would be possible.

To examine the apparently contradictory observations of laminar flow (hence wide valve opening) and small amount of reversed flow (hence partial closure of the valve in late systole) and the rival explanations, a model aortic valve was built and studied using a pulsatile-flow rig.

The model valve (Fig. 1) consisted of a rigid Perspex case into which the cusps (A) were glued. The sinuses (B) were also made of Perspex and could be detached. The cusps, 0·1 mm thick, were made of nylon net coated with silicone rubber and were attached to the Perspex aortic root so that they assumed their fully open position when no forces were applied to them.

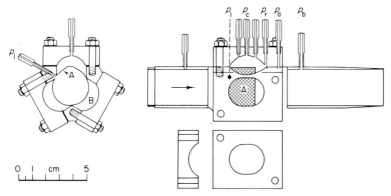

FIG. 1. Scale drawing of model aortic valve: at left, end-on; at right, side-on.

The cusps were shorter, in the axial direction, than the sinuses, and in their open position they projected into the sinuses. The scale drawing in Fig. 1 shows the valve end-on on the left, and side-on on the right. The positions of the pressure tappings are shown and marked p_l, p_a, p_b, p_c and p_r.

The dimensions of the model valve matched those of the aortic root in man (Fig. 2). The aorta is marked A, the ventricle V, one cusp is marked C,

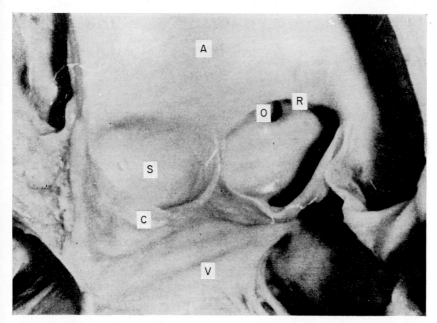

FIG. 2. Photograph of aortic root. A: aorta; C: cusp; O: orifice of coronary artery; R: sinus ridge; S: sinus; V: outflow tract of left ventricle.

a sinus ridge R and a coronary ostium O. The ostium is on the sinus ridge, but within the sinus; the advantage of this position is discussed below.

The main differences between the model valve and the physiological one were that the model root was transparent (so that flow patterns in the sinuses could be seen from outside) and rigid so that elastic recoil of the sinuses could be excluded as a contributory to valve closure mechanism. (The effect of elastic walls was studied at a later stage.)

A. DYE STUDIES

The model valve was perfused with a pulsatile water flow, and the flow patterns were made visible by injecting dye. At the start of systole the valve was closed, it opened rapidly and, as the cusps moved into the sinuses, vortices formed between the cusps and the sinus walls; the cusps then moved quickly back to a position with the centres of the free margins projecting slightly into the sinuses. The cusps did not flutter, and flow entered each sinus at the middle of the ridge (Fig. 3), curled back along the sinus wall, then along the

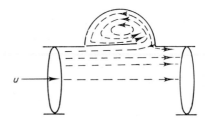

FIG. 3. Streamlines in aortic root at peak systole.

cusp to flow out into the main stream at the points of attachment of the cusp free margins. In steady flow the same description applied, with the cusps projecting slightly into the sinuses, and balanced between the main stream in the aorta and the trapped vortices in the sinuses.

After peak systole the cusps could be seen to move away from the sinuses, with gathering speed, and the valve was almost closed before the end of systole. The trapped vortices reached maximum strength at peak systole but decayed only slowly during the latter part of systole. The amount of back-flow was measured to be less than 5 per cent of forward flow, and the flow distal to the valve was laminar.

When the sinuses were occluded, the cusps opened early in systole until they touched the wall of the aorta, and no vortices formed behind them. The valve closed suddenly and unevenly by reversed flow alone, and back-flow was increased by a factor of five, to 25 per cent of forward flow, as described by Bellhouse and Bellhouse (1968a).

The sinuses were then replaced by flexible ones made of silicone rubber and of the same dimensions as the rigid sinuses. No alteration in valve performance was observed, and elastic recoil of the sinuses as a closure mechanism is discounted.

To examine more carefully the role of the sinus vortices and the unsteady nature of aortic flow in the closure mechanism of the aortic valve, simultaneous measurements were made of velocity and pressure distribution together with cusp position.

B. CINÉ FILM OF VALVE MOTION

The model valve was perfused with a pulsatile reversing flow, and aortic velocity was measured with a heated-element needle gauge (Bellhouse and Bellhouse, 1968b), placed on the axis of the aorta two diameters distal to the valve ring. A traverse of the probe across the lumen of the aorta showed that the velocity profile was flat.

A ciné camera was placed downstream of the valve so that an end-view of the cusps was obtained. The output of the velocity probe was displayed on an oscilloscope placed level with the valve, and was filmed simultaneously with the valve cusps. Twelve successive frames at 1/24 second intervals are reproduced in Fig. 4, with forward flow towards the camera. The needle velocity probe enters at six o'clock, with the element at the centre of the circle. Systole begins after (a), the valve is fully open at (c), closure begins at (i) and systole ends just after (j). Closure is completed [(k) and (l)] by reversed flow (Bellhouse and Talbot, 1969; Bellhouse and Bellhouse, 1969a).

Frame-by-frame analysis of the ciné film gave measurements of valve opening area and aortic velocity as functions of time. These are plotted non-dimensionally in Fig. 5. The time scale is such that the beginning of systole is at −1, the end at +1 and mid-systole at 0. Aortic velocity is divided by its value at peak systole, and the area defined by the cusp free margins is divided by the area of the aorta. The flat top of the curve of valve opening-area occurs because the cusps project into the sinuses, and are out of sight of the camera. The measurement, when the valve is wide open, is therefore an underestimate. In early and late systole, there is no such inaccuracy, and it may be seen that when systole ends (when the aortic velocity is zero), the valve is 72 per cent closed.

At the beginning of systole, valve opening lags behind the aortic velocity, because the cusps are pushed back towards the ventricle when loaded during diastole.

As the cusps relax at the beginning of systole, they displace fluid in the aorta before being swept aside by the accelerating flow. As the cusp free margins approach the circumference of the aorta, part of the aortic flow is intercepted by the sinus ridge, and the sinus vortices are formed. After

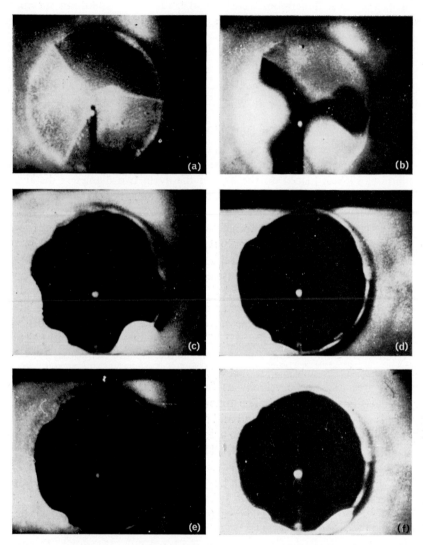

FIG. 4. Photographs of one cycle of the model aortic valve at 1/24 second intervals, with forward flow towards the camera. Systole begins after (a), the valve is open at (c), closure begins at (i), and systole ends just after (j). Closure is completed [(k) and (l)] by reversed flow.

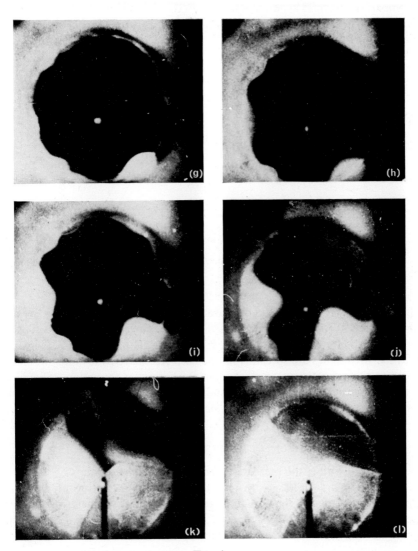

FIG. 4.

peak systole, the aortic flow decelerates under an axial pressure gradient (comparing pressures at two points on the axis of the aorta, the distal pressure will be higher to decelerate the aortic flow). The pressure in the sinuses depends on the pressure of the incoming fluid (that is, the pressure level with the sinus ridge) and the vortex strength. The effect of deceleration of

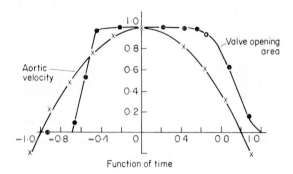

Fig. 5. Aortic velocity and valve opening area as functions of time (all non-dimensional).

the aortic flow is to make the pressure on the sinus side of the cusps exceed that on the aortic side, so the cusps start to move towards their closed position. The flow pattern established in the middle part of systole persists, and the streamlines are spread from the cusp-free margins towards the sinus ridge as the valve begins to close, thus preventing jet formation. (Should a jet form, sinus pressure would fall and the valve would tend to open again, as was seen with the stenosed valve described below.)

C. PRESSURE DIFFERENCES IN THE AORTIC ROOT

In a parallel pipe, the pressure difference between two points on the axis, distance $2a$ apart, necessary to give the flow an acceleration of du/dt, is $2\rho a(du/dt)$, where t is time and ρ fluid density. The increment in pressure produced by bringing fluid of velocity u to rest is $\frac{1}{2}\rho u^2$ (differences between end-hole and side-hole catheters). If the effect of cusp movement on pressure distribution is neglected, and if the peak velocity in the vortices is taken equal to aortic velocity, then the pressure differences between the ridge, p_r, the ring, p_l, and the sinus centre, p_c, taken in pairs (Fig. 1) are

$$p_r - p_c = \tfrac{1}{2}\rho u^2 \tag{2.1}$$

$$p_c - p_l = -2\rho a \frac{du}{dt} \tag{2.2}$$

and

$$p_r - p_1 = \tfrac{1}{2}\rho u^2 - 2\rho a\,\frac{\mathrm{d}u}{\mathrm{d}t}.\tag{2.3}$$

For three combinations of peak velocity and duration of systole, measurements of $p_r - p_c$, $p_c - p_1$, $p_r - p_1$ were made, together with aortic velocity. The experimental points are shown in Fig. 6, and calculations using (2.1), (2.2) and (2.3) are given as heavy lines. The broken lines are derived from an

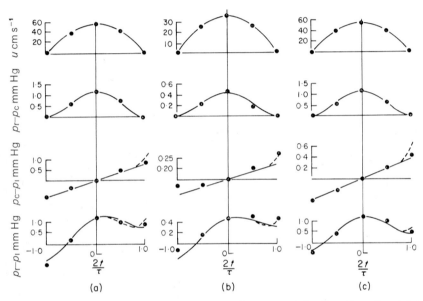

FIG. 6. Pressure and velocity measurements for a range of τ (duration of systole) and systolic velocities (u). (a) $\tau = 0\cdot575$ s, $u_{\max} = 56\cdot7$ cm s^{-1}; (b) $\tau = 0\cdot91$ s, $u_{\max} = 35\cdot0$ cm s^{-1}; (c) $\tau = 1\cdot170$ s, $u_{\max} = 56\cdot7$ cm s^{-1}. The continuous line is derived from equations (2.1), (2.2) and (2.3).

improved theory (Bellhouse, 1969). Even the simple theory accounts for the variation of pressure differences within the aortic root when heart rate and peak ejection velocities are varied. This shows that at higher heart rates, when the valve has to close quicker, the forces which close the valve are correspondingly higher.

D. STENOSED VALVE AND SYSTOLIC CORONARY FLOW

The cusps of the model aortic valve were glued together to form a central, circular stenosis of about half the aortic diameter. In steady flow, a turbulent jet was formed, and no vortices were observed in the sinuses, since the jet was not intercepted by the sinus ridge. In pulsatile flow also, the vortices were absent, and the pressure in the sinuses at peak systole was measured to be more than 30 mmHg below the pressure at the valve ring. The peak systolic velocity in the aorta, far downstream from the jet, was 62·4 cm s^{-1}, and the measured systolic pressure difference is shown in Fig. 7. This should

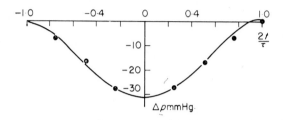

FIG. 7. Measurements of pressure difference, Δp, between a coronary ostium and the ventricle compared with theory (continuous line) for a valve with a 78·8 per cent stenosis; $\tau = 1\cdot0$ s, $u_{max} = 62\cdot4$ cm s^{-1}.

be compared with the measurements of systolic $p_r - p_l$ in Fig. 6, for the normal model valve. In diastole, of course, the pressure in the aorta is uniform, and if all coronary filling took place in diastole, then the pressure difference between the coronary ostia and the myocardium of the left ventricle during systole would be of no significance.

However, Gregg (1963) has shown that systolic left coronary flow does occur, and can equal, and even exceed, diastolic left coronary flow in exercise. This requires that the pressure at the coronary ostia exceeds the pressure in the left ventricular myocardium for at least part of systole. The coronary ostia are always placed within the sinuses (Bellhouse and Bellhouse, 1969a), where the highest pressures in the aortic root are recovered, but this increment is only about 4 mmHg at an aortic velocity of 100 cm s^{-1}. The most important effect is probably due to the unsteady nature of the flow. Early in systole, the aortic flow is accelerating, and ventricular pressures will be higher than aortic, but later in systole, aortic flow is decelerating and ventricular pressure will be lower than aortic. Since myocardial pressure is related to the blood pressure in the lumen of the ventricle, this could explain why left coronary flow occurs in systole with a normal aortic valve.

When the aortic valve is stenosed, the velocity at the stenosis is greatly increased, with a corresponding drop in pressure (venturi effect). The pressure at the coronary ostia is also reduced (by more than 30 mmHg in the experiment), and retrograde systolic coronary flow is probable. The jet emerging from the stenosed valve will expand to fill the whole aorta a few diameters downstream from the valve, and some of the kinetic energy in the jet will be converted back to potential energy in the form of a pressure increase. Since the jet is turbulent, some energy will be dissipated by turbulence and the ventricle will have to develop a higher pressure than it would have had to if the valve had been normal. Thus the stenosed aortic valve causes reduction of pressure at the coronary ostia by eliminating the stagnation points in the sinuses, and by the venturi effect at the stenosis. It also increases ventricular pressure because of energy losses in the jet. All three effects will tend to eliminate coronary artery flow to the left ventricle during systole. They could be a cause of angina pectoris associated with effort, in cases where the coronary arteries are normal but the aortic valve is stenosed.

3. The Mitral Valve

There are significant differences in anatomy and function between the aortic and mitral valves. The aortic valve is in a duct, and each cusp is supported out of the plane of the ring in an axial direction. The mitral valve is in an orifice, and in order to prevent prolapse of the flexible cusps, chordae tendineae connect the free margins of the two cusps to the papillary muscles on the opposite wall of the ventricle, near the apex. Since the distance between the apex and the mitral ring shortens in systole, the papillary muscles must contract in systole to prevent prolapse of the mitral valve.

Henderson and Johnson (1912) demonstrated that when their model mitral valve was closed by reversed flow alone considerable regurgitation occurred, but if forward flow preceded backflow, less regurgitation resulted. They argued that the inertia of the moving blood produced in its wake a negative pressure, and called this effect the "breaking of the jet". This might be supplemented, they thought, by eddies behind the cusps. Dean (1916) recorded mitral valve movements in isolated, perfused hearts, which showed that the valve started to close during atrial systole.

Rushmer et al. (1956) attached silver clips to the mitral valve, and showed that cusp movements were small in diastole. They suggested that the cusps were drawn towards apposition by the traction exerted by the papillary muscles. When the heart was functioning at abnormally small dimensions, the cusps opened wider than usual. This could be due to too much slack in the chordae tendineae during diastole as Rushmer and his co-authors suggest, or it could be due to a reduced stroke volume altering a fluid mechanic control system. Padula et al. (1968) obtained ciné film of valve action in a beating heart, using a clear blood-substitute, and showed that the mitral valve leaflets remained in a mid-position towards the end of diastole, with the orifice of the valve approximately half the diameter of the valve annulus. Movements of the cusp free margins during diastole were observed. These movements would seem to conflict with Rushmer's hypothesis that the cusps are tethered in diastole. Taylor and Wade (1970) used ciné-angio-graphy in dogs and sheep to show that a vortex formed in the left ventricle, and that the mitral valve closed with negligible reversed flow. Their findings were in agreement with the model experiments of Bellhouse and Bellhouse (1969b).

As a secondary experiment Padula *et al.* (1968) studied the case of a pulsatile pump attached to the apex of a passive left ventricle. Their observations that the mitral cusps remained wide open during diastole is consistent with poor valve closure because the vortex was absent.

As with the aortic valve, there would appear to be three components of mitral valve closure: unsteady flow, vortex and backflow. The relative importance of these is evaluated in the following sections.

A. THE UNSTEADY FLOW EFFECT

Henderson and Johnson's concept of the "breaking of the jet" may be made less mysterious with the analysis of a simple model. Experiments were performed with a large glass container filled with water, and a Perspex tube immersed a distance L into the water (Fig. 8). Water was sucked up the tube

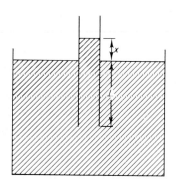

FIG. 8. Diagram of experiment to study unsteady pipe flow.

and then released, and the resulting oscillations were timed with a stop watch. The experiment was repeated for a range of immersion depths L and for two bores of tube (12·7 mm and 6·35 mm).

The oscillation is caused by the difference in levels of water in the tube and tank being matched by the inertia of the moving fluid and its weight. For small oscillations, and ignoring viscosity, a simple solution may be found. The pressure at the end of the tube in the tank will be close to tank pressure at that level, $\rho g L$ above atmospheric pressure (ρ density of water, g acceleration due to gravity).

The mass times acceleration (inertial force) of the slug of fluid in the tube is $A\rho(L+x)(d^2x/dt^2)$ where A is tube area, t time, and x differences in fluid levels. The vertical force on the slug is $A\rho gL$ (due to the pressure difference) — $A\rho g(L+x)$ (its weight).

Thus

$$(L+x)\frac{d^2x}{dt^2} + gx = 0. \tag{3.1}$$

Since $x \ll L$, (3.1) has a simple harmonic solution

$$x = x_0 \cos \omega t \tag{3.2}$$

where $\omega = \sqrt{g/L}$ and the period of oscillation is $\tau = 2\pi\sqrt{L/g}$. (This is identical to the solution for a simple pendulum, length L.)

The experimental results, together with the solutions of (3.2), marked A, are shown in Fig. 9. When skin friction on the tube wall is taken into account,

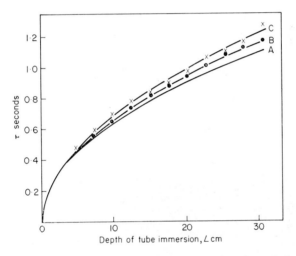

FIG. 9. Measurement of oscillation period τ as a function of depth of tube immersion, L, compared with theory. A: inviscid; B: viscous, large tube; C: viscous, small tube.

the calculated curve of oscillation time against depth of immersion is shifted upwards. The curve B is for the 12·7-mm diameter tube, and C is for the 6·35-mm diameter tube. The scatter in the measurements for the smaller tube is due to the viscous damping which reduced the number of oscillations that could be timed in sequence. For the larger tube, agreement between theory and experiment is good.

In the same way that (2.1) was derived, the pressure differences between outside and inside the tube, Δp, (distance l above the bottom of the tube) may be calculated

$$\Delta p = \rho l \frac{d^2 x}{dt^2} = \frac{-\rho l g x_0}{L} \cos \omega t. \qquad (3.3)$$

Starting with the level in the tube above that in the tank, Δp is negative until the levels are equal, then becomes positive. Hence if a flexible rubber sleeve with an open end were attached to the bottom of the pipe, the sleeve would begin to close down as soon as the fluid in the pipe started to decelerate. Since the pressure difference is proportional to the distance from the lower end of the sleeve, the base of the sleeve would begin to close first, and the edge last.

It would appear, therefore, that the "breaking of the jet" effect is identical to the axial pressure gradient associated with decelerating flow, which has been shown to be a feature of the aortic valve mechanism.

B. MODEL LEFT VENTRICLE

To see if a vortex filling the whole left ventricle could improve mitral valve performance, and to examine the effect of atrial systole on mitral valve closure, a model of the left ventricle was built. It consisted of a rigid base made of Perspex incorporating a mitral and an aortic valve (Fig. 10). The remainder of the ventricle was simulated by a transparent rubber bag. The

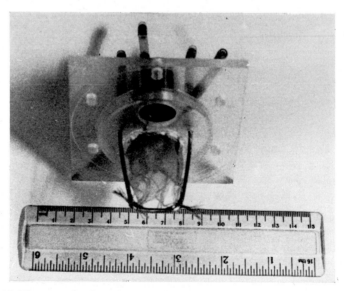

FIG. 10. Photograph of model ventricle showing the rigid base and mitral and aortic valves.

model ventricle was fixed inside a Perspex tank, which was filled with water and attached to a pulsatile pump to actuate the ventricle (Fig. 11). The aortic valve was connected by a pipe to a header tank, which overflowed to a lower tank, which discharged through a viewer to the mitral valve

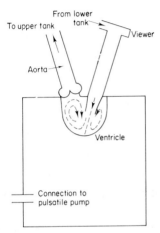

FIG. 11. Diagram of model left ventricle showing diastolic flow patterns.

(Bellhouse and Bellhouse, 1969b). The mitral valve consisted of a sleeve of nylon net coated with silicone rubber, shaped to make two cusps 0·1 mm thick and 28 mm long. The sleeve was shaped on a divergent cone (semi-angle 14°) with the narrower end forming the mitral ring. The free margins of the cusps were connected by threads to a fixed support 45 mm from the mitral ring.

C. FLOW PATTERNS IN THE MODEL LEFT VENTRICLE

When the ventricle was pumped, the mitral valve opened rapidly at the start of diastole, but it did not open to its fullest extent, and the chordae tendineae were slack. After the mitral valve had opened, the incoming jet struck the apex of the ventricle and spread out to flow up the walls to the base of the ventricle, then turned back behind the cusps towards the apex again, to form a ring vortex. The vortex was asymmetrical, with the greatest strength concentrated in the outflow tract, behind the anterior cusp. The pump actuating the ventricle produced a sinusoidal flow, one half for diastole, the other for systole. After peak diastole, the anterior cusp moved steadily towards closure, and just before ventricular filling was complete, the posterior cusp also started to close. Only a small amount of reversed flow was required to seal the mitral valve. This could be estimated from solid particles suspended in the water (tea leaves were found to be easily visible).

When the ventricle was filled slowly, and when all fluid motion had died down and the mitral cusps lay open, the external pump was switched on and the ventricle was contracted. The amount of reversed flow through the mitral valve increased by about a factor of five.

The next experiment was to increase the size of the ventricle, without altering stroke volume or pulse rate, so that the stroke volume was small compared with the end-systolic volume of the ventricle. Early in diastole, the valve opened as with a small ventricle, and a small starting vortex was formed, similar in appearance to a smoke ring. This ring moved towards the apex of the ventricle, but the remainder of the fluid in the ventricle remained stagnant. No movement was seen behind the cusps.

After peak diastole, both cusps began to move towards closure simultaneously and at the same speed. Reversed flow was less than when the ventricle was filled slowly, but more than when the ventricle was small.

D. MEASUREMENTS IN THE MODEL LEFT VENTRICLE

The amount of backflow when a valve closes is one measure of efficiency. However, much of the measured backflow is caused by stretching of the valve cusps as they seal against each other, so small differences in efficiency could go undetected by this means. For this reason, the techniques used with the aortic valve were preferred. Velocity was measured upstream of the mitral valve in a parallel pipe of cross-sectional area equal to that of the mitral ring; pressure was measured in the input tube to the mitral valve, 19 mm from the mitral ring, and on the anterior and posterior sides of the mitral cusps (Fig. 10). The cusp positions were recorded on ciné film, using the viewer shown in Fig. 11. The view of the cusps was therefore from the atrial side.

Two types of mitral valve were used. The first had an elliptical ring; this made measurement of valve opening area difficult when the valve was wide open, because the viewer tube was circular and obstructed a part of the orifice. The second valve had a circular ring so that the mitral valve could be rotated, so that the anterior and posterior cusps could be interchanged. With this mitral valve, also, the field of view of the camera was limited by the viewing tube. In both valves, therefore, measurements of valve opening area tend to be underestimates when the valve is wide open.

Using the elliptical-ring type of mitral valve, four different situations were examined. With a slow pulse rate and small ventricle, velocity in the mitral ring and three pressure differences were measured. In addition, the valve was filmed at 50 frames per second from the atrial side, and the film was synchronized with the other measurements by means of a flashing light actuated by a trigger on the pulsating pump.

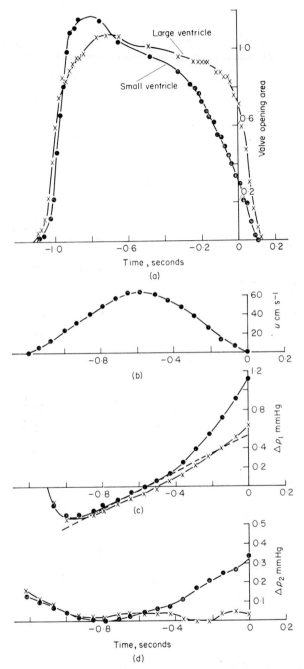

FIG. 12. Measurement of valve opening area (a), velocity through the mitral ring (b), and pressure differences (c), Δp_1 (pressure behind the anterior cusp–pressure in atrium) and (d), Δp_2 (pressure behind anterior cusp–pressure behind posterior cusp). Low frequency case for small ($\bullet$) and large ($\times$) ventricles, $f = 0.46$ Hz.

The measurements were repeated for a fast pulse rate, but with no change in stroke volume, and then the ventricle was increased in size (to eliminate the ventricular vortex) and the measurements were repeated for fast and slow pulse rates. In Fig. 12 measurements for the slower pulse rate are shown for a small ventricle (●) and a large ventricle (×). The end-systolic ventricular volumes were 107 and 1216 cm^3 respectively. At mid-diastole, the cusps were almost parallel, and it has been convenient to divide the measured cusp opening area by the mid-diastolic value averaged over the four cases plotted in Figs. 12(a) and 13(a). The difference in closure rate between the small ventricle, when a strong vortex was formed, and the large ventricle when no vortex was seen, is apparent in Fig. 12(a). The velocity through the mitral ring for both cases is shown in Fig. 12(b). The pressure difference, Δp_1, between behind the anterior cusp, in the ventricle, and the pressure tapping on the atrial side of the mitral ring, 19 mm from the ring, is shown in Fig. 12(c). The broken line is calculated from the velocity curve 12(b) and the formula $\Delta p_1 = -\rho L(\mathrm{d}u/\mathrm{d}t)$, where ρ is fluid density, L a length and $\mathrm{d}u/\mathrm{d}t$ acceleration through the mitral orifice. The value of L was chosen to be 33 mm to agree with the pressure difference measured when the ventricle was large. The same value of L was used to calculate the broken line in Fig.

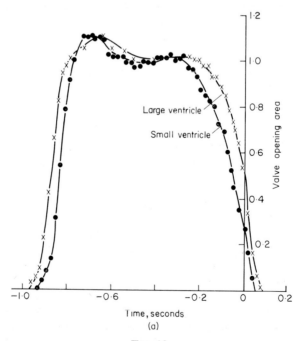

Fig. 13.

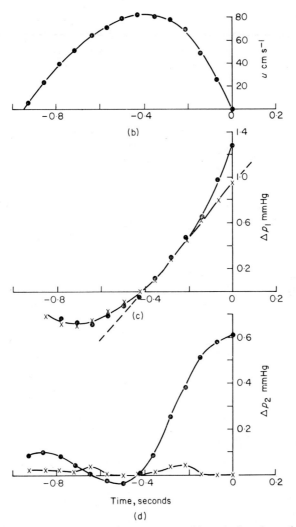

Fɪɢ. 13. Measurement of valve opening area (a), velocity through the mitral ring (b), and pressure differences (c), Δp_1 and (d), Δp_2 (see Fig. 12). High frequency case for small (●) and large (×) ventricles, f = 0·53 Hz.

13(c), which demonstrates that when the vortex is absent, Δp_1 is proportional to the deceleration of the flow through the mitral ring.

Fig. 12(d) gives the pressure difference, Δp_2, measured between the positions behind the anterior and posterior cusps. Negligible difference was obtained for the large ventricle, and a significant difference occurred for a small ventricle.

Figure 13 is similar to Fig. 12, but with an increased pulse rate, and the same remarks apply. From these measurements, it is seen that deceleration of the flow through the mitral ring produced about 30 per cent of the closure, and the vortex and deceleration together accounted for 70 per cent of the valve closure. The remaining 30 per cent of closure was achieved by backflow.

E. DIFFERENCES IN ANTERIOR AND POSTERIOR CUSP MOVEMENT

The elliptical mitral valve was replaced with a circular valve which could be rotated in position, so that the anterior and posterior cusps could be

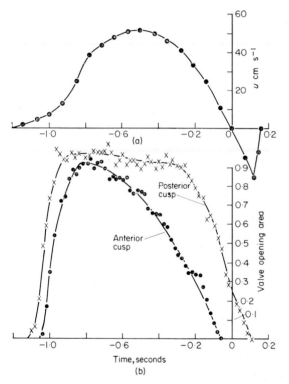

FIG. 14. Difference in closure rate between anterior (●) and posterior (×) cusps for small ventricle. There is no difference when the ventricle is large.

interchanged without dismantling the model. Measurements of valve opening area were made for the anterior and posterior halves separately; these measured values were divided by half the area of the valve ring, and plotted as functions of time in Fig. 14. Velocity through the mitral ring is shown at the top of the figure. The more rapid closure of the anterior cusp was because the main vortex strength was in the outflow tract.

When the mitral valve was rotated through 180°, the new anterior cusp (which had been the posterior) moved first towards closure. This excluded the possibility that differences in cusp stiffness, size or attachment could be responsible for the differences in closure rate. The asymmetry of the vortex,

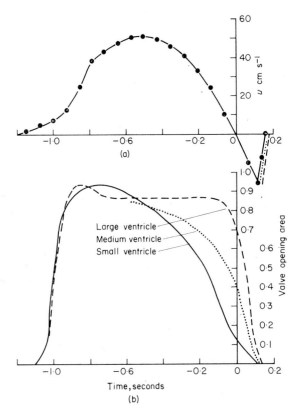

Fig. 15. Effect of ventricle volume on valve closure rate. (Large 1216 cm³, medium 207 cm³, small 107 cm³ at end of systole.)

demonstrated by the motion of suspended particles, was seen to be the cause of the differences in cusp movement when the ventricle was reshaped (unphysiologically) so that the main vortex strength lay behind the posterior cusp. In this case, the posterior cusp closed first.

To see if ventricle size, and hence vortex strength, affected the circular mitral valve as much as the elliptical valve, valve closure rate was measured for three end-systolic ventricular volumes (107, 207 and 1216 cm³) for the same stroke volume (169 cm³) and pulse rate. The substantial differences are shown in Fig. 15. The differences in anterior and posterior cusp movements decreased with increasing ventricular volume (decreasing vortex strength) until they vanished with the largest ventricle.

F. SIMULATION OF ATRIAL SYSTOLE

To simulate atrial systole, a balloon pump was used. It was inserted in the Perspex tank of Fig. 11, and was expanded and contracted in a wire cage by compressed air, which was controlled by two solenoid-operated air valves

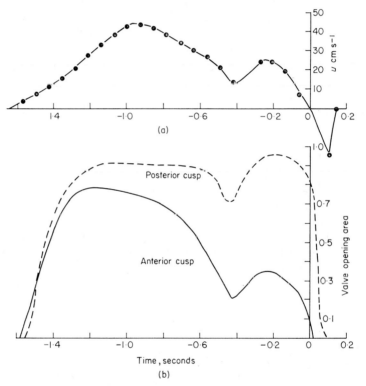

(a)

(b)

FIG. 16. Effect of atrial systole on valve closure. Anterior cusp full line, posterior cusp broken line (early atrial systole).

triggered by the sinusoidal pump used for the work described above. The balloon could be exhausted during diastole to increase the ventricular volume, and simulate atrial systole. The balloon was filled during systole. By varying the trigger mechanism, the timing of atrial systole could be altered. Two cases are shown in Figs. 16 and 17. In both, the mitral valve begins to close at the first velocity peak and continues towards closure until the onset of atrial systole, when the valve responds to the accelerating flow and begins to open again. At the next peak in velocity at the mitral ring the valve starts to close again. The difference in closure rate of the anterior and posterior cusps is evident.

The experiments were limited to short periods of slow ventricular filling between passive filling and atrial systole. One extension of the work would be to study longer periods of slow filling, when vortex strength could be expected to decrease because of frictional losses, and the mitral valve might require more reversed flow to close it.

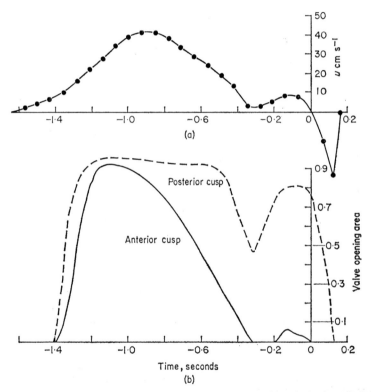

Fig. 17. Effect of atrial systole on valve closure. Anterior cusp full line, posterior cusp broken line (delayed atrial systole).

4. Conclusion

In a model of the aortic valve strong vortices were shown to form in the aortic sinuses, with a ridge at the distal end of the sinuses maintained at free-stream stagnation pressure during systole. At peak systole, the cusps projected slightly into the sinuses and were held in a stable position by the trapped vortices. After peak systole, axial deceleration in the aorta caused a pressure imbalance across the cusps, which moved towards the closed position, and the valve was three-quarters closed by the end of systole. The persistence of the vortices was responsible for spreading streamlines through the cusps and maintaining the pressures closing the valve during systole. Reversed flow, less than 5 per cent of stroke volume, was required to seal this valve.

Using a model of a stenosed aortic valve, pressures in the aortic sinuses were found to be more than 30 mmHg below the pressures measured in the model of a normal valve. Since the coronary ostia lie within the sinuses, a fluid mechanic explanation of angina pectoris associated with effort, when the aortic valve is stenosed, was proposed.

The action of the mitral valve was studied with the aid of a model of the left ventricle, consisting of a rigid base incorporating a bicuspid mitral valve and an aortic valve, and a thin rubber diaphragm for the remainder of the ventricle. The mitral valve was shown to achieve most of its closure during diastole and that a ring-vortex filled the ventricle. When the ventricle was increased in size, without increasing stroke volume or pulse rate, the vortex decreased in strength and the mitral valve closed later. The vortex was found to be asymmetrical and caused the anterior cusp to close earlier in diastole than the posterior cusp.

Closure of the mitral valve during diastole depended on two effects: vortex strength and flow deceleration through the mitral ring. These two effects were varied independently for a single peaked filling curve (velocity at the mitral ring), and were shown to be of nearly equal importance.

Atrial systole was simulated by introducing a second surge in the ventricular filling curve. The mitral valve opened at the beginning of the first surge, the ventricular vortex was established and the valve began to close after the first velocity peak, with the anterior cusp moving more than the posterior. At the onset of the second surge, the valve reopened slightly, with the posterior cusp responding more than the anterior. After the peak in the second surge the valve began to close again.

REFERENCES

Bellhouse, B. J. (1969). Velocity and pressure distributions in the aortic valve. *J. Fluid Mech.* **37**, 587–600.
Bellhouse, B. J. and Bellhouse, F. H. (1968a). Mechanism of closure of the aortic valve. *Nature, Lond.* **217**, 86–87.
Bellhouse, B. J. and Bellhouse, F. H. (1968b). Thin-film gauges and the measurement of velocity or skin friction in air, water or blood. *J. Sci. Instr.* Series 2, **1**, 1211–1213.
Bellhouse, B. J. and Bellhouse, F. H. (1969a). Fluid mechanics of model normal and stenosed aortic valves. *Circulation Res.* **25**, 693–704.

Bellhouse, B. J. and Bellhouse, F. H. (1969b). Fluid mechanics of the mitral valve. *Nature, Lond.* **224,** 615–616.

Bellhouse, B. J. and Talbot, L. (1969). The fluid mechanics of the aortic valve. *J. Fluid Mech.* **35,** 721–735.

Bellhouse, B. J., Schultz, D. L., Karatzas, N. B. and Lee, G. de J. (1967). *In* "Blood Flow through Organs and Tissues" (W. H. Bain and A. M. Harper, eds.), pp. 43–54. Livingstone, Edinburgh.

Davila, J. C. (1961). Mechanics of the cardiac valves. *In* "Prosthetic Valves for Cardiac Surgery" (K. Merendino, ed.), Thomas, Illinois.

da Vinci, L. (1513). *Quaderni d'Anatomica* II, 9.

Dean, A. L. (1916). The movements of the mitral cusps in relation to the cardiac cycle. *Amer. J. Physiol.* **40,** 206–217.

Gregg, D. E. (1963). Physiology of the coronary circulation. *Circulation* **27,** 1128–1137.

Henderson, Y. and Johnson, F. E. (1912). Two modes of closure of the heart valves. *Heart* **4,** 69–82.

McMillan, I. K. R., Daley, R. and Matthews, M. B. (1952). Movement of aortic and pulmonary valves studied post mortem by colour cinematography. *Brit. Heart J.* **14,** 42.

Padula, R. T., Coran, G. S. M. and Camishion, R. C. (1968). Photographic analysis of the active and passive components of cardiac valvular action. *J. Thor. Cardiovasc. Surgery* **56,** 790–798.

Rushmer, R. F., Finlayson, B. L. and Nash A. A. (1956). Movements of the mitral valve. *Circulation Res.* **4,** 337–342.

Schultz, D. L., Tunstall-Pedoe, D. S., Lee, G. de J., Gunning. A. J. and Bellhouse, B. J. (1968). Velocity distribution and transition in the arterial system. *In* "Circulatory and Respiratory Mass Transport" (G. E. W. Wolstenholme and J. Knight, eds.), CIBA Foundation Symposium, Churchill, London.

Taylor, D. E. M. and Wade, J. D. (1970). The pattern of flow around the atrioventricular valves during diastolic ventricular filling. *J. Physiol.* **207,** 71–72.

Chapter 9

Pressure and Flow in Large Arteries

D. L. SCHULTZ

Fellow of St. Catherine's College, Oxford:
Department of Engineering Science, Oxford, England

1. INTRODUCTION

A knowledge of the velocity with which the ventricles eject blood into the arterial system is equally as important as information on the pressures produced by the contracting ventricles in various sectors of the arterial bed. To some extent the emphasis in most published work on arterial blood flow has been on the relationship of pressure gradient to flow, influenced no doubt by the earlier theoretical studies of Witzig (1914) and Womersley (1957) which were then available. The proper function of organs is, however, affected by the volumetric flow with which they are perfused and information on local pressures or pressure gradients is inadequate by itself for the determination of the efficiency of perfusion. Admittedly the measurement of pressure posed less problems than that of volumetric flow and with experience it has become possible to recognize malfunction in the heart, lungs and other organs from measurements of pressure alone. This relative success is rendered possible by the nature of the source impedance of the ventricles themselves, which being relatively high tends to generate a constant flow irrespective, to a large extent, of the load presented to it. While such conclusions about organ perfusion are relatively straight-forward in cases in which the ventricular function is normal or only slightly abnormal, our understanding of the mechanical function of the failing heart is as yet insufficiently complete to enable pressure measurements alone to yield completely unambiguous information. Although a great deal of research has been done on the mechanical function of the ventricles, this pioneering work has not yet been coupled to the equally extensive studies of the arterial bed, the effective load which is presented to the ventricles. Until such an amalgamation is made our insight into the behaviour of the complete system must remain minimal. Although the catheter technique for pressure measurement only predated the first use of the electromagnetic flowmeter by a few years the former gained for itself fairly widespread understanding, use and hence confidence. The inherent technical difficulties associated with electromagnetic flowmeters and the need to cannulate the arteries in early models retarded its widespread use although recent developments, in particular the appearance of the cuff and catheter tip flowmeters (Mills and Shillingford, 1967) have substantially altered this position. There have been of course many other arterial flowmeters, either volumetric or strictly velocity meters, in use for some time before the appearance of the electromagnetic flowmeter and the development up to 1963 is well recorded by Kramer et al. (1963). Many of these developments, such as the bristle flowmeter, pitot probes and others, were ingenious and in the hands of experienced workers could yield surprisingly good results, which although sometimes lacking in accuracy, produced qualitative ideas about the waveform of ejection or the mean flow rate.

The electromagnetic flowmeter developed by Kolin (1945) and the hot wire anemometer used by Machella (1936) were forerunners of the miniaturized instruments suitable for use on or in small vessels which in quite recent years have begun to yield quantitative results. The thin film anemometer, which will be discussed in more detail later in this chapter and also by Mills (Chapter 3) uses essentially the same transducing action as the hot wire, the heat transferred from a small element to a flowing fluid is related to the velocity of the fluid past the element, if the fluid density is constant, whether it be a fine wire or a metallic film on the surface of an insulator. Serious interest in detailed studies of velocity distribution in blood vessels did not arise until Hale et al. (1955) following Richardson and Tyler (1929), Sexl (1930), Schonfeld (1948) and Lambossy (1950) tabulated the solution of the equation:

$$\frac{\partial U}{\partial t} = -\frac{1}{\rho}\frac{\partial p}{\partial x} + \nu\left(\frac{\partial^2 U}{\partial r^2} + \frac{1}{r}\frac{\partial U}{\partial r}\right) \tag{1.1}$$

which describes the behaviour of the axial velocity U as a function of radius r and time t, when the fluid is subjected to an oscillatory pressure gradient $p = Ae^{i\omega t}$. The geometric form of the oscillatory profile is now well known from frequent publication and discussion. The historical development of these ideas has been well documented by McDonald and Taylor (1959), McDonald (1960), Noordergraaf (1969) and Bergel and Schultz (1971), and has been discussed in detail by Fry et al. (1964) and Rudinger (1966).

Those aspects which are more relevant to the present review are, however, the origins of the radial distribution of velocity, i.e. the velocity profile in the ascending aorta and its alteration through the aortic system. In so far as the pressure and velocity waveforms are coupled by the elastic nature of the vessel walls it will be necessary to consider both phenomena. The effect of the non-linear terms such as $U(\partial U/\partial x)$ which arise in the equations describing both fluid motion and pressure wave propagation have been discussed by Wiener et al. (1966), Whirlow and Rouleau (1965), Rideout and Sims (1969) and Fry et al. (1964). It is not proposed to enter into a detailed comparison of linear versus non-linear analyses in the present exposition since these have been treated in great detail but when such effects are found to be significant they will be remarked upon. The general conclusions at present would appear to be that as far as pressure wave propagation is concerned the effects are small, barely within the range of current measuring techniques, but the effect on velocity waveforms may be somewhat greater (Rideout and Sims (1969), Vander Werff (1971). Skalak (1966, and see Chapter 19) has given a useful review of the status of the non-linear effects on pressure wave propagation up to 1966 and in the same year Wylie (1966) presented some numerical results of pressure and discharge wave distortion in tapered tubes with non-linear wall properties. More recently there have been two more detailed studies by Vander Werff (1971) and Anliker et al. (1970) of both pressure and velocity waveform modification in arterial systems.

2. Velocity Distribution in the Aortic System of Dogs

The physical arrangement of the left ventricle with respect to the aorta resembles the equipment used in classical fluid dynamic experiments to investigate the nature of the transition process from laminar to turbulent flow. In these a bell mouth entry section connects a large reservoir with the tube and it is found that the velocity distribution is virtually constant over the cross section near the entrance to the tube. The velocity at the wall is, however, zero and a boundary layer is formed which gradually grows in thickness until the flow in the whole of the tube is influenced by this viscous phenomenon and the velocity distribution assumes a parabolic form. The flow velocity in the centre of the tube is then greater than at the inlet, in order to preserve continuity, and the distance from the inlet to the first location at which the velocity profile is independent of the entrance distribution, is known as the entrance length. This length has been calculated several times by different authors and the results range from 0.058 to $0.13 UD/\nu$.

When, however, the entrance velocity is periodic the entrance length will also fluctuate. This phenomenon has been studied by Atabek and Chang (1961) and Atabek et al. (1964) who found that the ratio of "pulsatile" inlet length to steady inlet length varied by $\pm 36\cdot5$ per cent at a value of $\alpha\,(= R\sqrt{\omega/v})$ of 4, appropriate to the iliac artery of a dog. Thus taking an average Re of 465 for a dog with mean velocity $12\cdot5\,\mathrm{cm\,s^{-1}}$ and aortic diameter $1\cdot5$ cm we would expect to find a mean flow inlet length/diameter ratio of 27 giving possible locations of flow profile development at about 55 cm during ejection and 25 cm during diastole. Although it is not possible to relate the theoretical work (which was concerned with sinusoidal disturbances on inlet velocity) of Atabek and Chang to the waveforms found in the physiological case there is nevertheless some indication that the development of the profile may be observable in man and animals.

This profile development is sufficiently interesting in its own right to merit closer study. For instance it might be expected that the details of the division of flow at major branches in the aorta would be influenced by the velocity profile in the main vessel although, as we shall see later, the dominant feature must be the driving pressure gradient and the impedance of the branching structure. Atabek et al. (1964) have made observations along a tube to test their theoretical predictions and the results appear to be in fair agreement with theory although the measurements were made in regions where one would not expect major departures from blunt profiles caused by viscous effects. Florio and Mueller (1968) have extended this work and have also shown that the inlet phenomenon can be regarded as the superposition of a developing steady flow and a fully developed oscillatory flow. A reasonable average for the diameter of a 20-kg dog's aorta is $1\cdot5$ cm and the mean ejection velocity about $25\,\mathrm{cm\,s^{-1}}$. The velocity profile would be expected to show more or less complete development to parabolic profile at lengths of about 40 cm using the steady flow criterion and over a range of 30 to 70 cm under oscillatory conditions. Signs of departure from bluntness should be expected before this and it is therefore not unreasonable that in the descending aorta of dogs we do in fact find the profile departing from its shape at the inlet. In a series of experiments on dogs Tunstall-Pedoe (1970) made velocity measurements across the diameters of the ascending arch and descending aorta of dogs. Although the weights and sizes of the dogs varied to some extent the general geometry remained similar and it is not therefore unreasonable to expect that the normalized results will be comparable from one experiment to another. The velocity was determined by means of a thin film anemometer mounted in the angled foot of a hypodermic needle of 8 mm diameter. The technique has been described in detail in several papers, by Ling et al. (1968), Schultz et al. (1969) and Seed and Wood (1970) for instance, and is discussed in Chapter 3.

A small metallic film baked on to the surface of a glass substrate is heated to a temperature about 5 °C above that of blood. Heat is transferred to the flowing liquid by forced convection and conduction and a feedback system is used to maintain the element at constant resistance (hence constant temperature). The power required in this feedback circuit is monitored and by calibration can be related to the fluid velocity. For detailed velocity studies,

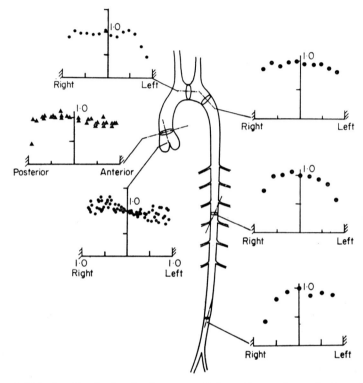

FIG. 1. Velocity distribution in the aorta of dogs. For each graph the ordinate shows $\overline{U}/\overline{U}_{C.L.}$, mean velocity at each station normalized to the mean centre-line velocity, and the abscissa is R/R_W, the radial location of the measuring station normalized on the internal luminal radius.

which are closely allied to those of thermistor bridges (Grahn *et al.*, 1969), the advantages of the technique are that point measurements of velocity are obtained and the sensor has a sufficiently high frequency response to detect turbulence when it is present. The electronic circuitry used to control the heated element is available commercially and is extensively used in fluid dynamics research. The approximate locations at which the traverses in dogs were made by Schultz *et al.* (1969) are shown in Fig. 1 and the velocity

11*

profiles are superimposed. The profiles are shown as $\bar{U}/\bar{U}_{C.L.}$, the bars denoting time-averaged values normalized to the centreline time averaged velocity. Radial locations are also shown as R/R_W, i.e. normalized to the inside vessel wall radius. It should be noted that this presentation, although illustrating in a compact manner the general nature of the velocity distribution does not enable the time history of the profile to be shown. Before illustrating this additional feature of the profile it is worth noting one or two points from Fig. 1. Firstly in the ascending aorta it will be seen that there is a slight asymmetry across the vessel diameter with higher velocities on the inner wall and on the right lateral walls. Similar observations of asymmetry have been reported by Amyot et al. (1970). This asymmetry has apparently disappeared at about the mid-point of the aortic arch and subsequently in the mid- and lower thoracic aorta the profile begins to exhibit signs of development towards the parabolic form. This symmetrical form of the profile in the descending thoracic aorta has been confirmed by Ling et al. (1968). These observations are consistent with the approximate estimations made earlier where a figure of about 30 to 70 cm was expected to represent the region of the first appearance of developed flow during acceleration in uniform bore tubes.

The evolution of the profile in the lower thoracic aorta demonstrates that viscous effects are present and cannot be neglected although it will be seen subsequently that the actual waveform is dominated by inertial effects. It might be expected that impedance measurements made at similar locations would also give confirmation of this trend towards a viscous dominated flow. This information is contained in the phase angle of the impedance whose tangent is the compliance/resistance in the case of a negative phase angle and inertance/resistance in the case of a positive phase angle. Most of this work has been done with a view to the identification of reflecting sites and there is little reported work at a series of locations down the aorta. Even in the ascending aorta it is found (O'Rourke and Taylor, 1967) that this phase angle indicates a substantial resistive component in the impedance. For instance, at the first impedance minimum O'Rourke and Taylor have measured a phase angle of 1 radian indicating that losses of one sort or another are about $1/\sqrt{3}$ of the reactive or "recoverable" terms in the total input impedance. This fraction of losses to storage or inertance terms generally increases with frequency so that it should not be thought that viscosity plays a wholly unimportant role even in such major vessels as the ascending aorta. In the ascending aorta of dogs with heart rates from 150 to 200 min^{-1} and aortic diameters between 1·5 and 2·0 cm, the value of the frequency parameter α ranges between 13 and 22. These values are sufficiently high for the velocity profile to exhibit the blunt characteristics first illustrated by Richardson and Tyler (1929), Lambossy (1950), and Hale et al. (1955), although it must be emphasized that these earlier calculations were not concerned with entrance effects and were simply predictions of the velocity profile in a rigid tube subjected to a longitudinal pressure gradient. These studies indicated that the profile would be maintained with much the same shape throughout the whole of the oscillatory cycle. Ling *et al.* (1968), Schultz *et al.* (1969) and Amyot *et al.* (1970) have reported measurements of this oscillatory profile in animals.

Figure 2 illustrates the instantaneous profile at progressive phases throughout the cardiac cycle in a dog's ascending aorta. This profile was obtained

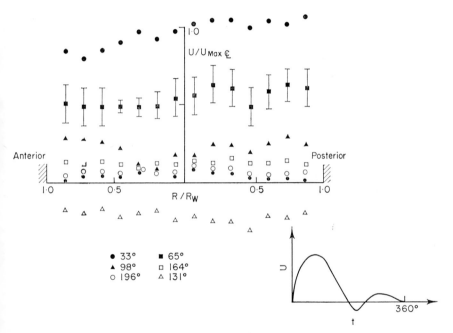

FIG. 2. Fluctuating velocity profile in ascending aorta of dog. 1 cardiac cycle = 360°. Maximum divergence from the average velocity at each location occurs during the deceleration phase at 65°. Maximum and minimum values observed during 10 cycles shown.

by recording 10 velocity waveforms at 14 diametral locations across the aorta of a dog with an aortic diameter of 1·6 cm. The value of α calculated from the fundamental of the cardiac frequency was 14·2. It will be seen that the slightly skewed profile shown in the time-averaged velocities of Fig. 1 is repeated in the instantaneous profile and the shape of this profile is maintained during acceleration and reverse flow. Due to the finite size of the velocity sensing probe (0·8 mm diameter) it was not possible to observe the profile very close to the wall but there is no clear evidence of local flow reversal near the wall which would be expected from simple pressure gradient theory, neglecting inlet effects. Unfortunately it would be quite difficult to check the existing theory *in vivo* since the descending thoracic aorta at a site where developed flow appears is too narrow to enable adequate spatial resolution, at least in dogs, to be obtained. Ling *et al.* (1968) have used a thin film anemometer to confirm the predicted waveforms in a rigid tube subjected to a sinusoidal pressure gradient and the results of this test

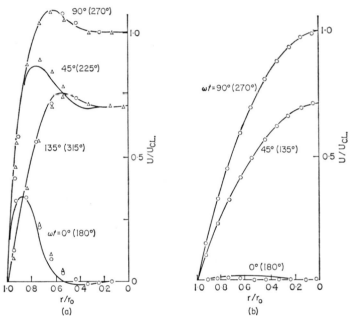

FIG. 3 (a) Predicted and experimental waveforms of velocity in a rigid tube at an α of 10 obtained in dog blood (△) and in glycerin and water (○). (b) Predicted (—) and experimental (○) velocity profiles in a rigid tube at an α of 1·0 in glycerin. Redrawn from Ling *et al.* (1968).

carried out at a value of α of 1 and 10 are shown in Fig. 3. The closeness of agreement of theory and experiment in these tests shows, at the same time, that blood behaves as a Newtonian fluid within the range of α relevant to animals and man.

3. VELOCITY PROFILES IN HUMAN SUBJECTS

Although in man there are important differences in vascular geometry when compared with the dog, it is possible to make some haemodynamic comparisons. If we take a mean value of the ascending aorta diameter within the range 2·5 to 4·5 cm and of distance to lower thoracic aorta of 35 cm, the length/diameter ratio of 10 can be compared with the value of 20 in the dog. The value of α for the fundamental frequency in the aorta of man ranges from 13 to 17 compared with the range of 5 to 10 in the aorta of dogs, so that similar behaviour from the point of view of the oscillatory

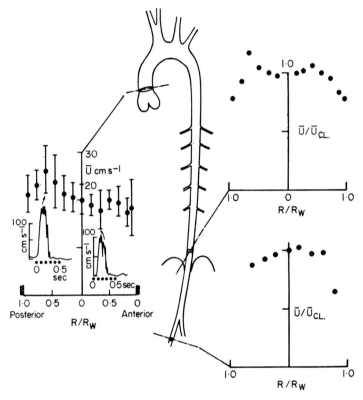

FIG. 4. Velocity distribution in the ascending aorta, lower thoracic aorta and femoral artery of man. Data obtained from three patients.

velocity and its development might be expected (for larger diameters at least). There are greater differences in the arterial input impedance in the two species but this will not affect the velocity distribution. Time-averaged velocity profiles in the ascending and descending aorta and femoral artery of man are shown in Fig. 4. These results were obtained in three separate subjects during surgery for aortic valve replacement and although two of the patients studied had cardiovascular disorders (mitral incompetence in the case of the study made in the ascending aorta, and aortic stenosis in the case of the femoral artery traverse) these were not expected to have any noticeable effect on the profile at the sites available. From Fig. 4 it will be seen that the profile in the ascending aorta is indeed quite similar to that found in the animal experiments. There is a slight increase in average velocity near the posterior wall although the variable heart rate resulted in quite large standard deviations in the mean velocity determined at any one radial location. In this particular case the flow is disturbed from peak systole onwards throughout the ejection cycle. This patient had mitral incompetence and X-ray studies revealed a degree of left ventricular enlargement. The disturbances in the flow could have been due either to the high ejection velocities (peak Re 7800) or there may have been some damage to the aortic valve. Alternatively, though less likely, the disturbances could have arisen from wall vibrations transmitted from the

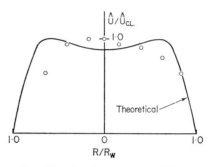

Fig. 5. Comparison of predicted and experimental ($\bigcirc$) velocity profiles at peak forward velocity in femoral artery of man. The profile is more developed than expected from simple theory.

left atrium. None of these effects would, however, be expected to influence the time-averaged profile. In the descending aorta traverse 2 cm above the diaphragm the profile is still relatively blunt although showing signs of development, and at the site of the femoral artery there is an increasing tendency towards developed flow. The observations at this location were made on a patient with aortic stenosis and all traces of the turbulent flow from the stenosed valve had decayed. The value of α for the fundamental at this location is 7 and the peak centreline velocity reached 34 cm s^{-1} with a corresponding Re of 850. The reduction in α from 15 in the ascending aorta to 7 in the femoral artery is a factor, additional to viscosity, in affecting transition to a more parabolic waveform. However, a comparison of the theoretical and observed velocity profiles under conditions of maximum forward flow show considerable discrepancies, Fig. 5, the observed profile being more developed than one would expect from simple theory.

4. THE EVOLUTION OF THE WAVEFORMS OF PRESSURE AND VELOCITY IN THE AORTA

In addition to the changes in the radial velocity distribution down the aorta there are variations in waveform both of velocity and pressure which reveal different aspects of the function of the cardiovascular system. The propagation of the pressure wave originating in the left ventricle has received extensive treatment and there is a substantial literature which will not be reviewed in the present chapter. Ideas on the reasons for the observed pressure peaking in the descending aorta and femoral artery have undergone extensive changes since as recently as 1963 when Spencer and Denison were able to quote support for the existence of a standing wave in the aorta, which would have the effect of causing localized regions of high pulse pressure. McDonald and Taylor in 1959 pointed out that this approach was much less fruitful than one which resolved the initial pulse into harmonics whose propagation and attenuation were considered as steady-state phenomenon. Bergel and Schultz in 1970 reviewed progress in this field since the McDonald and Taylor paper, and Noordergraaf (1969) has given a useful survey of the development of the windkessel theory and its subsequent modification by Jones (1969).

Most of the recent work by Streeter *et al.* (1963), Wylie (1966), Barnard *et al.* (1966) and Rudinger (1966) has been concerned with variations in the pressure pulse although Anliker *et al.* (1970), Rideout and Sims (1969) and Wiggert and Keitzer (1964) have paid particular attention to changes in the velocity waveform. Attempts to relate the travelling pressure and velocity waves are complicated by several factors which make rigorous analytical treatment impossible and at present the most rewarding line of attack has been by numerical techniques using the method of characteristics. The complexity of the analysis arises from the need to take into account the following aspects:

(a) The variation in the elasticity of the aorta from inlet to the branches at the femoral artery.
(b) The variation in area.
(c) The effects of flow into the intercostal arteries and other branches.
(d) The variation of the elastic modulus with pressure.

In any numerical technique such as the method of characteristics it is possible to include all of these effects but an understanding of their relative contributions to the overall behaviour can only come from a systematic study of test cases in which one parameter at a time is varied. It is this systematic study which has been lacking in much of the work so far published and which has reduced the value of the results obtained by this otherwise powerful technique.

The two basic equations governing the fluid dynamics in the aorta, the continuity equation:

$$\frac{\partial A}{\partial t} + \frac{\partial (UA)}{\partial x} = 0 \tag{4.1}$$

and the momentum equation:

$$\rho \frac{\partial U}{\partial t} + \rho U \frac{\partial U}{\partial t} + \frac{\partial p}{\partial x} = 0 \tag{4.2}$$

are non-linear forming a pair of hyperbolic partial differential equations, and therefore cannot be solved as they stand above in closed form with existing mathematical techniques. Using the method of characteristics a fine grid is established which specifies the pressure and velocity in space and time. At each point two characteristic curves are determined which define a forward and backward running wave. The curves are loci of propagation paths for small disturbances and since the actual pressure and velocity waveforms are formed by superimposing the two waves, forward and reverse, they inherently contain information on the nature of the terminating impedances although the quotient pressure/flow is not used as such, and it is not possible to specify an impedance as a boundary condition. It must be emphasized that the pressure and flow waveforms are related via the wall elasticity equation and the geometry of the system which must be obtained from the same preparation at the same instant in time. This close connection has not always been appreciated in the past by those using this technique.

The usual application of the method of characteristics is to define a set of initial conditions along the tube at time zero and to compute continually new parameters at each tube location until a stable distribution is obtained. The approach of Vander Werff (1971) has been to take advantage of the periodicity of the event so that only two proximal conditions, pressure and velocity need be specified. The fact that the process repeats after one cardiac cycle enables a set of boundary conditions to be regenerated continuously as the solution seeks new values of pressure and velocity down the tube. At present one of the difficulties associated with this method is that of the correct manner in which to allow for fluid viscosity since radial variations in velocity are not easily taken into account. Barnard et al. (1966) did in fact base their analysis on the two dimensional Navier Stokes equations and retained the non-linear terms which they did not consider negligible. They considered the problem of how best to describe a system whose total cross-sectional area including branches increased although the main channel, the aorta, did constrict distally. It was concluded that it would be valid to use a straight tube with an inset section whose stiffness increased by a factor of five over 40 cm. Their solution does in fact exhibit a peaking in the pressure waveform but it is now known that the velocity also increases distally due to geometric taper (Vander Werff, 1971; Schultz *et al.*, 1969) which is not predicted by their model. Anliker *et al.* (1970), Vander Werff (1971), Streeter *et al.* (1963) and Wiggert and Keitzer (1964) have all attempted to include the effects of viscosity by calculating an equivalent pressure drop in the momentum equation, postulating either a Poiseuille type flow or

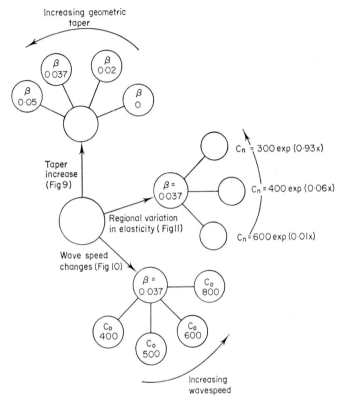

Fig. 6. Diagram showing systematic changes made in taper, mean wave speed and regional variation in wave speed to assess relative importance of each of the three variables in determining distal properties. The effects of taper alone are shown in Fig. 9, those of mean wave speed alone in Fig. 10 and those of a regional variation in wave speed in Fig. 11.

turbulent slug flow. Streeter *et al.* (1963) in fact used both laminar and turbulent pressure drop calculations during forward and reverse flow regimes respectively although this does not seem at all likely in the physiological case especially in the femoral artery. Anliker *et al.* (1970) were able to demonstrate numerically that the predicted pressure waveforms were in close agreement for both $v = 0$ and $v = 0.049 \, \text{cm}^2 \, \text{s}^{-1}$ and only by increasing the kinematic viscosity tenfold was it possible to produce marked changes in pressure, such as the distal increase, which would be expected. The same general results have been found by Vander Werff (1971) who found that over a short length of the descending aorta a factor of 100 in kinematic viscosity was required to produce appreciable changes in both pressure and velocity waveforms. These conclusions do not wholly agree with the observations made earlier in this chapter concerning the relative magnitudes of the resistive and inertial terms in the characteristic impedance of the aorta where it was noted that

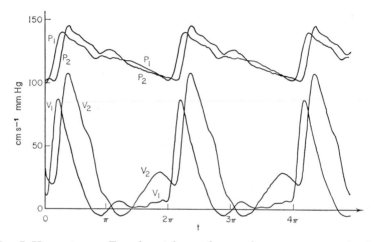

Fig. 7. Upper traces. Experimental waveforms of pressure at proximal (P_1) and distal locations (P_2) used as basis for theoretical predictions illustrated in Figs. 9, 10 and 11. Lower traces. Experimental waveforms of velocity at proximal (V_1) and distal locations (V_2). Control conditions: Pulse period $= 0\cdot39$ s. Mean aortic pressure $= 119$ mmHg. Mean cardiac output $= 46\cdot4$ ml s^{-1}. 30 kg dog. Taper factor of aorta $\beta = 0\cdot037$. Separation of sites 14 cm. From Vander Werff (1971).

although the former terms were small they were not so negligible that a factor of 10 would have been unnoticed.

The effect of flow into the intercostal arteries may be included in characteristics solutions by employing a modified continuity equation which matches the selected run-off. There have been several attempts at mathematical statements of the overall effect of branches by, for instance, Skalak and Stathis (1966) who were concerned with the dichotomously branching pulmonary system, and Streeter et al. (1963). Consider for the present only the aortic system where in the descending thoracic aorta the major branches are the intercostal arteries which themselves branch rapidly and whose terminal capillaries are not too far distant. In these circumstances a uniformly "porous" wall with pressure dependent flow is probably the closest approximation justified in our present state of knowledge. Vander Werff (1971) has made a systematic analysis of the pressure and flow waveforms in the thoracic aorta of dogs using two simultaneously recorded pressures and centreline fluid velocities a distance 14 cm apart. Employing the actual arterial taper and wave-speed-pressure relationship and an estimate of the intercostal flow based on the relative distribution of body mass the proximal pressure and velocity data were used to predict the equivalent distal parameters. These predictions were then compared with measurements and a systemic series of calculations were performed to show how sensitive the distal predictions were to variations in such parameters as geometric taper, wave speed variation, etc.

A diagram illustrating the parameter variations which were used for comparison with experiment is shown in Fig. 6. A typical series of proximal and distal pressure and velocity waveforms which were used as a basis for comparison with calculation is shown in Fig. 7.

A. THE EFFECT OF AREA CHANGES

The internal area change along the aorta was measured *in vivo* to be closely approximated by $A = A_0 \exp(-0.036x/R_0)$ where A_0 and R_0 are the area and vessel internal radius at the proximal site. There is very little information available on area taper in dogs and Table 1 below indicates that there is a considerable variation in observed values of the exponent among different investigators.

TABLE 1

Taper factor β in the aorta of dogs

Weight of dog (kg)	β	Remarks	Source
20	0·0121	From cast	Vander Werff (1971)
27	0·046	*In vivo*	Vander Werff (1971)
30	0·0367	*In vivo*	Vander Werff (1971)
23·5	0·0533	*In vivo*	Vander Werff (1971)
31	0·0202	—	Ling et al. (1968)
22·1	0·0328	—	Patel et al. (1963)

Although the area of the aorta changes in an exponential manner, measurements on a cast by Vander Werff (1971) including intercostals shows that the total area is very nearly constant (Fig. 8). The effect that a variation in taper alone would be expected to have is shown in Fig. 9 in which taper exponents β of 0·01, 0·02 and 0·05 covering the range in Table 1 are plotted for comparison with the actual taper value β of 0·0367. The general effect

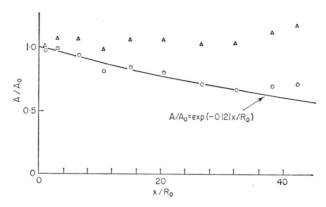

FIG. 8. Aortic area A expressed as a fraction of mean proximal aortic area A_0 versus distance down descending aorta expressed as ratio of distance/mean aortic radius at proximal location, x/R_0. Obtained from aortic cast. $\bigcirc$, Aorta. $\triangle$, Aorta plus intercostals. From Vander Werff (1971).

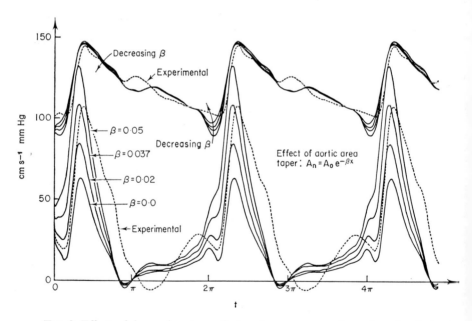

FIG. 9. Effect of increasing taper factor β on pressure (upper) and velocity (lower) waveforms in descending aorta of dog. The experimental results (- - - - - -) fit the predicted curves for the maximum velocity at the value of β corresponding to the aorta. Note that the pressure waveforms are very insensitive to large changes in β. Mean wave speed 650 cm s^{-1}. From Vander Werff (1971).

appears to be to increase (or decrease) the magnitude of the velocity waveform proportionally without altering the shape substantially. A value of β
of 0·05 does eliminate the slight notch in the velocity prior to systolic
acceleration phase but with $\beta = 0·0367$, the peak experimental velocity
appears to agree satisfactorily with measurement. Anliker *et al.* (1970) in
their analysis of changes in pressure and flow waveforms used $\beta = 0·0225$,
scaled from the Patel data for a hypothetical dog weighing 30 kg, but it can be
seen from Fig. 9 that the peak velocity is quite sensitive to β and the wide
variation in β from one dog to another makes it necessary to specify the area
taper quite accurately if detailed comparisons of theory and experiment
are to be made. The values obtained from plastic casts should be used with
caution unless great care is taken to employ the correct filling pressure when
the cast is made.

B. CHANGES IN WAVE SPEED

There are two ways in which wave speed variations can effect the
propagation of disturbances. Firstly the wave speed is known to be pressure
dependent, the higher the aortic pressure the higher the wave speed. Secondly
the wave speed in the aorta increases with distance from the aortic valve.
From the limited data currently available it is difficult to summarize the
variations in regional wave velocity which have been observed, although the
data of McDonald (1968) shows a more or less linear variation with
distance down the descending aorta, rising from about $4·2 \text{ m s}^{-1}$ just distal
to the arch to $7·5 \text{ m s}^{-1}$ at the bifurcation. McDonald reported that there
was only a slight change in wave speed within this region when the mean
pressure was lowered. Taylor (1967) has reported similar measurements in the
rabbit showing substantially smaller changes in wave velocity ($4·5 \text{ m s}^{-1}$
rising to $6·0 \text{ m s}^{-1}$ from arch to bifurcation). For mathematical convenience
it is preferable to express the wave speed in the form $C_n = C_0 e^{kx/R_0}$ and over
a limited range this exponential form is a valid approximation. Returning
to the first mode of variation, Fig. 10 shows the effect of simply varying the
wave speed C_0 in the entire aorta without allowing for any regional increases.
It will be seen that a wave speed of 5 m s^{-1} shows the best general agreement
with experiment although a quite large discrepancy occurs during deceleration. There is a substantial change in the general wave shape during late
diastole between the case for $C_0 = 4 \text{ m s}^{-1}$ and 5 m s^{-1}, and at 8 m s^{-1},
well above the experimental value of $6·5 \text{ m s}^{-1}$, the diastolic phase has altered
completely. It might be argued that it would be worth while to allow for the
known change of wave speed with pulse pressure particularly in view of the
fact that the wave speed–pressure relationship used by Vander Werff in the
present studies, based on Bergel's (1961) compilation, differs from that used
by Streeter *et al.* (1963).

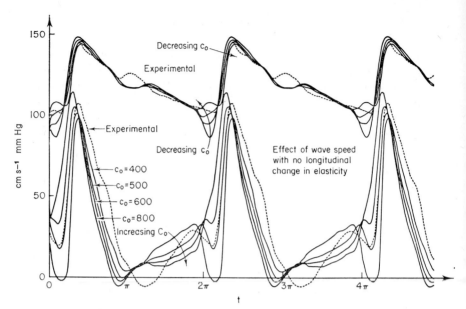

FIG. 10. Effect of changes in mean wave speed C_0 on predicted waveforms and of pressure (upper) and velocity (lower) at distal location in descending aorta of dog. The peak values of pressure and velocity which are predicted agree with the experimental curves for the measured mean wave speed of 650 cm s^{-1}. From Vander Werff (1971).

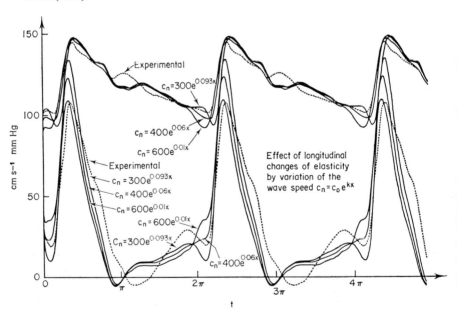

FIG. 11. Effect of longitudinal variations of wavespeed on waveforms of pressure (upper) and velocity (lower) in descending aorta of dog. From Vander Werff (1971).

Vander Werff has shown, however, that because of the relatively small pressure variation in the aorta there is almost no observable difference between the pressure and velocity waveforms based on any of the above state equations for the wall. The effect of regional variations, on the other hand, is quite large and is shown in Fig. 11 for three types of wave speed increase. Firstly with an initial low speed, 3 m s^{-1} rising to 10 at $x/R_0 = 13$, and secondly a wavespeed of 4 m s^{-1} rising to 8·75 and thirdly 6 m s^{-1} rising to 6·8 again at $x/R_0 = 13$. This mode of variation results in a wave

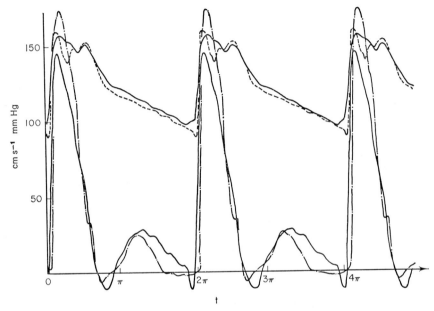

FIG. 12. Comparison of pressure and velocity waveforms predicted at distal location from input waveforms measured at proximal location. Isoprenaline infusion, mean wave speed 510 cm s^{-1}, $\beta = 0·0533$. Predicted (——). Experimental (– – – –). Redrawn from Vander Werff (1971).

speed in the central region of the aorta of approximately $6·50 \text{ m s}^{-1}$. It can be seen that the theoretical model is capable of predicting the general waveform changes in distal pressure from the input boundary conditions of pressure and velocity. The increase in pulse pressure and fluid velocity over even the relatively short length of aorta is predicted quite well. The peak velocities match reasonably well although the diastolic and deceleration phases of the cycle again show differences; this being due to some extent to the need in the theory to preserve continuity of mass flow at the end of each cycle.

One further stringent test of the validity of such theoretical models is the ability to predict pressure and velocity waveforms when agents such as iso-prenaline are used to affect the heart rate and contractile force of the ventricle. An example of this is shown in Fig. 12 where it will be seen that the general behaviour of both distal pressure and velocity is in quite good agreement with theory especially when the gross departure from the control state in Fig. 7 for instance is considered. In this last series of computations a mean wave speed, $5 \cdot 10 \text{ m s}^{-1}$ with no longitudinal variation was used and intercostal flow was neglected.

There are some general conclusions which can be drawn from this experimental-computational exercise. Foremost it is evident that both velocity (or volumetric flow) and pressure must be used as a test of the validity of any theoretical model of the aorta. From pressure waveforms alone it is impossible to distinguish between the linear frictionless and any of the various non-linear solutions. Simple change in geometric taper has a predictable result in that there is a proportional increase or decrease in fluid velocity which interacts only with the end diastolic phase of the pressure waveform.

5. LAMINAR AND TURBULENT FLOW

Clinical interest in the possible occurrence of turbulent flow arises from two sources. Cardiovascular murmurs, which still represent one of the main early identifying diagnostic techniques, can be caused by flow disturbances originating at the valves or by turbulence resulting from high Re flow in otherwise normal conditions. It is not proposed to review here the sources of other cardiovascular sounds resulting for instance from the closure of valves or from muscle contraction. The difficulty of conducting research into the sources of the random noises associated with turbulent flow in elastic pipes perhaps explains the relative scarcity of published work in this topic. It is necessary to generate an unstable or turbulent flow in a particular part of a system in such a way that pressure fluctuations are not transmitted through the wall to the test section from upstream or downstream for here they may produce spurious responses in wall mounted pressure gauges. One of the most interesting series of experiments designed to elucidate sound production by turbulent jets in liquid systems is that reported by Yellin (1966). In experiments in which a bounded turbulent jet was formed by a small diameter (0·125 or 0·375 inch) orifice in a 1·5 inch diameter pipe. Yellin found that the R.M.S. signal from a submerged phonocatheter (with a bandwidth of about 2 kHz) increased with distance from the jet, reaching a maximum at an L/D of about 5 or 10 depending on the Re, before decreasing. Figure 13 reproduced from Yellin's paper illustrates this feature. These results are in general agreement with fluid velocity and pressure fluctuation measurements made by Rouse (1959), Fig. 13 insets.

No signals were recorded by Yellin when the phonocatheter was placed upstream of the orifice suggesting strongly that the pressure fluctuations were radiated downstream only as is the case in a free jet in air. The process of fluid entrainment by the expanding jet finally results in the jet attaching to the wall. This process of pumping from the dead water region around the

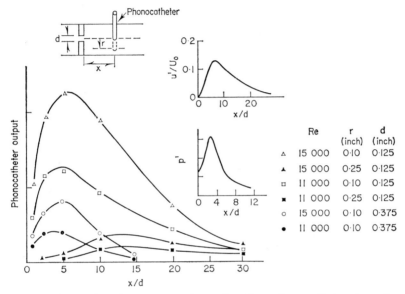

FIG. 13. Fluctuations in pressure observed with a phonocatheter downstream of a sharp-edged orifice simulating a stenotic aortic valve (redrawn from Yellin, 1966). Insets: velocity and pressure fluctuations observed by Rouse (1959).

orifice into the jet is a relatively slow and irregular one which was found by Yellin not to be symmetrical. The impingement of the jet on the wall gives rise to wall motions which can be detected and it is presumably these fluctuations which are finally transduced at the surface when a stethoscope is employed in clinical observations. It is particularly interesting to note that Yellin could not detect fully established turbulent flow with his phonocatheter and ascribes all the pressure fluctuations transduced by his phonocatheter to the mixing process in the expanding jet. It is perhaps fortunate that the region in which these fluctuations are most marked should also be accessible on the surface of the human chest.

Observations of the shape and spreading of turbulent jets caused by stenotic aortic valves have been reported by Schultz et al. (1969) and extensively by Tunstall-Pedoe (1970). The latter studies were made during surgery for valve replacement and employed the thin film anemometers similar to those used for velocity traverses in dogs. The orifice caused by the thickening and fusing of the valve cusps is very irregular, the ascending aorta just distal to the valve is generally dilated and its diameter may greatly exceed that expected under normal conditions. It is impracticable to make more than one or two traverses with the anemometer and therefore the data can be regarded as only indicative of the manner in which the jet spreads. In view of the lack of symmetry in the jet, recourse to theoretical predictions is unlikely to be profitable. It is probably valid, however, to conceive of three regimes in the jet, a potential core at the exit from the valve, a mixing region and a region

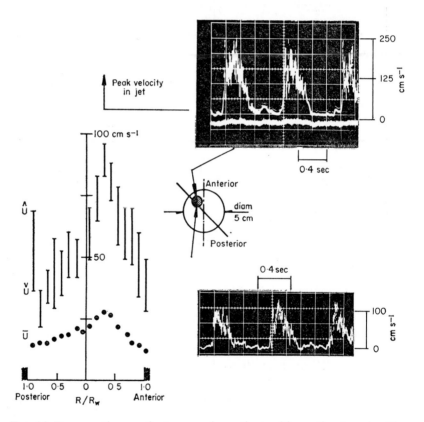

Fig. 14. Pre-operative aortic traverse in patient with aortic stenosis. Time-averaged velocities and maximum and minimum systolic instantaneous velocities shown. Aortic diameter 5 cm. Upper inset: Velocity waveform recorded in centre of jet with peak velocity 250 cm s^{-1}. Lower inset: Typical velocity waveform in high velocity region of jet. Note the turbulence on wavefront and during deceleration.

of similar velocity profiles. The locations at which traverses have been made is shown in Fig. 14. A traverse made at a distance of 35 mm from a stenosed valve is illustrated. Initially a posterior-anterior traverse was made perpendicular to the plane of the chest but no evidence of the expected jet was found. A second traverse at approximately 45° to the first showed that there was a quite narrow jet, whose approximate location is shown, with a velocity of about 250 cm s^{-1} at peak systole, which was found by manipulating the anemometer after the traverse. The velocity waveforms show rapid acceleration, large fluctuations of velocity in systole followed by a reasonably quiet period during diastole. The patient had an ejection systolic murmur at the left sternal edge radiating to the carotid artery but there was no diastolic murmur. The auditory information appears to agree quite well with the conclusions from the velocity traverses. The velocity rises rapidly and turbulence appears to occupy most of the systolic ejection period. The velocity during diastole is low and is consistent with the results of the aortic angiogram which revealed no evidence of aortic incompetence. The valve showed calcification and the opening had an area of approximately 5 mm × 2 mm.

Evidence that the jet formed at a valvular stenosis spreads rapidly was found from two traverses made at different distances from the valve ring. Figure 15 illustrates the jet profile 3·5 cm and 7 cm from the valve. This particular patient had an ejection systolic murmur heard in all areas but at a maximum in the aortic area. There was an early diastolic murmur and some valvular incompetence. It is apparent that the jet had been distorted very rapidly both by impact with the wall and by interacting with the surrounding fluid. The peak velocities in the jet of 100–150 cm s^{-1} during systole are reduced to 50 cm s^{-1} at the downstream station. Although the jet itself is distributed across the aorta apparently within a few diameters of the valve the turbulence may persist for distances greater than this.

The decay of turbulence must be looked at strictly from the point of view of a periodic flow. If the stroke volume ejected by the ventricle were, say, 100 cm^3 (based on a cardiac output of 6 litres min^{-1} in an aorta of diameter 2·5 cm at a heart rate of 60 min^{-1}), the leading edge of the ejected bolus would extend 20 cm into the aorta. This would imply that the primary ejected bolus supplies blood to the first major branches. During diastole there is a slight forward movement but for the most part diastole is a low or zero velocity phase during which the turbulence will decay due to viscous effects. The ejection bolus acts as a piston forcing the first bolus further into the systemic arteries. If, for example, the primary bolus remained still long enough for the eddies to decay completely, a stationary velocity sensor located one ejection stroke volume downstream would see, during the acceleration phase, a laminar flow with a "switch on" to turbulence as the

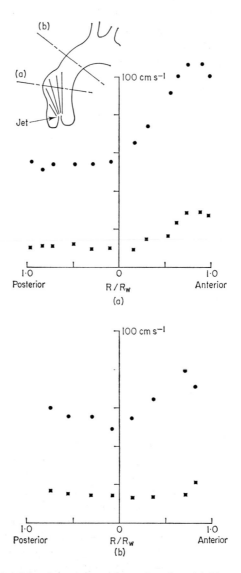

FIG. 15. Spread of jet from stenosed aortic valve. (a) Traverse 3·5 cm above aortic valve. (b) Traverse 7 cm above valve. The traverse at 4 cm made at the site of the post-stenotic dilatation shows a well-defined jet which is rapidly dissipated and barely discernible at the 7 cm distal location. Peak velocity, (●). Average velocity, (■). From Tunstall-Pedoe (1970).

leading edge of the following bolus passed over it. Figure 16 illustrates this feature and emphasizes the differences which would be observed in the output signals of velocity sensors located at different distances from the aortic valve. An example of this phenomenon from a dog is shown in Fig. 17.

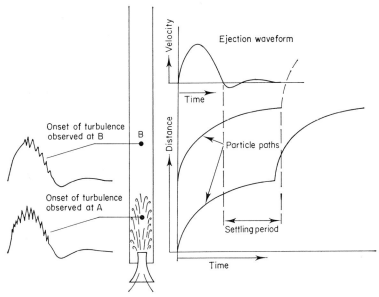

FIG. 16. To illustrate the delay in onset of transition observed in the aorta at a distal location, caused by decay of turbulence during the settling period. See also Fig. 17.

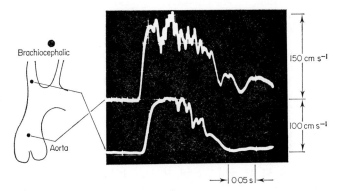

FIG. 17. Comparison of velocities in ascending aorta and brachiocephalic artery of dog. Turbulent flow had been induced by the use of intravenous isoprenaline. The turbulence at the distal site occurred at approximately mid-stroke whereas the turbulence in the ascending aorta was at peak velocity. See also Fig. 16.

Two velocity probes were located close to the aortic valve and in the brachio-cephalic artery respectively. Turbulent flow was induced by raising the ejection velocity through the action of intravenous isoprenaline. The "switch on" of turbulence as the leading edge of the bolus passes over the second probe is clearly seen. Turbulence is detected by the first, more proximal probe, much earlier in systole. It should be remembered that accelerating flows with positive pressure gradients have a stabilizing effect on the growth of instabilities while the reverse is true of decelerating flows. There is the expectation therefore that turbulence, if present during forward flow will tend to persist during deceleration and this is supported by the records shown in Figs 14 and 17. In man, turbulence has been observed as far down the aorta as T11, although in this case the flow below the diaphragm was wholly laminar.

REFERENCES

Amyot, J. W., Francis, G. P., Kiser, K. M. and Falsetti, H. L. (1970). Measurement of sequential velocity development in the aorta. Paper 70-WA/BHF-13. ASME, New York.

Anliker, M., Rockwell, R. L. and Ogden, E. (1970). Theoretical analysis of non-linear phenomena affecting the pressure and flow pulse in arteries. In "Fluid Dynamics of Blood Circulation and Respiratory Flow", Agard Conference Proceedings No. 65. Technical Editing and Reproduction Ltd., London.

Atabek, H. B. and Chang, C. C. (1961). Oscillatory flow near the inlet length of a circular tube. J. Appl. Math. Phys. 62, 185–201.

Atabek, H. B., Chang, C. C. and Fingerson, L. M. (1964). Measurement of laminar oscillatory flow in the inlet length of a circular tube. Phys. Med. Biol. 9, 219–227.

Barnard, A. L. C., Hunt, W. A., Timlake, W. P. and Varley, E. (1966). A theory of fluid flow in compliant tubes. Biophys. J. 6, 717–724.

Bergel, D. H. (1961). The dynamic elastic properties of the arterial wall. J. Physiol. 156, 458–469.

Bergel, D. H. and Schultz, D. L. (1971). Arterial elasticity and fluid dynamics. In "Progress in Biophysics and Molecular Biology" (J. A. V. Butler and D. Noble, eds.), Vol. 22, pp. 1–36, Pergamon, Oxford.

Florio, P. J. and Mueller, W. K. (1968). Development of periodic flow in a rigid tube. Paper 68-FE-8. ASME, New York.

Fry, D. L., Greenfield, J. C. and Griggs, D. M. (1964). In vivo studies of pulsatile blood flow: the relationship of the pressure gradient to the blood velocity. In "Pulsatile Blood Flow" (E. O. Attinger, ed.), pp. 101–114, McGraw-Hill, New York.

Grahn, A. R., Paul, M. H. and Wessel, H. U. (1968). Design and evaluation of a new linear thermistor velocity probe. J. Appl. Physiol. 24, 236–246.

Hale, J. F., McDonald, D. A. and Womersley, J. R. (1955). Velocity profiles of oscillating arterial flow, with some calculations of viscous drag and the Reynolds number. J. Physiol. 128, 629–640.

Jones, R. T. (1969). Blood Flow. Ann. Rev. Fluid. Mech. 1, 223–244.

Kolin, A. (1945). An alternating field induction flow meter of high sensitivity. *Rev. Sci. Instrum.* **16**, 109–116.

Kramer, K., Lochner, W. and Wetterer, E. (1963). Methods of measuring blood flow. *In* "Handbook of Physiology" (W. F. Hamilton, ed.), Vol. 2, Sect. 2, pp. 1277–1324, American Physiology Society, Washington, D.C.

Lambossy, P. (1950). Aperçu historique et critique sur le problème de la propagation des ondes dans un liquid incompressible enfermé dans un tube élastique. *Helv. Physiol. Acta* **8**, 209–277.

Ling, S. C., Atabek, H. B., Fry, D. L., Patel, D. J. and Janicki, J. S. (1968). Application of heated-film velocity and shear probes to hemodynamic studies. *Circulation Res.* **23**, 789–801.

McDonald, D. A. (1960). "Blood Flow in Arteries", Arnold, London.

McDonald, D. A. (1968). Regional pulse-wave velocity in the arterial tree. *J. Appl. Physiol.* **24**, 73–78.

McDonald, D. A. and Taylor, M. G. (1959). The hydrodynamics of the arterial circulation. *In* "Progress in Biophysics" (J. A. V. Butler and B. Katz, eds.), Vol. 9, pp. 105–173, Pergamon, Oxford.

Machella, T. B. (1936). The velocity of blood flow in arteries in animals. *Am. J. Physiol.* **115**, 632–644.

Mills, C. J. and Shillingford, J. P. (1967). A catheter tip electromagnetic velocity probe and its evaluation. *Cardiovasc. Res.* **1**, 263–265.

Noordergraaf, A. (1969). Haemodynamics. *In* "Biological Engineering" (H. P. Schwann, ed.), pp. 391–545, McGraw-Hill, New York.

O'Rourke, M. F. and Taylor, M. G. (1967). Input impedance of the systemic circulation. *Circulation Res.* **20**, 365–380.

Patel, D. J., De Freitas, F. M., Greenfield, J. C., Jr. and Fry, D. L. (1963). Relationship of radius to pressure along the aorta in living dogs. *J. Appl. Physiol.* **18**, 1111–1117.

Richardson, E. G. and Tyler, W. (1929). The transverse velocity gradient near the mouths of pipes in which an alternating or continuous flow of air is established. *Proc. Phys. Soc.* **42**, 1–15.

Rideout, V. C. and Sims, J. B. (1969). Computer study of the affects of small non-linearities in the arterial system. *Math. Biosciences* **4**, 411–424.

Rouse, H. (1959). "Advanced Mechanics of Fluids", Wiley, New York.

Rudinger, G. (1966). Review of current mathematical methods for the analysis of blood flow. *In* "Biomedical Fluid Mechanics Symposium", pp. 1–33, ASME, New York.

Schonfeld, J. C. (1948). Resistance and inertia of the flow of liquids in a tube or open canal. *Appl. Sci. Res.* **A, 1**, 169–197.

Schultz, D. L., Tunstall-Pedoe, D. S., Lee, G. de J., Gunning, A. J. and Bellhouse, B. J. (1969). Velocity distribution and transition in the arterial system. *In* "Circulatory and Respiratory Mass Transport" (G. E. W. Wolstenholme and J. Knight, eds.), pp. 172–199, J. and A. Churchill, London.

Seed, W. A. and Wood, N. B. (1970). Development and evaluation of a hot-film velocity probe for cardiovascular studies. *Cardiovasc. Res.* **4**, 253–263.

Sexl, R. (1930). Cited by Womersley (1957).

Skalak, R. (1966). Wave propagation in blood flow. *In* "Biomechanics" (Y. C. B. Fung, ed.), pp. 20–46, ASME, New York.

Skalak, R. and Stathis, T. (1966). A porous tapered elastic tube model of a vascular bed. *In* "Biomechanics" (Y. C. B. Fung, ed.), pp. 68–81, ASME, New York.

Spencer, M. P. and Dennison, A. B. (1963). Pulsatile blood flow in the vascular system. *In* "Handbook of Physiology" (W. F. Hamilton, ed.), Vol. 2, Sect. 2, pp. 839–864, American Physiology Society, Washington, D.C.

Streeter, V. L., Keitzer, W. F. and Bohr, D. F. (1963). Pulsatile pressure and flow through distensible vessels. *Circulation Res.* 13, 3–20.

Taylor, M. G. (1967). The elastic properties of arteries in relation to the physiological functions of the arterial system. *Gastroenterology* 52, 358–363.

Tunstall-Pedoe, D. S. (1970). Velocity distribution of blood flow in major arteries of animals and man. D.Phil. Thesis, University of Oxford.

Vander Werff, T. J. (1971). Studies in cardiovascular fluid dynamics. D.Phil. Thesis, University of Oxford.

Whirlow, D. K. and Rouleau, W. T. (1965), Periodic flow of a viscous liquid in a thick-walled elastic tube. *Bull. Math. Biophys.* 27, 355–370.

Wiener, F., Morkin, E., Skalak, R. and Fishman, A. P. (1966). Wave propagation in the pulmonary circulation. *Circulation Res.* 19, 834–850.

Wiggert, D. C. and Keitzer, W. F. (1964). Pulsatile flow in cylindrical and tapered rubber tubing. Paper 64-WA/HUF-1, pp. 1–8, Annual Meeting, ASME, New York.

Witzig, K. (1914). Über erzwungene Wellenbewegungen zäher, inkompressibler Flussigkeiten in elastischen Röhren. Ph.D. Thesis, University of Bern.

Womersley, J. R. (1957). An elastic tube theory of pulse transmission and oscillatory flow in mammalian arteries. WADC technical Report TR-56-614. Wright Air Development Center, Dayton, Ohio.

Wylie, E. B. (1966). Flow, through tapered tubes with non-linear wall properties. *In* "Biomechanics" (Y. C. B. Fung, ed.), pp. 82–94. ASME, New York.

Yellin, E. L. (1966). Laminar-turbulent transition process in pulsatile flow. *Circulation Res.* 19, 791–801.

Chapter 10

Vascular Input Impedance

U. GESSNER

Department of Biomedical Engineering,
Hoffmann-La Roche & Co., A.G., 4002 Basel, Switzerland

SYMBOLS USED IN THE TEXT

A_i Modulus of cosine component (in Fourier series of a signal) at frequency i

B_i Modulus of sine component at frequency i

c or c_i Phase velocity of wave (at frequency i)

$\hat{C}_{p\dot{q}}$ Estimate of cospectral power density

E Young's modulus of elasticity

h Thickness of arterial wall

Im   Imaginary part of . . .

j $\sqrt{(-1)}$

K Kinetic energy

L Distance from origin of vessel to site where reflections occur

M_i Modulus of ith Fourier component

N Number of samples

$p(t)$ Pressure signal, a function of time

p Pressure signal in complex notation (Re $p = p(t)$)

p_f, p_r Sinusoidal pressure waves propagating peripherally and retrograde, respectively

P Magnitude of sinusoidal component of pressure pulse or of pressure at a particular time

$\dot{q}(t)$ Flow velocity signal (ml s^{-1}), a function of time

$\dot{q}$ Flow signal in complex notation (Re $\dot{q} = \dot{q}(t)$)

$\dot{Q}$ Magnitude of sinusoidal component of flow pulse or of flow at a particular time

$\hat{Q}_{p\dot{q}}$ Estimate of quadrature spectral power density

R Correlation function

Re   Real part of . . .

r_i, r_o Inner and outer radius of blood vessel, respectively

S Lumen area of artery

t Time

T Duration (period) of cardiac cycle

v Flow velocity (cm s^{-1}) averaged over lumen area of artery

V Volume

W Energy, $\dot{W} =$ Power

x Spatial coordinate along artery

X Coherence

Z_i Impedance at frequency i

Z_0 Characteristic impedance

Z_{long} Longitudinal impedance

$\hat{Z}$ Estimate of impedance

γ Propagation constant of wave

Γ Reflection coefficient

λ Wavelength

ξ_i Phase angle of impedance at frequency i

ξ_0 Phase angle of characteristic impedance

ρ Density of blood

τ Time at which correlation function is computed

φ Phase angle of sinusoidal pressure component

ϕ Power spectral density

ψ Phase angle of sinusoidal flow component

ω Angular frequency $= 2\pi/T$

$||$ Magnitude (absolute value) of . . .

1. INTRODUCTION

For many years physiologists and physicians have used the concept of vascular resistance as a measure of the functional state of the peripheral parts of a vascular bed. Vascular resistance is computed as the ratio of the average pressure difference across the bed to the average flow through it.

Thus, vascular resistance defines the pressure-flow relationship. The concept has been most useful in clarifying the behaviour of circulatory systems, e.g. with respect to regional flow distributions, although many factors are known to complicate its interpretation. In most beds, vascular resistance depends on pressure, i.e. the pressure-flow relationship is non-linear. Furthermore, changes in vascular dimensions with pressure, anomalous viscosity of blood, and the possible existence of a critical opening pressure in some beds influence vascular resistance. Nevertheless, vascular or peripheral resistance is an important system property. It finds its analogy in electric network theory (resistance = steady voltage/steady current), in the theory of diffusion (diffusion constant = concentration gradient/particle flux), as well as in other sciences.

The concept of vascular resistance cannot be used when taking into account the pulsatile nature of pressure and flow. The ratio of oscillatory pressure to oscillatory flow is termed hydraulic impedance, or vascular input impedance, again by analogy with the impedance of electrical networks. In spite of the great complexity of oscillatory pressure-flow relationships in arteries, the study of vascular impedance has led to further clarification of the influence of geometry and properties of vascular systems on the circulation of blood. In addition, input impedances in the aorta and main pulmonary artery can be used to estimate the external work of the heart.

The impedance is defined only for sinusoidal waveforms, i.e. it can only be computed as the ratio of a sinusoidal pressure and a sinusoidal flow, both of the same frequency. If the frequency changes, the impedance generally changes also. Formally, such signals are (see Fig. 1):

$$\text{pressure} \quad p(t) = P_i \cos{(\omega_i t + \varphi_i)} \qquad (1.1)$$

$$\text{flow} \quad \dot{q}(t) = \dot{Q}_i \cos{(\omega_i t + \psi_i)} \qquad (1.2)$$

where

P_i = amplitude or modulus of pressure, at frequency ω_i
φ_i = phase of pressure oscillation
$\dot{Q}_i$ = amplitude of flow oscillation
ψ_i = phase of flow oscillation
ω_i = angular frequency = 2π.frequency i
t = time

As indicated in Fig. 1(a), pressure and flow are not generally in phase, i.e. their maxima do not occur simultaneously. For example, when oscillatory pressure is applied to an elastic chamber, the flow rate increases (for the volume within the chamber must increase significantly) before pressure reaches its peak. In this case $\psi_i > \varphi_i$. The time origin ($t = 0$) can often be chosen arbitrarily; it has no effect on the value of the impedance.

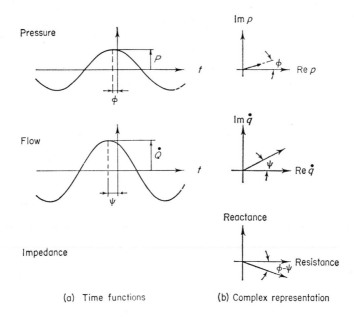

(a) Time functions   (b) Complex representation

Fig. 1. (a) Quantities characterizing sinusoidal pressure and flow signals needed to compute impedance. Amplitudes (P_i, $\dot{Q}_i$) and phases (φ_i, ψ_i) must be determined from which the magnitude of impedance $|Z_i| = P_i/\dot{Q}_i$ and its phase $\xi_i = \varphi_i - \psi_i$ follow. In the case shown it is assumed that flow leads pressure and ξ_i is a negative angle. The sinusoids may be the Fourier components, at frequency ω_i, of compound pressure and flow pulses. (b) Phasor representation of sinusoids. The sinusoid $M_i(\cos \omega_i t + \varphi_i)$ is represented as a complex number. Its real part is $M_i \cos \varphi$ (i.e. real part of $\exp(j\omega t + \varphi)$ at $t = 0$) and its imaginary part is $M_i \sin \varphi$. The phasors in the upper two diagrams represent the same pressure and flow waves as shown in (a). The impedance can be obtained by forming the quotient of the two complex numbers. The diagram at the bottom shows the result. Z is a complex number whose real part is resistance, its complex part is reactance (i.e. elastance or inertance). Note that Z is a function of frequency. The units in these diagrams are arbitrary. In the example shown, ξ_i is negative since pressure lags flow.

With the above definitions we can define the impedance Z_i. Impedance has an amplitude, or absolute value, $|Z_i|$ and phase angle ξ_i, as follows:

$$\text{amplitude} \quad |Z_i| = \frac{P}{\dot{Q}_i} \tag{1.3}$$

$$\text{phase} \quad \xi_i = \varphi_i - \psi_i \tag{1.4}$$

A formally more elegant method of computing Z_i involves the use of the concept of complex numbers (Fig. 1(b)).

Let

$$p = P_i \exp\left[j(\omega_i t + \varphi_i)\right]; \quad \text{i.e. } p(t) = \text{real part of } p$$
$$\dot{q} = \dot{Q}_i \exp\left[j(\omega_i t + \psi_i)\right]; \quad \text{i.e. } \dot{q}(t) = \text{real part of } \dot{q} \tag{1.5}$$

where $j = \sqrt{(-1)}$,
then

$$Z_i = \frac{p}{\dot{q}} = \frac{P_i}{\dot{Q}_i} \exp\left[j(\varphi_i - \psi_i)\right] \tag{1.6}$$

In this expression note the modulus $P_i/\dot{Q}_i$ and in the exponent the phase $(\varphi_i - \psi_i)$. Z_i as a complex number has real and imaginary parts, thus:

$$\text{real part} \qquad \frac{P_i}{\dot{Q}_i} \cos(\varphi_i - \psi_i) = \text{resistance} \tag{1.7}$$

$$\text{imaginary part} \qquad \frac{P_i}{\dot{Q}_i} \sin(\varphi_i - \psi_i) = \text{reactance} \tag{1.8}$$

The resistance is always zero or positive (i.e. energy is lost); hence the phase angle of the impedance cannot be larger than 90° or smaller than −90°. Reactance can be positive or negative. When flow leads pressure (as in elastic chamber) then $(\varphi_i - \psi_i) < 0$.

Note that Z_i, as calculated above, is found from the two signals at a particular frequency ω_i. The calculation must be repeated for all frequencies of importance or interest, and the impedance is found as a function of frequency. One may then talk of an impedance spectrum. The value at zero frequency (or d.c. = direct current) is, of course, the peripheral resistance.

Since impedance is a function of frequency, the frequency components of blood pressure and blood flow must be determined by Fourier analysis, as explained in the next section.

The decomposition of pulsatile signals into sinusoidal components is always (mathematically) possible, provided certain conditions are fulfilled (*vide infra*). Whether or not one gains insight into the system studied by this is a different question. Strictly, Fourier analysis should only be applied to signals observed in linear systems. A hydraulic system is linear if an imposed sinusoidal flow signal causes one sinusoidal pressure only (or vice versa) and if, when the flow amplitude is increased by a certain amount, the resulting pressure increases by the same relative amount, with no change in the phase. In such a linear system, two or more components at different frequencies can be imposed simultaneously to create independent pressure waves which sum to give the observed response. Conversely, in non-linear systems, a sinusoidal input at one frequency causes a complicated output usually containing several harmonic (i.e. sinusoidal) waves. Doubling the input does not generally result in doubling of the output if the impedance is non-linear. Most real systems are in fact non-linear. One can, however, separate those systems which are slightly non-linear and those with inherently strong non-linearities. An example of the latter is found in the nerve membrane near threshold: a small disturbance renders the system unstable and an action potential results. Conversely, slightly non-linear impedances are those in which large pressure signals are distorted and in which small stimuli are distorted very little. In fact, in most cases the response to small sinusoidal signals can often be considered sinusoidal because measurement errors prevent unequivocal detection of distortions due to non-linearities. This applies to the vascular system which is effectively linearized when small signals are studied.

The concept of hydraulic impedance was introduced into haemodynamics by Randall and Stacy (1956). Its particular usefulness in describing and analysing the state of a vascular system (and wave reflections) was recognized by McDonald (1960), Taylor (1957) and Womersley (1957). Direct evidence for the applicability of the concept despite the known non-linearities due to hydraulic phenomena and to pressure-dependent vessel characteristics, has been obtained by Bergel and Milnor (1965) and Dick *et al.* (1968). The former determined that the impedance spectra (canine pulmonary artery) are essentially independent of heart rate, i.e. that the harmonics do not interact detectably. Dick *et al.* (1968) used sinusoidal waves generated by pumps and did not observe significant distortions. Clearly, whether or not the system can be treated as linear depends both on the amplitudes of pressure and flow occurring, and on the measurement errors. At the time of writing, "small signal analysis" seems to be satisfactory and particularly powerful when the determinants of impedance (e.g. spatial non-uniformity of visco-elasticity of arterial walls) are examined (see last section of this chapter). Linearization is feasible partly because of the difficulty of obtaining highly reliable measurements. For example, O'Rourke (1968) has argued that total pressure (the "head-on" pressure seen by an open-ended catheter facing the flow) should be used in (1.6). However, this pressure varies from point to point within the vessel and it does not seem feasible to obtain an appropriate average over the lumen. Experimentally, lateral or static pressures (obtained through side holes in a catheter with a closed tip) are more easily measured. The difference between the two pressures, the dynamic pressure ($\rho v^2/2$, where ρ = density of blood, v = local velocity of flow) is generally small except during early systole in the ascending aorta. Other errors in pressure signals are due to noise and non-linearity in the transducers. In addition, the inaccuracies in present-day flow measurements are still fairly large (± 5–7 per cent). When using magnetic tape recorders additional noise and errors are introduced.

We therefore treat, in the following, the vascular system as approximately linear, in which case the concept of the impedance spectrum becomes very useful. It is also called the input impedance (into the distal part of the vessel tree) or the driving point impedance (i.e. the impedance measured at the point where pressure is applied and flow is "driven" into the vessel system).

2. WAVE REFLECTIONS AND IMPEDANCE IN AN ARTERIAL SEGMENT

In general, the signals measured in an artery result from waves travelling simultaneously both peripherally and in retrograde direction. The impedance therefore depends also on the two waves. The relation between forward (orthograde, centrifugal, or incident) and reflected (retrograde) waves depends, however, on the properties of the arterial system. We must therefore discuss first the interdependence of wave components, impedance and system properties to prepare the grounds for the interpretation of arterial impedance.

The general form of a forward pressure wave, at a particular frequency i (cf. 1.5), is

$$\text{forward wave:} \quad p_{if}(x, t) = P_{if} \exp\left[j(\omega_i t - \varphi_i) - \gamma x\right] \qquad (2.1)$$

where

$x =$ distance from beginning of the vessel to site x,
$\gamma =$ propagation constant.

The propagation constant γ is a complex number. Its real part determines the change in wave amplitude with distance travelled. It is a logarithmic measure of attenuation or damping, since the (peak) amplitude distribution of $p(x, t)$ is given by $\exp(-x \operatorname{Re} \gamma)$, where $\operatorname{Re} \gamma =$ real part of γ. $\operatorname{Re} \gamma$ gives the wave attenuation in Nepers cm^{-1} (where 1 Neper $= 8.96$ dB). The imaginary part of γ ($\operatorname{Im} \gamma$) determines the phase shift, or delay of the wave, over the distance travelled; it is related to the phase velocity (c_i) of the wave as follows:

$$\operatorname{Im} \gamma = \frac{\omega_i}{c_i} \qquad (2.2)$$

At the distal end of the arterial segment under consideration (e.g. at the site of a major bifurcation) where, say, $x = L$, the pressure due to the forward wave is

$$p_{if}(L, t) = P_{if} \exp\left[j(\omega_i t - \varphi_i) - \gamma L\right] \qquad (2.3)$$

If reflections occur at $x = L$, as they always will at major discontinuities, a certain fraction of the incident wave travels, from $x = L$, in the retrograde direction. Let Γ_L be the fraction, then the pressure due to the reflected wave at $x = L$ is given by:

$$p_{ir}(L, t) = \Gamma_L P_{if} \exp\left[j(\omega_i t - \varphi_i) - \gamma L\right] \qquad (2.4)$$

Thus the pressure due to the reflected wave at any distance x is:

$$p_{ir}(x, t) = \Gamma_L P_{if} \exp \left[j(\omega_i t - \varphi_i) - \gamma L - \gamma(L-x) \right] \qquad (2.5)$$

Hence, the total pressure wave, the sum of orthograde and retrograde waves, becomes (2.3 and 2.5)

$$p_i(x, t) = P_{if} \exp \left[j(\omega_i t - \varphi_i) - \gamma x \right] \left\{ 1 + \Gamma_L \exp \left[-2\gamma(L-x) \right] \right\} \qquad (2.6)$$

This equation expresses the total pressure wave in terms of the forward wave and Γ_L. Γ_L, the fraction reflected at the site of reflection, is called the terminal reflection coefficient. Although we assume Γ_L to be real in most examples to be discussed in the following, it is generally a complex number. At any point x, the total wave must be of the form

$$p_i(x, t) = \text{forward wave} \left[1 + \frac{\text{retrogr. wave}}{\text{forw. wave}} \right] \qquad (2.7)$$

Hence, a general reflection coefficient $\Gamma(x)$ can be defined as the quotient in the above bracket, i.e.

$$\Gamma(x) = \Gamma_L \exp \left[-2\gamma(L-x) \right] \qquad (2.8)$$

where $(L-x) = $ distance over which reflected wave has travelled.

It can be shown (using energy considerations) that the flow wave, at x, is described by an equation similar to (2.6)

$$\dot{q}_i(x, t) = \dot{Q}_{if} \exp \left[j(\omega_i t - \psi_i) - \gamma x \right] \left\{ 1 - \Gamma_L \exp \left[-2\gamma(L-x) \right] \right\} \qquad (2.9)$$

The impedance is the ratio of pressure and flow; thus it is a function of x. At frequency ω_i:

$$Z_i(x) = \frac{P_{if}}{\dot{Q}_{if}} \exp \left[j\xi_0 \right] \frac{1 + \Gamma_L \exp \left[-2\gamma(L-x) \right]}{1 - \Gamma_L \exp \left[-2\gamma(L-x) \right]} \qquad (2.10)$$

where $\xi_0 = \psi_i - \varphi_i$.

From this expression, several conclusions follow. If there is no discontinuity at the point $x = L$, no reflections occur and $\Gamma_L = 0$. The impedance Z_i then equals $P_{if}/\dot{Q}_{if} \exp(j\xi_0)$ which is independent of x. This special impedance, measured only if there exists one (orthograde) wave, is called the characteristic impedance Z_0. It is determined entirely by the properties of the arteries under consideration (lumen area, wall thickness, viscoelasticity of wall material, mode of hydraulic oscillation) and not by any boundary or end conditions.

From this we find a general relation for the impedance at any point in terms of the properties of the arterial segment (γ, Z_0) and the nature of the termination (Γ_L)

$$Z_i(x) = Z_0 \frac{1 + \Gamma_L \exp \left[-2\gamma(L-x) \right]}{1 - \Gamma_L \exp \left[-2\gamma(L-x) \right]} = Z_0 \frac{1 + \Gamma(x)}{1 - \Gamma(x)} \qquad (2.11)$$

The impedance at $x = L$, the termination, becomes

$$Z_i(L) = Z_0 \frac{1+\Gamma_L}{1-\Gamma_L} \tag{2.12}$$

or

$$\Gamma_L = \frac{Z_i(L)/Z_0 - 1}{Z_i(L)/Z_0 + 1} \tag{2.13}$$

These two equations show how load impedance and terminal reflection coefficient are related. For example, if a vessel were open at the end, the pressure at the termination would become zero, and $Z_i(L) = 0$ (or near zero). But from (2.13), $\Gamma_L \cong -1\cdot0$. This means that the reflected pressure wave is equal and opposite to the forward wave at $x = L$. Conversely, if a vessel is occluded at $x = L$, $Z_i(L) = \infty$ (no flow); hence, $\Gamma_0 \cong +1\cdot0$. In this case, the reflected wave is equal in magnitude, and in phase with, the incident wave. In fact, in the circulation, reflections from peripheral sites are generally of the latter type. Γ_L may be about $0\cdot6$; and impedances near the periphery are thereby increased. Note that both $Z(L)$ and Γ_L are functions of frequency. Using (2.11) we may compute Z_i at any point x. In particular, we are interested in the input impedance $(x = 0)$. Then

$$Z_i(0) = Z_0 \frac{1+\Gamma_L \exp(-2\gamma L)}{1-\Gamma_L \exp(-2\gamma L)} \tag{2.14}$$

At the input, the relation between Γ_L and Z_i is obviously more complex. Consider first the case where Γ_L is real, positive and close to unity. It may happen, however, that at a certain frequency, $\Gamma_L \exp(-2\gamma L)$ is a negative real number. This will occur when $2 \operatorname{Im} \gamma L = \pi$. It then follows that $2\omega L/c = \pi$, or $4\pi L/\lambda = \pi$ (where $\lambda = $ wavelength $= c/$frequency); and thus, $L = \lambda/4$. This may be called the $\lambda/4$ condition for which $Z_i(0)$ is smaller than the characteristic impedance Z_0, and in fact is at a minimum even though at the periphery $Z_i(L)$ is much larger than Z_0 (2.12). The reflected pressure wave, in this example, additive at the end of the arterial segment, is delayed so much over the distance L that it is out of phase with the forward wave at $x = 0$. The pressure wave amplitude has a minimum at the input when $L = \lambda/4$, and conversely the flow oscillations have a maximum. Early workers in this field who observed minima in the input impedance spectra attempted to compute the distance L to the "site of reflection" (see McDonald, 1960) in the systemic circulation. However, the laws described above apply only to uniform (homogeneous) vessels, or transmission lines. If a major reflection site in the dog is computed to be in the region of the femoral artery, this can only indicate an apparent termination. The wave velocity, and therefore γ, changes significantly between the aorta and femoral artery. The single "transmission line" model is not satisfactory, as will be explained in more detail later.

The relation between Z_i and Z_0 (2.14) is useful in that it allows the estimation of Z_0 from an observed Z_i. At high frequencies $\Gamma_L \exp(-2\gamma L)$ is usually small. Waves at high frequencies are attenuated or damped more than those at low frequencies. If reflections travel some distance from the site of reflection to point $x = 0$ and are attenuated, $\Gamma(0)$ is reduced and $Z_i \approx Z_0$. In addition, if waves are reflected at many sites along the line, the reflections will tend to cancel each other at the input if they all travel over some distance comparable to their wavelength. This may occur, as the following example shows, in the circulation.

A pressure wave at 8 Hz may propagate at an average velocity of 600 cm s^{-1} in the thoracic and abdominal aorta. The wavelength is $\lambda = c/f = 600/8 = 75 \text{ cm}$. Hence, in man, an 8 Hz wave travels nearly one wavelength before it reaches the iliac arteries.

Before discussing reflections further it is useful to relate the characteristic impedance and the properties of the arterial system. First we define the longitudinal impedance: this is the ratio of axial pressure gradient and flow:

$$Z_{\text{long}} = -\frac{\partial p}{\partial x}\frac{1}{\dot{q}} \tag{2.15}$$

Z_{long} clearly has the dimensions of impedance per distance. It allows the calculation of the pressure drop along an artery if the flow is known, or vice versa. Note, however, that $\partial p/\partial x$ may be a function of position x.

If no reflections are present and there exists only one wave in a vessel, as defined by (2.1), we find

$$\frac{\partial p_{if}}{\partial x} = -\gamma p_{if} \tag{2.16}$$

and from (2.15), $Z_{\text{long}} = \gamma p_{if}/\dot{q}_{if}$. But the characteristic impedance is $p_{if}/\dot{q}_{if}$, and therefore

$$Z_0 = \frac{Z_{\text{long}}}{\gamma} \tag{2.17}$$

It can be shown (McDonald, 1960) that in large arteries Z_{long} is approximately equal to $j\omega\rho/S$ where $\rho = $ density of blood and $S = $ lumen area of vessel. Furthermore, in large arteries the imaginary part of γ is much larger than the real part, i.e. $\gamma \cong j\omega/c$, as stated above. Hence

$$Z_0 \cong \frac{\rho c}{S} \quad \text{(large arteries)} \tag{2.18}$$

For these large arteries, the wave velocity c may be approximately related to the vessel properties by the Moens–Korteweg or Bramwell–Hill equation

$$c \cong \sqrt{\frac{(Eh)}{(2r_i\rho)}} = \sqrt{\frac{(\Delta PV)}{(\Delta V\rho)}} \tag{2.19}$$

where

E = Young's modulus of elasticity of wall material,
h = wall thickness of vessel,
r_i = inside radius of vessel,
ρ = density of blood,
$\Delta PV/\Delta V$ = relative volume elasticity of vessel segment.

We therefore find that the characteristic impedance may be described in terms of vessel properties,

$$Z_0 = \frac{1}{S}\sqrt{\left(\rho\frac{\Delta PV}{\Delta V}\right)} \tag{2.20}$$

Another application of transmission line theory concerns the reflections from vessel junctions or bifurcations. The example is largely theoretical for it is known that flow profiles must reform in the distal vessels and that such inlet length conditions probably prohibit the use of transmission line theory. It is of interest, however, to be able to separate the effects of the branching itself from those due to other factors. We therefore assume, for the sake of the argument, that so little energy is lost by entrance length effects within the two daughter vessels that their input impedances can be described by transmission line theory. Furthermore, assume that the characteristic impedances of the two daughter vessels are the same and also that the reflections from both peripheries are the same (purely symmetrical bifurcation). Then one may write the formula for $Z_1(B)$, the load impedance of the parent vessel (subscript 1) in terms of the conditions in the two distal arteries (subscript 2). $Z_1(B)$ is one half of the input impedance of each of the parallel daughter vessels:

$$Z_1(B) = \tfrac{1}{2}Z_{02}\frac{1+\Gamma_2}{1-\Gamma_2} \tag{2.21}$$

where

$Z_1(B)$ = impedance in parent vessel at bifurcation,
Z_{02} = characteristic impedance of each daughter vessel,
Γ_2 = reflection coefficient at the junction in daughter vessels.

The terminal reflection coefficient of the parent vessel, at the junction is therefore

$$\Gamma_1(B) = \frac{\dfrac{1}{2}\dfrac{Z_{02}}{Z_{01}}\dfrac{1+\Gamma_2}{1-\Gamma_2} - 1}{\dfrac{1}{2}\dfrac{Z_{02}}{Z_{01}}\dfrac{1+\Gamma_2}{1-\Gamma_2} + 1} \tag{2.22}$$

where Z_{01} = characteristic impedance of parent vessel.

This equation can be discussed to a certain extent since some typical values of Z_{02}/Z_{01} are known. From (2.18) we have

$$\frac{Z_{02}}{Z_{01}} = \frac{c_2}{S_2} \frac{S_1}{c_1} \tag{2.23}$$

The ratio of the cross-sectional areas, S_1/S_2, is smaller than 2·0 at most vessel junctions, generally about 1·67. The sum of the lumen areas of the daughter vessels is approx. 1·2 times the lumen area of the parent vessel (McDonald, 1960). However, the ratio of the wave velocities, c_2/c_1, is generally larger than unity. (Approximate values for c are: in femoral artery: 10–11 m s^{-1}; in iliac artery: 9–10 m s^{-1}; in abdominal aorta: 7–8 m s^{-1}). If c_2/c_1 were equal to $2S_2/S_1$, $\Gamma_1(B)$ would simply be equal to Γ_2 (cf. 2.22). This would mean that there existed, at this bifurcation, no change in reflection content although there would be an increase in impedance. There is no experimental evidence available to indicate what is the case in nature. It should also be remembered that we assumed perfect symmetry at the junction which probably applies rarely, if ever.

Another simple situation was studied in detail by Womersley (1957). If $\Gamma_2 = 0$, (2.22) reduces to

$$\Gamma_1(B) = \frac{\dfrac{1}{2}\dfrac{Z_{02}}{Z_{01}} - 1}{\dfrac{1}{2}\dfrac{Z_{02}}{Z_{01}} + 1} \tag{2.24}$$

This is the case when no reflections exist in the daughter vessels, which again is not very likely in nature. However, Womersley studied the influence of changes in cross-sectional areas $(2S_2/S_1)$ on $\Gamma_1(B)$. Strictly this is not just a matter of introducing a variable area ratio into (2.23) and then into (2.24). The wave velocity also depends, especially in smaller vessels, on the geometry and on the frequency; see Womersley (1957) and McDonald (1960). The findings are interesting since the reflection coefficient computed for the "Womersley mode" of fluid oscillation, at symmetric junctions whose daughter vessels are assumed to be very long, exhibits a minimum ($\Gamma_{min} \cong 0\cdot03$) at a $2S_2/S_1$ ratio of approximately 1·2. This again suggests that reflections from bifurcations are probably small so long as reflections from more peripheral sites are also very small. However, there is very little experimental data relating to these questions.

The above is only a cursory summary of transmission line theory. (See Taylor, 1957, 1959; or Noordergraaf, 1969, for a complete treatment.) The simple relations presented here allow the understanding of phenomena such as the superposition of orthograde and reflected waves and the influence of reflections on local impedance. They are formulated so generally that they apply to any mode of wave propagation. Once a mode of fluid oscillation is established, waves propagate at a certain velocity c and certain γ typical for that mode. As we will see later, for the treatment of entire vessel systems, transmission line theory alone does not suffice. Transmission line theory mostly concerns uniform structures. Arteries branch and change their properties as a function of distance. Hence, the spatial distribution of pressure, flow, etc. have to be explained and predicted by more complex models.

3. METHODS OF DETERMINING IMPEDANCE

It is obvious that phasic (instantaneous) pressure and flow must be measured simultaneously at the site of interest if one wishes to compute impedance spectra. Techniques of obtaining flow and pressure signals are discussed in Chapters 2 and 3. We therefore can concentrate here on the processing and analysis of the signals.

The necessity also frequently occurs to measure the average arterial diameter or circumference in addition to flow and pressure. This is because many flowmeters actually measure flow velocity (v, cm s^{-1}). Volume flow ($\dot{q}$, cm^3 s^{-1}) is of course found when the area of the lumen is known. This may be obtained with satisfactory accuracy from the external circumference U

$$S = \pi r_i^2 = \frac{U^2}{4\pi} \left(1 - \frac{h}{r_o}\right)^2 \tag{3.1}$$

where

r_i = inside radius of artery,

h/r_o = wall thickness to outside radius ratio which can be considered constant: $h/r_o \cong 0\cdot13$. Therefore $(1 - h/r_o)^2 \cong 0\cdot76$.

It would be even more desirable to measure phasic changes of diameter together with pressure and flow. This would yield independent estimates of Z_0 and c. In the future, ultrasonic methods may render this possible in the intact animal (see Chapter 4).

A. IMPEDANCE SPECTRA FROM FOURIER SERIES OF $p(t)$ AND $\dot{q}(t)$

It was stated in the previous section that every periodic signal can be decomposed into a series of sinusoidal components, the so-called harmonics. In other words, the pressure pulse signal $p(t)$ can be built up or represented by a sum of the following form (the following remarks, of course, also apply to flow signals):

$$p(t) \cong A_0 + M_1 \cos(\omega t - \varphi_1) + M_2 \cos(2\omega t - \varphi_2) + M_3 \cos(3\omega t - \varphi_3) +$$
$$+ \ldots + M_{m-1} \cos[(m-1)\omega t - \varphi_{m-1}] + M_m \cos(m\omega t - \varphi_m) \tag{3.2}$$

where

M_i, φ_i = modulus and phase of ith harmonic, respectively; $i = 1, 2, \ldots, m$,

A_0 = steady or mean pressure component (the component at "zero frequency"),

m = number of highest harmonic which is, in practice, limited (*vide infra*),

ω = the fundamental frequency, i.e. $2\pi/T$, where T = duration of record analysed.

Note that all the frequencies occurring are integer multiples of ω, the fundamental frequency. The individual harmonic terms can be split into a sine and a cosine term (since $\cos(\alpha-\beta) = \cos\alpha\cos\beta + \sin\alpha\sin\beta$), so that (3.2) is equivalent to the following Fourier series:

$$p(t) \cong A_0 + A_1 \cos \omega t + A_2 \cos 2\omega t + \ldots A_m \cos m\omega t +$$
$$+ B_1 \sin \omega t + B_2 \sin 2\omega t + \ldots B_m \sin m\omega t \qquad (3.3)$$

where

$$\begin{aligned} A_i &= M_i \cos \varphi_i \\ B_i &= M_i \sin \varphi_i \end{aligned} \qquad i = 1, 2, \ldots, m \qquad (3.4)$$

or, conversely

$$\begin{aligned} M_i &= \sqrt{(A_i^2 + B_i^2)} \\ \varphi_i &= \arctan (B_i/A_i) \end{aligned} \qquad i = 1, 2, \ldots, (m-1) \qquad (3.5)$$

Before it is shown how the A_i and B_i terms can be obtained from a given $p(t)$, some remarks concerning (3.2) and (3.3) are in place.

In the first place (3.2) presupposes that the pressure signal is obtained from an animal whose vascular system is in a steady state and not undergoing any change, for example, of peripheral resistance. The mathematical form of the right hand term makes this obvious: the cosine functions are defined for $-\infty \leqslant t \leqslant +\infty$, and their sum is a periodic function over the same time span. However, we want to represent $p(t)$ over some fixed interval, i.e. $t_0 \leqslant t \leqslant t_1$, for which we know that a steady state exists and during which consecutive heart cycles exhibit great similarity. In fact, we may select just one cardiac cycle as representative of a series of beats, if there is a steady state, as shown in Fig. 2. Then $(t_1 - t_0) = T$ = the period of the cardiac cycle. It is possible to represent a sequence of heart cycles by a sum of the form of (3.2), e.g. all the cycles during one respiratory cycle. It must be remembered, however, that the approximating Fourier series is always periodic:

Let
$$\hat{p}(t) = \text{Fourier series} \cong p(t)$$
$$\hat{p}(t+T) = \hat{p}(T)$$

where T = duration of record analysed, which contains one or several complete heart cycles.

Pressure $p(t)$

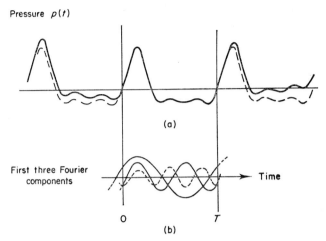

(a)

First three Fourier
components

Time

O T
(b)

FIG. 2. The Fourier series of a pressure pulse. (a) The upper trace (heavy line) shows a pressure signal of which one heart cycle is selected whose beginning and end are at the same pressure level. This pulse can be represented by the sum of several sinusoidal waves. (b) The first three harmonics are shown below. The fundamental has the same period as the duration T of $p(t)$ analysed. The frequencies of the higher harmonics are integer multiples of the fundamental frequency. Their amplitudes and phases are obtained from (3.7) to (3.10). The sum of all harmonics is a periodic function which approximates $p(t)$ very closely from $0-T$ (provided a sufficient number of sinusoids are used). The Fourier series is used to represent any chosen section of a curve. It may differ from the observed $p(t)$ for $t < 0$ and $t > T$, as is indicated by the interrupted curve in the upper panel. This does not matter so long as the vascular system is in steady state. The durations of the cycles preceding those analysed should be nearly constant.

This consideration has bearings on the choice of the record analysed. The part of $p(t)$ subjected to Fourier analysis must fulfil the same condition:

$$p(t+T) = p(t).$$

It may be possible to proceed, even if the above condition is not exactly fulfilled, for example if pressure changes slightly, by analysing not $p(t)$ but an artificial signal $p^*(t)$ obtained from $p(t)$ as follows

$$p^*(t) = p(t) - \frac{p(t_0+T)-p(t_0)}{T}(t-t_0) \tag{3.6}$$

where

$p^*(t)$ = signal corrected for baseline drift, subjected to Fourier analysis,
t_0 = time of beginning of fraction of signal processed,
T = duration of fraction of signal processed.

In (3.6) it is assumed that the mean pressure was changing at a steady rate.

In the second place the $\cong$ signs in (3.2) and (3.3) show that the sums on the right are always approximations to $p(t)$. Were this an ideal signal known to contain only m harmonics, we could determine the coefficients A_i and B_i and synthesize $p(t)$ exactly according to (3.3). In practice, however, the signal $p(t)$ contains unknown noise (irregular catheter motion, noise in the electronic circuitry, noise on the record on the magnetic tape). For this reason one should take as many sinusoids as are thought necessary to approximate $p(t)$ by their sum to within the experimental error due to uncertainties of calibration and the effects mentioned above, while ensuring also that all significant harmonics contained in the pressure wave are taken into account. This must be remembered when the coefficients are determined.

The cosine and sine coefficients of the Fourier series A_i and B_i in (3.3), are determined by multiplying the signal $p(t)$ by cos $i\omega t$, and by sin $i\omega t$, respectively, and by averaging the resulting time functions over the period T. The term A_0, the mean pressure, is of course found by averaging $p(t)$ over T. These computations are generally done by computer, after $p(t)$ has been measured, i.e. converted from analog form (as on magnetic tape or paper chart) into digital form, at discrete times spaced by equal intervals (Δt). The analog-to-digital conversion replaces the continuous function $p(t)$, $t' \leqslant t < (t'+T)$ by a set of N numbers $P(k\Delta t)$, $k = 0, 1, 2, \ldots, (N-1)$, where $\Delta t = $ sampling interval, $N = $ number of samplings obtained, $N\Delta t = T$, period analysed. Note that we do not include $p(N\Delta t)$ since, by definition, $P(N\Delta t) = P(0)$.

Multiplication by the sinusoidal functions must now be done at all times $k\Delta t$. The Fourier coefficients are computed from the N samples available, using the following equations:

$$A_0 = \frac{1}{N} \sum_{k=0}^{N-1} P(k\Delta t) \tag{3.7}$$

$$A_i = \frac{2}{N} \sum_{k=0}^{N-1} P(k\Delta t) \cos\left(\frac{2\pi}{N} ik\right) \tag{3.8}$$

$$B_i = \frac{2}{N} \sum_{k=0}^{N-1} P(k\Delta t) \sin\left(\frac{2\pi}{N} ik\right) \tag{3.9}$$

where $i = $ number of harmonic.

The moduli and phases of the pressure Fourier coefficients are computed from (3.5):

$$M_i = \sqrt{(A_i^2 + B_i^2)}; \quad \varphi_i = \arctan \frac{B_i}{A_i} \tag{3.10}$$

The moduli and phases of the flow harmonics are obtained in the same way. Then the impedances are readily calculated from (1.3) and (1.4) for all values of ω_i. Examples of pressure, flow and impedance spectra are shown in Fig. 3.

Before discussing another way to measure impedance four important points ought to be raised.

(a) If a (pressure) signal is digitized at N instants in time, it is impossible to obtain more than $N/2$ cosine coefficients and $(N/2)-1$ sine coefficients.

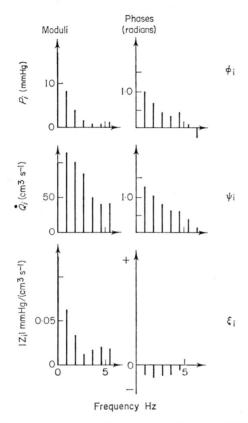

Fig. 3. Typical frequency spectra of pressure (top), flow (middle) and impedance (bottom) observed in the pulmonary artery (unpublished data). The diagrams on the left represent moduli, the ones on the right the corresponding phases, both as a function of frequency. Only the first six harmonics are shown since the higher ones of the pressure signal are very small and noisy, and therefore not useful for the determination of impedance. The upper two rows represent the Fourier series of signals, such as those in Fig. 2. The impedance spectrum is obtained at each frequency by dividing the moduli of pressure and flow, and by subtracting flow phase from pressure phase. Note the typical impedance pattern: A large d.c. value (mean pressure divided by mean flow) and much smaller moduli for the oscillatory terms. The phase of impedance, ξ, below 5 Hz is negative.

For example, with 24 samples of a pressure pulse, one can compute only the mean pressure (A_0), $A_1 \rightarrow A_{12}$, and $B_1 \rightarrow B_{11}$.

(b) If m harmonics are to be evaluated, because we believe they are significant, the minimal number of samples is fixed by the so-called sampling theorem:

$$N \geqslant 2m \qquad (3.11)$$

If this requirement is violated, i.e. if N is chosen to be smaller than $2m$, the calculated Fourier coefficients are wrong, and the so-called aliasing or folding errors are introduced (Bendat and Piersol, 1966). This must be avoided by choosing a sufficiently high sampling rate. It is known that there is very little energy in the harmonics of a pressure or flow pulse above the tenth. Therefore, one pressure pulse must be sampled at least 22 times; 40–50 readings per heart beat are recommended which gives a good safety margin. When digitizing at a rate much above the likely folding-frequency, which is easy by electronic means, one is in a position to judge in each case how many Fourier terms are significant (see Lanczos, 1956, for the necessary criteria) and at how many frequencies the impedance can be reliably computed.

(c) We have tacitly assumed in the above that the signals $p(t)$ and $\dot{q}(t)$ directly represent pressure and flow, respectively. This is not necessarily so. Fluid-filled catheter-manometer systems may exhibit poor dynamic responses such that the true pressure waveform is distorted—although this is less of a problem with catheter-tip pressure transducers. Moreover, most electro-magnetic flowmeters, the instruments best suited for this type of work (Bergel and Gessner, 1966), do not reproduce flow waveforms with high fidelity. In both cases remedy is possible. The frequency responses of mano-meter systems can be obtained fairly simply (McDonald, 1960) from their step responses, and flowmeter characteristics are either available from the literature or can be established (Bergel and Gessner, 1966). The frequency response of an instrument describes the ratio of output to input amplitude, and the phase delay between output and input signals, as a function of frequency. Thus, the calculated pressure (or flow) moduli and phases $(M_i$ and $\varphi_i)$ can be corrected for the errors introduced by the apparatus. These corrections are necessary, particularly in animal work (high heart rates) and for accuracy in the impedance values for the high harmonics.

(d) Some additional corrections may be necessary if the distance between the sites where flow and pressure are observed is considerable. Even if this is a few centimetres only it may become considerable in terms of wavelengths for the high harmonics. The following calculation is based on (2.6). Assume that pressure is measured just distal to a flowmeter transducer; this is usually done so that the impedance of the arterial section at the flowmeter site is not included in the measurement. If the pressure at site x is defined as the sum of forward (p_f) and reflected (p_r) waves, we have

$$p(x) = p_f + p_r \tag{3.12}$$

The flow, measured upstream by the distance Δx, is

$$\dot{q}(x + \Delta x) = \frac{1}{Z_0} \left[(p_f \exp (\Delta x \gamma) - p_r \exp (-\Delta x \gamma) \right] \tag{3.13}$$

The approximate impedance $\hat{Z}$ is then (using the reasonable approximation $\exp (\pm \Delta x \gamma) = 1 \pm \Delta x \gamma$)

$$\hat{Z}(x) = Z_0 \frac{1 + \Gamma(x)}{1 - \Gamma(x) + \Delta x \gamma [1 + \Gamma(x)]} \tag{3.14}$$

After some manipulation one finds that the true value of Z_i can be obtained from the estimate $\hat{Z}_i$ by

$$Z_i(x) \cong \hat{Z}_i(x) \left(1 + \Delta x \gamma \frac{Z_i}{Z_0} \right) \tag{3.15}$$

In practice, the correction term will be small except at high frequencies where $\hat{Z}_i \sim Z_0$: the correction term then becomes $(1 + \Delta x \gamma)$ which may contribute significantly to the phase of the impedance. This, (3.15), is a more precise expression than the one published by Westerhof and Noordergraaf (1970).

B. Impedance Spectra from Auto- and Cross-Correlation Functions of $p(t)$ and $\dot{q}(t)$

There exists a useful relation between the autocorrelation function of a signal and its Fourier amplitude spectrum which often allows a better estimation of $Z(\omega)$ than the approach described above. We will state the relation as it applies to known functions of time, such as observed pressure and flow signals. We refer the reader to the literature on random processes (Davenport and Root, 1968) for discussions of the application of these mathematical tools to noisy signals.

The autocorrelation function $R_p(\tau)$ of any signal $p(t)$ is defined by

$$R_p(\tau) = \frac{1}{2T} \int_{-T}^{+T} p(t) p(t + \tau) \, dt \qquad \text{as } T \to \infty \tag{3.16}$$

R_p is maximal for $\tau = 0$, and for all values of τ it is a measure of the similarity of $p(t)$ and the shifted $p(t + \tau)$. If $p(t)$ is periodic, R_p is also periodic. It can be shown that the Fourier transform of R_p (rather than the Fourier series), generally termed the power spectral density ϕ, depends directly on the square of the magnitude of the frequency components of the signal. The Fourier transform is calculated as

$$\phi_p(\omega) = \int_{-\infty}^{\infty} R_p(\tau) \exp (-j\omega\tau) \, d\tau = 2 \int_{0}^{\infty} R_p(\tau) \cos \omega\tau \, d\tau \tag{3.17}$$

If $p(t)$ is periodic the relation to the Fourier spectrum is

$$\phi_p(\omega) = \sum_{i=-\infty}^{\infty} M_i^2 \delta(\omega - i\omega_0) \tag{3.18}$$

where

M_i = magnitude of frequency components of $p(t)$,
δ = Dirac impulse,
$\omega_0 = 2\pi/T$.

The cosine transform only appears in (3.17) since $R_p(\tau)$ is an even function: $R_p(\tau) = R_p(-\tau)$. Note that the integral in (3.17) is a function defined at all values of ω, i.e. the power distribution in theory is computed at all frequencies and not just at the harmonic frequencies. In practice, that is by numerical computation, this property is lost. Note that $\phi_p(\omega)$ has the units of amplitude^2/Hz; this is why it is the power spectral density. Note also that information on the phase of the harmonics is lost. In the case shown above ($p(t)$ periodic), ϕ_p consists of a series of Dirac impulses whose strengths are equal to the power of the component frequencies (M_i^2). The relation between R and power density also holds for non-periodic functions under conditions which need not concern us. We assume in the following, however, that the signals analysed have zero average, (i.e. the mean pressure is first subtracted) and that the first reading $P(0)$ equals the last $P(N\Delta t)$.

In practice, one only obtains estimates of R and ϕ. Furthermore, the integrals are replaced by sums, as shown in the following, where the approximate $\hat{R}$ and $\hat{\phi}$ are computed numerically from the digitized signal:

$$\hat{R}_p(n\Delta t) = \frac{1}{N} \sum_{k=0}^{N} P(k\Delta t)P[(k+n)\Delta t] \tag{3.19}$$

where $n = 0, 1, 2, \ldots, n_{max} < N$,

$$\hat{\phi}_p(i\Delta\omega) = 2\Delta t \left[\hat{R}_p(0) + 2 \sum_{k=1}^{n_{max}} \hat{R}_p(k\Delta t) \cos \frac{\pi i k}{n_{max}} \right] \tag{3.20}$$

These expressions are applicable if we deal with a periodic signal (for which $n_{max} = N-1$) or for a signal which we assume to be periodic. In both cases the product of the signal with the shifted signal (3.19) is obtained, when $(k+n) > N$, by introducing $P[(k+n)\Delta t] = P[(k+n-N)\Delta t]$. There may be cases in which periodic repetition of the signal is not satisfactory, however. Then, the product in (3.19) is zero for all k's larger than $(N-n)$, i.e. (3.19) becomes

$$\hat{R}_p(n\Delta t) = \frac{1}{N-n} \sum_{k=0}^{N-n} P(k\Delta t)P[(k+n)\Delta t] \tag{3.21}$$

In other words, when n increases, the number of terms in the sum decreases and so does the reliability of the estimate $\hat{R}_p$. In fact, n_{max} must be limited for non-periodic signals: $n_{max} \approx 0.1N$. Then, however, we must analyse a signal of longer duration, e.g. 40 heart cycles or more. $\hat{\phi}_p(i\Delta\omega)$ must often be computed by (3.20) using smoothed values of $\hat{R}_p$, as discussed at the end of this section.

$\hat{\phi}_p(i\Delta\omega)$ is an estimate of the power distribution function of pressure. The equivalent $\hat{\phi}_{\dot{q}}(i\Delta\omega)$ can be obtained for the flow signal. Hence the spectrum of the impedance moduli follows

$$|Z_i| = \left[\frac{\hat{\phi}_p(i\Delta\omega)}{\hat{\phi}_{\dot{q}}(i\Delta\omega)}\right]^{\frac{1}{2}} \tag{3.22}$$

The cross-correlation function $\hat{R}_{p\dot{q}}$ between pressure and flow is needed to estimate the phase (ξ) of the impedance. By analogy with (3.21) for $0 \leqslant n \leqslant n_{max}$:

$$\hat{R}_{p\dot{q}}(n\Delta t) = \frac{1}{N-n} \sum_{k=0}^{N-n} P(k\Delta t)\dot{Q}[(k+n)\Delta t] \tag{3.23}$$

and for $-n_{max} \leqslant n < 0$:

$$\hat{R}_{p\dot{q}}(n\Delta t) = \frac{1}{N-n} \sum_{k=n}^{N} P(k\Delta t)\dot{Q}[(k+n)\Delta t] \tag{3.24}$$

The Fourier transform of this contains sine and cosine terms because $\hat{R}_{p\dot{q}}$ is not an even function. Using the definition for the cosine (cospectral) density:

$$\hat{C}_{p\dot{q}}(i\Delta\omega) = 2\Delta t \sum_{k=-n_{max}}^{n_{max}} \hat{R}_{p\dot{q}}(k\Delta t) \cos\left(\frac{\pi ik}{n_{max}}\right) \tag{3.25}$$

and for the sine or quadrature spectral density

$$\hat{Q}_{r\dot{q}}(i\Delta\omega) = 2\Delta t \sum_{k=-n_{max}}^{n_{max}} \hat{R}_{p\dot{q}}(k\Delta t) \sin\left(\frac{\pi ik}{n_{max}}\right) \tag{3.26}$$

one computes the impedance phase spectrum

$$\xi(i\Delta\omega) = \tan^{-1} \frac{\hat{Q}_{p\dot{q}}(i\Delta\omega)}{\hat{C}_{p\dot{q}}(i\Delta\omega)} \tag{3.27}$$

The information obtained in this way leads also to a useful statistical measure of the interdependence of pressure and flow. The coherence is a type of correlation coefficient (being a function of frequency) for p and $\dot{q}$. It is computed as follows

Coherence

$$X(i\Delta\omega) = \frac{[\hat{C}_{p\dot{q}}(i\Delta\omega)^2 + \hat{Q}_{p\dot{q}}(i\Delta\omega)^2]^{\frac{1}{2}}}{[\hat{\phi}_p \hat{\phi}_{\dot{q}}]^{\frac{1}{2}}} \tag{3.28}$$

X is unity if the signals are as directly related as possible, as they would be for example in an absolutely linear system. Non-linearities and inherently uncorrelated random components of the signal lower the coherence. Thus it is useful to consider coherence alongside $|Z_i|$ and ξ_i in order to recognize those impedance values which are not contaminated by noise.

If one analyses many consecutive heart cycles one obtains the impedance values not only at frequencies which are multiples of the (average) heart rate but also at subharmonics, the lowest of which is determined by the total duration of the signals. The technique involving correlation functions has the advantage over the direct Fourier analysis that the impedance spectra are also estimated quite accurately, even if the heart cycle duration changes from beat to beat. The longer the record analysed, the more satisfactory the result. In fact there exists the following relation between N (total number of samples), n_{max} (maximum shift used in correlating the signals), and σ^2, the variance of the estimate of power density (Bendat and Piersol, 1966):

$$N = \frac{n_{max}}{\sigma^2}. \tag{3.29}$$

On the other hand, the lowermost frequency at which impedance can be computed and the frequency resolution in the impedance spectrum is $(n_{max}\Delta t)^{-1}$, while the highest frequency is $1/(2\Delta t)$. Thus, the number of samples to be analysed, if we require for example $1/(2\Delta t) = 20$ Hz, $(n_{max}\Delta t)^{-1} = 0\cdot25$ Hz, $\sigma^2 = 0\cdot1$, is $N = 1600$, i.e. the duration of the signal analysed is 40 s. Even when such long records are analysed, the correlation functions $\hat{R}$ exhibit considerable irregularities which do not represent high frequency components present in the original signals and which may, in fact, be due to noise and the sampling procedure. Therefore the correlation functions are usually smoothed to avoid spurious components in the spectral densities due to aliasing. A number of possible smoothing routines are available in the literature (Bendat and Piersol, 1966); and Taylor (1966b) discusses the effects and the physical meaning of smoothing.

It should be noted that the above is true only for the pulsatile components of pressure and flow, and only if the baseline is steady. Bendat and Piersol (1966) discuss the general case and show how d.c. components or drift must be treated. Randall (1958) was the first to use these methods in haemodynamics and Taylor (1966b) and his co-workers (e.g. O'Rourke and Taylor, 1967) have published several papers demonstrating the power of this approach.

4. ARTERIAL INPUT IMPEDANCE

The publication of the first estimate of femoral impedance by Randall and Stacy (1956) was followed by a series of papers from the McDonald school (Bergel et al., 1958; McDonald and Taylor, 1959; McDonald, 1960).

These authors dealt with the fundamentals of physical haemodynamics in physiological terms. The hydrodynamics of pulsatile flow were studied so that verifiable relations could be established between the properties of blood and the arterial wall and the mode of oscillatory flow, on the one hand, and wave propagation and characteristic impedance, on the other. Having determined the propagation constants and characteristic impedance of different arteries, questions relating to the spatial distribution of pressure, flow and impedance could be investigated. Although the theories developed were relatively simple they did include the dominant factors such as the visco-elasticity of both blood and vessel wall, pulsatile flow profiles, and reflections of waves. Thus many of the concepts necessary for the understanding of the design of vascular systems were defined which proved indispensable to later developments. The impedance and its alterations between the centre and the periphery, and its dependence on the spatial distribution of vascular properties and of reflections are important parts of the whole theory.

We will not cover the entire history of these developments. An excellent and spirited review has been written by McDonald (1968). In the following some highlights will be mentioned, together with such interpretations as are possible and useful at the time of writing.

Early studies concerned mostly the dog's femoral impedance; Patel *et al.* (1963) reported measurements of aortic and pulmonary input impedance, and discussed the relative importance of the resistive and reactive components. Bergel and Milnor (1965) carried out careful investigations of the pulmonary input impedance. The first observations in man were made by Gabe *et al.* (1964) in the aorta, and by Milnor *et al.* (1969) in the pulmonary artery. The general features of the impedance spectra were similar in all cases (Figs. 3 and 4). The impedance modulus is high at very low frequencies and approaches the peripheral resistance for steady flow (d.c.); it drops precipitously over the first few harmonics, and remains nearly constant at the higher harmonics, with relatively small oscillations. It will be shown later that the frequencies at which the maxima and minima occur, and the mean impedance at high frequencies, are of significance. These features are different at different sites in the circulation, as shown by the extensive animal studies of O'Rourke (1967) and O'Rourke and Taylor (1967) (Fig. 4). The phase of the impedance is always negative and about $-50°$ to $-60°$ in the low frequency range (though always $0°$ at zero frequency). In the aorta it approaches zero near the frequency of the first $|Z|$ minimum, and probably remains near zero at higher frequencies. Figure 4 shows the impedance patterns as functions of frequency and position in the systemic circulation of a dog. At more distal points in the circulation the first $|Z|$ minimum occurs at higher frequencies. The phase remains negative over a broader range the nearer the periphery is approached.

Several conclusions can be drawn: It is obvious that the average levels of the impedance moduli are much below the zero frequency values (5–10 per cent of peripheral resistance in the ascending aorta; 2–5 per cent in the femoral artery). The power required to maintain oscillatory flow is therefore only little greater than that which would be needed if the heart were a steady flow source. This is explained, in a very simplified way, by the large elastic

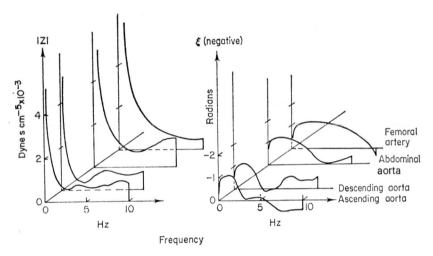

Frequency

FIG. 4. Impedance spectra (moduli: left panel; phases: right panel) in the systemic circulation, observed at four different locations. Measurements in the dog, redrawn from O'Rourke (1967). These impedance values were obtained by correlation and Fourier integral methods, which gives values at many more frequencies than does the Fourier series. The calculated values are therefore connected by smooth curves. Note the typical impedance pattern, particularly at the input (the ascending aorta) which shows a rapid decrease in $|Z|$, from the peripheral resistance, to a nearly constant level at the higher frequencies which is close to the characteristic impedance of the aorta. The first minimum in $|Z|$ is found at 2–3 Hz in the aorta and at 9–10 Hz in the femoral artery. The phase in the aorta is negative (near $-57°$) below 2 Hz and close to zero or positive at higher frequencies. Nearer the periphery, phase remains negative up to 10 Hz.

or capacitive component of the impedance which causes the negative phase angle. Clearly, the ventricle does not pump directly into the peripheral resistance, for only a fraction of the stroke volume is displaced peripherally into the arterioles during ventricular ejection. The rest is taken up by the large central distensible arteries. The same considerations apply to any part of the vascular system (which is another way of saying that we are dealing with a distributed-parameter system).

The input impedance of the pulmonary circulation shows the same basic characteristics as that of the aorta. The difference lies in the ratio of d.c. resistance and the mean level of $|Z|$ above 2 Hz. This value of $|Z|$ which approximates to Z_0, is about 30 per cent of the pulmonary resistance (Milnor et al., 1966). The oscillations in $|Z|$ above 2 Hz are somewhat larger than in the aorta. The phase is also negative at low frequencies (below 3 Hz) although with a rather smaller angle than in the aorta. Above the frequency of the first $|Z|$ minimum the phase is about zero or slightly positive. Much the same picture emerges from observations in man (Milnor et al., 1969).

Taylor (1964) pointed out that the heart rate at rest is generally at a frequency below the one at which the first aortic impedance minimum occurs. It appears that there is some reserve: if the heart rate goes up, the impedance goes down. This is true at least for the fundamental frequency, which contains the most energy. Some energy saving may be achieved (even though the total external work is approximately 10 times that of the pulsatile components), unless the stroke volume increases together with the heart rate.

The above remarks apply equally well to the human systemic system, as shown by Gabe et al. (1964) and by Mills et al. (1970).

The effect of changes in peripheral resistance on aortic impedance in dogs was studied by O'Rourke and Taylor (1967) who induced changes with norepinephrine, acetylcholine, and isoproterenol. The mean level of the aortic impedance changed remarkably little, as Fig. 5 shows. Vasoconstriction shifted the first minimum from 3 Hz to 5 Hz. $|Z|$ at 2 Hz changed by approximately 60 per cent but much less so at the higher frequencies, even though the mean blood pressure rose to 190 mmHg. Vasodilation (mean pressure 60 and 75 mmHg after acetylcholine and isoproterenol, respectively) caused the first impedance minimum to shift to 2 Hz, while the mean level of $|Z|$ did not change significantly. These are remarkable findings. The aortic impedance is in fact highly insensitive to changes in the periphery. The pulsatile energy requirements of the ventricle may change because waveforms change (more rapid acceleration of flow in early systole), but not when the peripheral vascular controls alone adapt to new requirements.

Very similar findings were obtained by Gabe et al. (1964) in man. They compared normal impedances with those after noradrenaline. As they pointed out, however, these studies do not reveal to what extent changes in distensibility (due to changes in mean pressure) and changes in peripheral resistance interact. It is not clear, for example, whether changes in peripheral resistance cause proportional changes in terminal wave reflection because the latter depends on small variations of pressure and flow, and the local slope of the pressure-flow relationship does not extrapolate through the origin.

A further comment concerns reflected waves in the ascending aorta. From (2.14) we know that $\Gamma(0)$, the reflection coefficient, can be calculated provided Z and Z_0 are known. If we assume, for the moment, that the aortic impedance is the input impedance of a uniform transmission line (as is normal in electrical engineering), we obtain the following results. Near

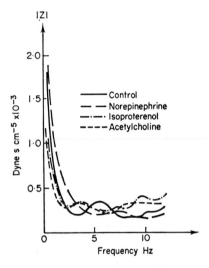

FIG. 5. The decoupling of peripheral resistance from input impedance. In the graph of $|Z|_{\text{aorta}}$ vs. frequency, the effects of vasoconstriction (norepinephrine, mean pressure 190 mmHg) and vasodilation (acetylcholine, 60 mmHg mean pressure; isoproterenol, 75 mmHg mean pressure) are very small. The impedance moduli, in the frequency range covered change very little, although the peripheral resistance changed from $3 \cdot 4 \times 10^3$ to $10 \cdot 7 \times 10^3$ dyne s cm^{-5}. The ventricle faces an almost constant oscillatory load which is much smaller than the d.c. resistance. See text for implications concerning the power output of left ventricle. Data from O'Rourke (1967).

zero frequency, the impedance is about $15Z_0$; hence $\Gamma \cong 0 \cdot 85$. At approximately 4 Hz, $|Z|/Z_0 \cong 0 \cdot 5$, hence $\Gamma = -0 \cdot 33$. Above 6 Hz, $|Z| \cong Z_0$, hence Γ is very small. Such rapid changes cannot occur in a uniform transmission line segment with attenuating properties comparable to those in arteries. Thus we have obtained the first strong indication that a single section of a uniform transmission line is a very poor model of the systemic vascular tree, which is hardly surprising. This, however, does not mean that the basic relations between impedance, characteristic impedance, and reflection coefficient do not apply locally, at any particular point in the arterial system.

5. Hydraulic Power

Investigations on the impedance are not only of interest to those studying the haemodynamics of whole vascular beds but also to those investigating the pumping performance of the heart. One measure of the mechanical output of a ventricle, that is, its capacity to maintain flow at a certain pressure, is the hydraulic power delivered to the vascular system. This is the external work of the heart per unit time. In principle, power can be computed if flow and pressure are known, but if the impedance is known several stages in the calculations can be simplified, as the following development will show. In addition the impedance allows some prediction of the relation between power and heart rate, provided the waveform of pressure is known or can be predicted. Clearly, if the pressure and impedance are known, the same information is available as when pressure and flow are known.

When the pressure is raised within an elastic vessel, the vessel walls are deformed. This requires energy; it is potential energy which is stored in and can be regained from the vessel walls. The fluid acts, in this case, as a transmitter for the energy. When fluid is made to flow through the vessel, a certain pressure is needed at the inlet. This pressure in turn again deforms the vessel walls. Thus, to maintain fluid flow, energy is delivered to the system at a certain rate. This is the product of pressure and flow and may be called flow work rate (see Chapter 19). The sum of the flow work rate and the kinetic energy of the fluid flowing into the vessel represents the power input. The kinetic energy (K) per unit volume is $\rho v^2/2$; if an average inflow $\dot{Q}_0$ is maintained the following power (kinetic energy per time) is flowing into the system. For the steady flow component:

$$\dot{K}_0 = \tfrac{1}{2}\rho v^2 \dot{Q}_0 = \frac{1}{2}\frac{\rho}{S^2}\dot{Q}_0^3 \qquad (5.1)$$

where

ρ = density of blood,
$\dot{Q}_0$ = mean blood flow (cm^3 s^{-1}),
v = flow velocity averaged over lumen and time (cm s^{-1}),
S = lumen area of vessel.

Therefore, with average flow $\dot{Q}_0$ at mean pressure P_0, the total, steady, inflow of power ($\dot{W}$) is

$$\dot{W}_0 = P_0 \dot{Q}_0 + \frac{1}{2}\frac{\rho}{S^2}\dot{Q}_0^3 \qquad (5.2)$$

While this is interesting from the viewpoint of the flow source, it does not tell us what happens to the energy within the system (see Chapter 19).

For the oscillatory pressure and flow terms we must also consider the inflow of flow work and kinetic energy. The flow work rate is again obtained from the product of pressure and flow. For one particular harmonic we have

$$p_i(t) = P_i \cos (\omega_i t + \varphi_i)$$
$$\dot{q}_i(t) = \dot{Q}_i \cos (\omega_i t + \psi_i)$$

(5.3)

which may be rewritten as

$$p_i(t) = P_i \cos (\omega_i t')$$
$$\dot{q}_i(t) = \dot{Q}_i \cos [\omega_i t' - (\varphi_i - \psi_i)] = \dot{Q}_i \cos (\omega_i t' - \xi_i)$$

(5.4)

where

$$t' = \varphi_i / \omega_i + t$$
$$\xi_i = \varphi_i - \psi_i = \text{phase of impedance.}$$

Hence the product

$$\dot{W}_i(t) = P_i \dot{Q}_i [\cos \xi_i \cos^2 \omega_i t' + \sin \xi_i \sin \omega_i t' \cos \omega_i t']$$

(5.5)

The two terms in the bracket represent the in-phase or resistive power and the quadrature or apparent power, respectively. The time average of the former is $0.5 \cos \xi$. The latter is zero in the average while its amplitude is $0.5 \sin \xi$. Apparent power is manifest either in the form of elastically stored energy or as inertially stored energy; the stored energy is not lost to the vascular system. However, this additional energy must be supplied by the ventricle and, from the viewpoint of the source, it constitutes additional power expenditure. The preferred mathematical forms for the two types of power, using impedance moduli, are, for frequency i:

pulsatile power, in phase

$$\dot{W}_{ri} = \tfrac{1}{2} P_i \dot{Q}_i \cos \xi_i = \tfrac{1}{2} |Z_i| \dot{Q}_i^2 \cos \xi_i$$

(5.6)

pulsatile apparent power

$$\dot{W}_{ai} = \tfrac{1}{2} P_i \dot{Q}_i \sin \xi_i = \tfrac{1}{2} |Z_i| \dot{Q}_i^2 \sin \xi_i$$

Note also that $P_i \dot{Q}_i = P_i^2 / |Z_i|$. Note further that these power terms may be obtained from the signals in their complex form (1.5)

$$\dot{W}_i = \tfrac{1}{2} p \dot{q}^* = \tfrac{1}{2} P_i \dot{Q}_i \exp [j(\varphi_i - \psi_i)] = \tfrac{1}{2} P_i \dot{Q}_i (\cos \xi_i + j \sin \xi_i)$$

(5.7)

where $\dot{q}^* = $ conjugate complex of $\dot{q}$.

Of particular interest is the total flow work delivered in unit time by the ventricle, which comprises the steady term and all harmonics:

real power

$$\dot{W}_T = P_0 \dot{Q}_0 + \sum_{i=1}^{m} \dot{W}_{ri} = \dot{W}_0 + \tfrac{1}{2} \sum_{i=1}^{m} |Z_i| \dot{Q}_i^2 \cos \xi_i$$

(5.8)

apparent power

$$\dot{W}_{aT} = \tfrac{1}{2} \sum_{i=1}^{m} |Z_i| \dot{Q}_i^2 \sin \xi_i$$

(5.9)

The kinetic power in the pulsatile flow terms is best obtained by subtracting $\dot{K}_0$ (5.1) from the total kinetic power $\dot{K}_T$, which is

$$\dot{K}_T = \frac{1}{2} \frac{\rho}{NS^2} \sum_{k=0}^{N-1} |\dot{Q}(k\Delta t)|^3 \qquad (5.10)$$

where

$\dot{Q}(k\Delta t)$ = flow signal sampled at time $k\Delta t$,
Δt = time interval between samplings.

$\dot{K}_P(= \dot{K}_T - \dot{K}_0)$ can, in principle, be obtained also from the Fourier series of the flow signal. One must use (3.2) or (3.3) (and not the exponential form) if this approach is chosen despite the fact that the calculation is very cumbersome. In practice, (5.10) should be employed.

It should be noted that the above equations apply strictly only if pressure and flow are measured at the aortic or pulmonary valve. This is not easily done. Bergel et al. (1970) therefore developed a correction term which takes the transient energy storage within the segment between valve and measuring site (length Δx) into account. The correction term is

$$\dot{W}_{\Delta x} = \frac{1}{2} \Delta x \rho \frac{d(v^2)}{dt} S \qquad (5.11)$$

where v = blood velocity, averaged over lumen area.

Milnor (see Chapter 18) has discussed the power output of the right ventricle and shown how the oscillatory requirements change with heart rate and with stroke volume. Similar studies on the systemic circulation (O'Rourke, 1967b) show that the pulsatile terms are relatively small since the impedance level in the range of the significant harmonics is smaller relative to the peripheral resistance than in the pulmonary bed (5–10 per cent as opposed to 20–35 per cent). In the anaesthetized animal the total power per kg body weight was approx. 30 mW kg^{-1} (10 mW/kg in the right ventricle). The pulsatile power was about 10 per cent of the total (as opposed to 30 per cent in the pulmonary artery, see Chapter 18). Furthermore, O'Rourke (1967b) showed that limitation of aortic distensibility, which might be taken to model changes seen in arteriosclerosis, leads to significant changes in the impedance pattern and significant increases in pulsatile energy requirements.

The power requirements and the impedance of the circulation are relevant to the design of ventricular assist devices. Artificial pumps must, of course, be capable at least of delivering power at the quoted rates. Secondly, the pulse waveforms should probably also be controlled, which is possible if the input impedance is known. It is preferable that the baroreceptors, sensitive both to pressure and to the rate of change of pressure, should be presented with pressure pulses resembling the natural ones.

The hydraulic power delivered to the input of a vascular bed is not entirely lost by friction in the arteries. Part is available in the venous circulation to maintain flow there. See, e.g. Chapter 18 on the pulmonary circulation for a detailed discussion of this aspect. No equivalent data are available for the systemic circulation.

6. FACTORS DETERMINING THE INPUT IMPEDANCE

Transmission line theory describes the local factors governing impedance: characteristic impedance and reflection coefficient (2.14). The geometry of the vascular system, the effect of distal reflecting sites, the attenuation of pressure waves in arteries, etc. must be considered in any explanation of the reflection coefficient, e.g. in the aorta. All the information available must be used. In particular, any model of the impedance must also explain the spatial distribution of pressure and flow, i.e. the changes in the pulse wave forms observed between aorta and periphery (McDonald, 1960). Furthermore, it is the aim to be able to predict the outcome of different experiments such as changes in peripheral resistance or of posture. Much of this is beyond the scope of this chapter. The results presented below only summarize what is known at present.

First, let us consider how the anatomy of the systemic vascular tree influences the aortic input impedance. The left ventricle supplies two clearly separable portions of the circulatory system in parallel: the posterior circulation with the aorta as the main trunk, including the circulation of the viscera, and the vascular beds of the hind limbs, on the one hand, and the anterior circulation to the forelimbs and head on the other. The former system, in man and in many animals, is much larger physically as well as in terms of wavelengths. The anterior system comprises vessels which are close to the heart and less distensible than the aorta. This geometrical fact suggests a simple model in the form of an excentric Tee (see insert in Fig. 6) to explain several features of the input impedance. The notion of the excentric Tee has a long and complicated history summarized by McDonald (1968).

The properties of the two arms of the model may be chosen as follows. The characteristic impedances are derived from the average values of the wave velocities c (at high frequencies this corresponds to the foot-to-foot velocity of the pressure pulse, McDonald and Taylor, 1959) in the main trunks of the two systems. Assume that in the larger arm $c = 560 \text{ cm s}^{-1}$, and in the short section 750 cm s^{-1}. The lengths of the arms, assumed to be lossy transmission lines, are assigned by lumping together all reflecting sites, as if all peripheral reflections originated at single effective terminations for each line. In the dog, the effective periphery of the posterior circulation may even be placed at the level of the iliac arteries (McDonald, 1960). Thus

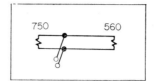

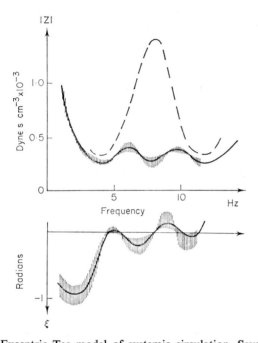

FIG. 6. Excentric Tee model of systemic circulation. Several features of aortic input impedance follow from the fact that the vascular system to trunk and hindlegs (of the dog) is larger and more distensible centrally than the vascular system of head and forelimbs. A simple model comprising two asymmetrically placed sections of homogeneous transmission lines (see insert) has an input impedance, shown here, which compares quite well with the input impedance measured in the dog's aorta (Fig. 4). The sections of the model are assumed to have characteristic impedances of 560 and 750 dyne s cm^{-3}, respectively, and an attenuation of 50 per cent per wavelength at all frequencies. Their lengths are such that the long arm has a length of $\lambda/4$ at 4 Hz, the short arm at 8 Hz. Terminal reflection coefficients are 0·5 (solid curve) in both lines. The impedance varies within the shaded area if terminal reflections vary from 0·4 to 0·6. The great insensitivity to changes in load is largely due to the fact that reflections cancel each other at the common input. Note that the impedance is here calculated as the ratio of pressure to blood velocity.

one arrives at a section of transmission line with length equal to one-quarter of the wavelength at 4 Hz. The length of the anterior section is chosen, more or less arbitrarily, so that the $\lambda/4$ frequency is 8 Hz. The $\lambda/4$ frequency is that at which the input impedance of a line shows the first minimum (i.e. magnitude minimal, phase zero), provided the peripheral resistance, or load, is greater than Z_0 and resistive (see Section 2).

Values for the terminal loads are chosen in the following manner. In many dogs, the first impedance minimum is approximately 50 per cent of Z_0 (O'Rourke and Taylor, 1967). The local or central reflection coefficient can therefore be computed, using (2.14) and typical attenuation values. The value of $\exp(-2\,\mathrm{Re}\,\gamma L)$ when $f = c/4L$ is approximately 0·7. This implies an attenuation of 50 per cent over a full wavelength, which is reasonable for large arteries. Hence, the effective peripheral reflection coefficient Γ_L may be found

$$\frac{Z_i(0)}{Z_0} = 0.5 = \frac{1-0.7\Gamma_L}{1+0.7\Gamma_L} \dots \Gamma_L = 0.47 \qquad (6.1)$$

The load is given by: $Z(\text{load})/Z_0 = (1+\Gamma_L)/(1-\Gamma_L) = 2.8$. This value is used, for want of a better one, for both arms of the Tee.

If we now compute the input impedances of the two arms and connect them in parallel, we obtain the result shown in Fig. 6. The typical features are seen: a rapid fall of the impedance amplitude at the low frequencies; two minima at approx. 4 and 8 Hz, little variation of $|Z|$ above 2·5 Hz. Furthermore, the phase spectrum simulates the one found in animals remarkably well (cf. Fig. 4). This impedance pattern is explained quite simply. The impedance of the posterior circulation has its minimum at 4 Hz, and a maximum at 8 Hz, as indicated by the interrupted line in Fig. 6. However, at 8 Hz the short arm of the Tee reaches its first minimum. The total impedance therefore is low with values close to the minimum for each line. (Note that this holds only up to 12 Hz.) Furthermore, the system is insensitive to peripheral reflections. The shaded area in Fig. 6 shows the effect of changing Γ_L from 0·4 to 0·6. This cancellation of reflected waves is an important factor in the decoupling of peripheral loads.

Obviously, many of the features of this model simply reflect the assumptions made. The model misbehaves in some respects, particularly with regard to the ratio of d.c. resistance to the mean impedance level above 4 Hz. However, it allows quantitative discussion of the aortic impedance in relation to the reflections from the two main arms. O'Rourke (1967) and O'Rourke and Taylor (1967) provided much evidence supporting the basic hypothesis. For example, the aortic input impedance exhibits a distinct maximum (at twice the frequency of the first minimum) when the brachio-cephalic and left subclavian arteries are occluded. Similarly, (see Fig. 4), the impedance of the descending aorta, representing the long arm only, is more oscillatory than the ascending aortic impedance, although the peaks and troughs are less pronounced than in the model (interrupted curve, Fig. 6). It is relevant here that the pulmonary impedance generally oscillates more than that for the systemic bed, and that the pulmonary bed is more symmetrical anatomically.

While the excentric Tee gives some insight into the nature of aortic input impedance, it fails to explain the changing pattern of impedance and of pulse waveform along the vessels. It is therefore necessary to introduce the geometric and viscoelastic non-uniformities. These represent many reflecting sites at many different distances from the heart. The resulting reflections tend to cancel at the input which makes the aortic impedance even less dependent on phenomena at the periphery. Furthermore, in this model (Taylor, 1966a) the amplitudes of all pressure harmonics increase, in the average, from centre to periphery, as they do in animals. (In a uniform transmission line the amplitude of pressure waves at frequencies above 5 Hz always decrease, in the average, even though local antinodes may be seen.) Taylor (1966a) demonstrated this in models containing many different transmission line sections arranged in dichotomous trees with random branch lengths. His results clearly show that randomly distributed reflection sites can make the input impedance almost completely independent of peripheral changes. Viscosity (of blood and the arterial wall) has little effect on Z but does play an important role in the spatial pressure distribution.

Thus, the input impedance is almost wholly determined by the characteristic impedance of the most proximal vessel. We have seen how the power requirements of the ventricle are thereby reduced. Robinson (1965) pointed to another consequence. If it were possible to estimate the effective internal source resistance of the left ventricle, this could be compared with the load, that is the aortic impedance. The internal pressure drop within the source could be estimated if the isovolumetric ventricular pressure were known. This is generally taken to be of the order of 300–350 mmHg. During a normal contraction, however, the ventricular pressure is about 100 mmHg, when the average systolic flow (in a dog) may be 50–100 cm^3 s^{-1}. Hence, the source resistance is approximately $225/75 = 3$ mmHg/(cm^3 s^{-1}) $\approx 4 \cdot 10^3$ dyn s cm^{-5}. This is 5 or 10 times the average level of the aortic input impedance, which suggests that the normal myocardium contracts as rapidly as allowed by its own rate-limiting mechanisms rather than by the hydraulic load it pumps into.

In summary, the concept of impedance is useful in characterizing the state of a vascular system, and in particular, the properties of the arteries near the site of measurement. Measurements of impedance in many different cases and at different positions in the arterial system gives insight into the functional roles of vascular geometry and vascular properties. The external work of the ventricles may be conveniently estimated from the input impedance. However, many questions remain unsolved. The known non-linearities (elasticity as a function of transmural pressure; non-linear hydrodynamic phenomena) seem to have little influence on the impedance, even allowing for measurement errors. We do not understand to what extent the peripheral load can be assumed to be purely resistive and linear. Furthermore, the problem of the optimum spatial distribution of vessel geometry and properties has not been solved. In other words, we do not know the criteria according to which the system has evolved although we believe that the decoupling of the normally high peripheral resistance undoubtedly plays an important role. In addition, and maybe most importantly at this stage, there is only relatively little data on impedance at present, and it is difficult to improve the existing quantitative models of vascular systems, so that we cannot explain fully the physiological significance of impedance variations.

REFERENCES

Bendat, J. S. and Piersol, A. G. (1966). "Measurement and Analysis of Random Data", John Wiley, New York.

Bergel, D. H., Clark, C., Schultz, D. L. and Tunstall-Pedoe, D. S. (1970). The determination of the mechanical energy expenditure during ventricular pumping. *J. Physiol.* **204**, 70–71P.

Bergel, D. H. and Gessner, U. (1966). The electromagnetic flowmeter. *In* "Methods in Medical Research" (R. F. Rushmer, ed.), Vol. 11, pp. 70–82, Year Book Medical Publishers Inc., Chicago.

Bergel, D. H., McDonald, D. A. and Taylor, M. G. (1958). A method for measuring arterial impedance using a differential manometer. *J. Physiol.* **141**, 17P.

Bergel, D. H. and Milnor, W. R. (1965). Pulmonary vascular impedance in the dog. *Circulation Res.* **16**, 401–415.

Davenport, W. P. and Root, W. L. (1958). "An Introduction to the Theory of Random Signals and Noise", McGraw-Hill, New York.

Dick, D. E., Kendrick, J. E., Matson, G. L. and Rideout, V. C. (1968). Measurement of nonlinearity in the arterial system of the dog by a new method. *Circulation Res.* **22**, 101–111.

Gabe, I. T., Karnell, J., Porjé, I. G. and Rudewald, B. (1964). The measurement of input impedance and apparent phase velocity in the human aorta. *Acta Physiol. Scand.* **61**, 73–84.

Lanczos, C. (1956). "Applied Analysis", Prentice Hall, Englewood Cliffs, N.J.

McDonald, D. A. (1960). "Blood Flow in Arteries", Williams and Wilkins, Baltimore.

McDonald, D. A. (1968). Hemodynamics. *Annu. Rev. Physiol.* **30**, 525–556.

McDonald, D. A. and Taylor, M. G. (1959). The hydrodynamics of the arterial circulation. *Progr. Biophys.* **9**, 105–173

Mills, C. J., Gabe, I. T., Gault, J. H., Mason, D. T., Ross, J. Jr., Braunwald, E. and Shillingford, J. P. (1970). Pressure-flow relationships and vascular impedance in man. *Cardiovasc. Res.* **4**, 405–417.

Milnor, W. R., Bergel, D. H. and Bargainer, J. D. (1966). Hydraulic power associated with pulmonary blood flow and its relation to heart rate. *Circulation Res.* **19,** 467–480.

Milnor, W. R., Conti, R. C., Lewis, K. B. and O'Rourke, M. F. (1969). Pulmonary arterial pulse wave velocity and impedance in man. *Circulation Res.* **25,** 637–649.

Noordergraaf, A. (1969). Hemodynamics. *In* "Biological Engineering" (H. P. Schwan, ed.), pp. 391–545, McGraw-Hill, New York.

O'Rourke, M. F. (1967a). Pressure and flow waves in systemic arteries and the anatomical design of the arterial system. *J. Appl. Physiol.* **23,** 139–149.

O'Rourke, M. F. (1967b). Steady and pulsatile energy losses in the systemic circulation under normal conditions and under simulated arterial disease. *Cardiovasc. Res.* **1,** 313–326

O'Rourke, M. F. (1968). Impact pressure, lateral pressure, and impedance in the proximal aorta and pulmonary artery. *J. Appl. Physiol.* **18,** 533–541.

O'Rourke, M. F. and Taylor, M. G. (1967). Input impedance of the systemic circulation. *Circulation Res.* **20,** 365–380.

Patel, D. J., de Freitas, F. M. and Fry, D. L. (1963). Hydraulic input impedance to aorta and pulmonary artery in dogs. *J. Appl. Physiol.* **18,** 134–140.

Randall, J. E. (1958). Statistical properties of pulsatile pressure and flow in the femoral artery of the dog. *Circulation Res.* **6,** 689–698.

Randall, J. E. and Stacy, R. W. (1956). Mechanical impedance of the dog's hind leg to pulsatile blood flow. *Amer. J. Physiol.* **187,** 94–98.

Robinson, D. A. (1965). Quantitative analysis of the control of cardiac output in the isolated left ventricle. *Circulation Res.* **17,** 207–221.

Taylor, M. G. (1957). An approach to an analysis of the arterial pulse wave. I. Oscillations in an attenuating line. *Phys. Med. Biol.* **1,** 258–269. II. Fluid oscillations in an elastic pipe. Ibid. 321–329.

Taylor, M. G. (1959). An experimental determination of the propagation of fluid oscillations in a tube with a viscoelastic wall; together with an analysis of the characteristics required in an electrical analogue. *Phys. Med. Biol.* **4,** 63–82.

Taylor, M. G. (1964). Wave travel in arteries and the design of the cardiovascular system. *In* "Pulsatile Blood Flow" (E. O. Attinger, ed.), pp. 343–372, McGraw-Hill, New York.

Taylor, M. G. (1966a). The input impedance of an assembly of randomly branching elastic tubes. *Biophys. J.* **6,** 29–51. Wave transmission through an assembly of randomly branching elastic tubes. Ibid. 698–716.

Taylor, M. G. (1966b). Use of random excitation and spectral analysis in the study of frequency-dependent parameters of the cardiovascular system. *Circulation Res.* **18,** 585–595.

Westerhof, N. and Noordergraaf, A. (1970). Errors in the measurement of hydraulic impedance. *J. Biomech.* **3,** 351–356.

Womersley, J. R. (1957). An elastic tube theory of pulse transmission and oscillatory flow in mammalian arteries. WADC Technical Report TR 56-614, Wright Air Development Center, Ohio.

Author Index (Volume 1)

Numbers in *italics* refer to pages where references are listed at the end of chapters.

Subject Index

S

Sampling theorem, 332
Sarcomere, G, 229
Sarcoplasm, G, 229
Sarcoplasmic reticulum, 229
Scanning photo-electric methods (see Transducers)
Second order system, G (see Control Systems)
Seepage through vascular wall (see Porous tubes)
Series elastic component (see Myocardium)
Servo manometer (see Transducers)
Set point (see Control systems)
Shear waves, 106
Sine wave (see Fourier analysis)
Single degree of freedom system (see Frequency Response)
Sliding filament hypothesis (see Muscle)
Smooth muscle (see Muscle)
Source impedance, 44
Source impedance or resistance of ventricle (see Ventricle)
Spectral analysis, 148, 333
Spectral density, 334
Stability of control loops (see Control systems)
Starling's Law (see Myocardium)
Stenosis, G, 269, 307
Step function (see Frequency response)
Stopcocks, 34
Strain, G
Strain gauge (see Transducers)
Strain function, G
Stress, G
Striated muscle (see Muscle)
Surfactant, pulmonary, G
Swept gain, 108
Sympathetic nerves (see Neural control of circulation)
Sympathomimetic drug, G
Systemic circulation, G
Systole, G

T

Taper elastic, 303
  geometric, 297, 301
Time derivative of pressure (see Pressure)

Temperature regulation, 214
Terminal load (see Impedance)
Tethered tube (see Elasticity)
Thermistor, 79
Thickness of the arterial wall (see Arterial wall)
Transducers, 12, 18, 91 (see Flowmeters)
  biological effects, 70 96
  calibration, 36 58, 81, 93
  capacitance, 30, 104
  differential transformer, 101
  inductance, 31, 100
  linearity, 12, 92
  mechanical effects, 95
  photoelectric, 31, 104, 109
  pressure, 11
    calibration, 36
    capacitance, 30
    catheters, 23, 34
    differential, 30, 37
    filling, 33
    frequency response, 18, 38
    inductance, 31
    optical, 31
    resistance, 29
    servo-manometer, 31
    volume elasticity, 19, 29, 32
  resistance, strain gauge, 29, 97
  ultrasonic, 71, 106
Transfer function (see Control systems)
Transfer ratio, 197
Transformer effect (see Flowmeters)
Transmural pressure (see Pressure)
Transmission line theory (see Impedance)
Transport of materials by bloodstream, 194
Transportation lag, G (see Control systems)
Traube-Hering waves, 156
Tropomyosin (see Muscle proteins)
Turbulence, G (see Flow)

U

Ultrasound
  in dimensional measurement (see Transducers)
  in flow measurement (see Flowmeters)